The Doctors' Doctor

The Doctors' Doctor

A Biography of Eugene A. Stead Jr., MD

John Laszlo, MD
and
Francis A. Neelon, MD

CAROLINA ACADEMIC PRESS
Durham, North Carolina

ISBN 1-59460-149-6
LCCN 2005933301

CAROLINA ACADEMIC PRESS
700 Kent Street
Durham, North Carolina 27701
Telephone (919) 489-7486
Fax (919) 493-5668
www.cap-press.com

Printed in the United States of America

CONTENTS

PREFACE

I never feel sorry for the doctor—the sick never inconvenience the well.

E. A. Stead Jr.

It seems a safe bet that you've never met anyone like Dr. Stead. Yet there may well be some unusual characteristic of his that you recognize or would like to develop in yourself or find in someone you know, a characteristic that calls for confirmation and exploration.

I began my residency at Duke Hospital in January of 1959, out of phase from almost all medical interns and residents, whose academic year of training typically starts on July 1. Dr. Stead always kept one or two residency slots open for a January 1 starting date, precisely to pick up people whose career development was out of synch with the norm. Having spent 2½ years in research at the National Cancer Institute, I was ready to complete my post-graduate specialty training in Internal Medicine and to sub-specialize in the diagnosis and treatment of blood disorders and cancer. Duke was one of the few top programs willing to accommodate my schedule. Furthermore (and this is most unusual for housestaff in training), Dr. Stead offered the use of a tiny laboratory in which to continue my cancer research in my "spare" time. A hand-me-down shaking incubator, some glassware and chemicals, and I was in heaven. The salary was $50 a month plus bed and board—about average for residents at that time.

In the late 1950s, Durham, North Carolina seemed just beyond the edge of the earth, at least to someone like me, educated at Ivy League institutions of the Northeast. But the grapevine had it that the medical training program at Duke was of the highest quality—if you could survive its rigors. It was run by the firm hand of E. A. Stead, Jr—"Doctor Stead" to all but a few select elders who called him "Gene." The housestaff sometimes referred to him as "Chief" or "Big Daddy" or "Daddy Blue Eyes" because of his penetrating gaze, but only when they were quite sure he wasn't around (and within the walls of Duke Hospital, day or night, it was difficult to be absolutely certain about this). He had far-reaching eyes and ears, so you worried lest he had an inkling that you had transgressed the code of total dedication.

To help me become acclimatized to Duke, and to break me in after a long absence from general medicine, I was assigned to work in the Medical Out-Patient Clinic during the day and to cover the inpatient wards on some nights and weekends. My first weekend at Duke was scheduled to be off-duty, but I stayed around the wards nonetheless. One of my co-residents chided me for this poor judgment and, sure enough, it was one of only two or three complete weekends that I had free of ward responsibility over the next 12 months. Eleven days after I started I got my next opportunity to leave the hospital. By this time the windshield of my car was plastered with tickets, because I hadn't found time to get a parking permit for the housestaff lot. (The Medical Department was not overly sensitive to human needs. One of my co-residents got married during the year and he managed to get an extra weekend off for the occasion, but he had to "pay back" other free nights for the privilege).

Being an intern or first-year (junior) resident meant being in the hospital five nights out of every seven; this meant that most nights off were spent catching up on sleep—before, sometimes during, or after dinner. Evenings in the hospital found us roaming the wards at all hours listening to heart murmurs, looking at unusual blood films, tuberculous sputums, or electrocardiograms. These were the days of the "iron interns and residents" that older doctors refer to wistfully. The expectation was one of total commitment; I heard the ironic "Welcome to the Duke Medical Service" long before I heard a football announcer describe a crunching tackle with a "Welcome to the N.F.L." In both instances, the statement conveyed nothing personal, just that there was a job to be done; no excuses; only maximum results acceptable. In getting professionals to perform at a level that was far beyond their own expectations, Chairman Stead, not Coach Lombardi, led the way. Of course, Stead strove for mental rather than physical toughness, but both go together at the moments of truth. Students and housestaff griped some (again when they were sure he wasn't around), but the quality of the experience made it the highlight of our professional lives.

Clearly the trend at present is away from this type of medical service. Young doctors now have (indeed, are required to take) more time away from the hospital for rest and for family life, but Dr. Stead believed that continuity of care best served both patients and trainees—the latter building a store of "intellectual learning capital" in the process. Participants in the Stead system of medical education didn't agree with the Chief in all things, but they wouldn't have changed a day of the learning experience.

Being a taskmaster is not difficult. There have always been supervisors who drive young people to the end of their endurance, often in a purposeless way. This is sometimes dressed up in the guise of "building character," which presumably would result from abundant sacrifice and suffering. Such harsh experiences often build the wrong kind of character among doctors, but for Dr. Stead and his pupils, medicine was fun, thinking was free in all ways, and each day was its own reward. To say that "they don't make them that way anymore" hardly explains the phenomenon. For almost everyone who knew him, Dr. Stead was "the most unforgettable person I've known." Each gathering of Stead-trained people generates wonderful stories about life in the arduous but rewarding days of the Stead Chairmanship.

In many ways, those were golden days for all of American medicine. In the 1950s and '60s, research funding and professional opportunities were available as never before to those who could cut the mustard. There were not yet the myriad review committees, government agencies and regulations that have smothered medical affairs, thereby changing forever the professional lives of doctors. There was not yet the proliferation of deans, or layers of hospital bureaucrats regulating bed occupancy, patient turn-over and financial bottom lines—goals often achieved at the expense of learning, service, and even honesty. Under Stead at Duke, young doctors could judge their progress and watch themselves grow professionally to achieve what Dr. Stead knew his pupils could achieve: skills and dedication and comprehension to meet the complex medical and psychological problems of the patients and families who came to them for help. It is often said that one could tell Stead-trained doctors by their philosophy, as well as their knowledge, of medicine. Not that Stead's trainees came out cut like identical cookies from a mold, for Stead's philosophy was based on realism, sometimes harsh realism, rather than cloudy goals of "service to humanity." Stead's young people brought their own value systems with them, and what they learned differed as a result. All of which was acceptable, as you can judge for yourself when you read Stead's story.

Stead's philosophy startled, persuaded, rambled, and cajoled people in the health professions, but it was always soothing to sick people. His ideas grew out of his experience in a changing world, and his language sounds rough and ready, even sexist in places. But few other leaders of modern medicine have been able to penetrate to the core of all manner of complex problems, using simple, quotable phrases that still reverberate more than 35 years after he stepped down as Chairman of Medicine. Stead was the person to whom competent professors and students and residents alike turned when they got stuck on a problem. Stead's wisdom, his message, his approach to the educational process, his single-minded insistence upon excellence, and a brief description of the man who met the highest test of leadership in American medicine are the subjects of this story about the doctors' doctor. This book is no plea for a return to good old days now lost; rather it is a recounting of what went on and why.

When I first approached Dr. Stead with the idea of doing a book about his life, he declined, saying that he "wouldn't cross the street for fame." He believed that the events and people of today would have no permanent effect on the history of the world. In geological time, the clock chimes to announce the comings and goings of glaciers, not individuals. Still, Dr. Stead knew full well that his ideas had a profound impact on the non-geological world of medicine, primarily during the mid-portion of the 20th century when he served as chairman of two departments of medicine. Still, he was convinced that the immediate world had no lasting significance, and that this was always the case. At first this seems at odds with his absolute passion for excellence. Scratching slightly below the surface of his motivation, however, one learns that he pursued his passions solely because of the fun they afforded him during the course of each day. We wanted to share with others what we could capture of this remarkable man, truly a national resource. He was kind enough to humor us, since we understand so little about geological time.

John Laszlo, MD

ACKNOWLEDGMENTS

We are grateful to the generosity of Dr. Stead in providing the many days of interviews needed to prepare background materials and for the hospitality of both Dr. and Mrs. Stead. The Steads also allowed us access to their personal photo albums, from which we selected the illustrations for this book. A number of his former students, associates, and colleagues provided their recollections and insights, including doctors Henry McIntosh, Jack Myers, Albert Heyman, Robert Whalen, John Romano, James Warren and Michael De Bakey. Three others, Drs. Paul B. Beeson, John B. Hickam, and George J. Ellis III, had written their recollections at the time of Stead's retirement as Chairman and these are included. Dr. Stead's wife Evelyn, his son, William W. Stead, MD, and his brother, William Stead, MD, helped illuminate the personal side of the Chief. A great many quotes from Dr. Stead were first published in a collection of Stead memorabilia entitled, *E. A. Stead, Jr.: What This Patient Needs Is A Doctor*, edited by Galen S. Wagner, MD, Bess Cebe, and Marvin P. Rozear, MD (Carolina Academic Press, 1978). That lovingly prepared collection of his sayings was a great resource for this book. Ms. Debbie Siebel was a tremendous help with the manuscript as was Ms. Mary Ellen Banisch, who not only transcribed tapes but also offered numerous helpful editorial suggestions. Betty and Ian Ballantine provided encouragement with the project and very skillful editing as the book took shape. The Rockefeller Foundation gave John Laszlo the valuable opportunity of working at its residence for scholars in Bellagio, Italy

Eugene Stead read the final draft of this book and gave it his imprimatur. He felt that the material recorded here reflected his life and his vision of the world as well as or better than any prior attempt to capture him in print. Most of the recorded material was obtained during the early 1990s, but Stead was still providing more information through 2004. Dr. Stead's personal philosophy of medical care, particularly at the end of life, is expressed in several areas of this book. Lest anyone doubt that he lived by the words he uttered, it is worth noting that when Evelyn Selby, his beloved wife of 63 years, suffered a lethal stroke, Stead did not rush her to a hospital. Recognizing that death was a hoped-for conclusion to her long life, he kept her at their rural home and held her to comfort her until she died. Stead, too, was determined not to leave his lake home, except finally. Two years later, on June 12, 2005, Eugene Anson Stead Jr died peacefully in his sleep, in his own bed in the house he had built with his own hands. He wanted and asked for no memorial; may this book then, the testimony and recollections of many of his friends and colleagues, provide at least a hazy portrait of this remarkable doctor and teacher.

The Doctors' Doctor

CHAPTER 1

PERMISSION TO BE DIFFERENT

Dripping water wears away rocks.

Eugene Anson Stead Jr. was born in Atlanta, Georgia in 1908, the second of five living children of Emily White and Eugene A. Stead. Gene Sr. had moved with his family from Ohio to Georgia when he was a boy, but Emily's family was steeped in the tradition of the South, with roots winding back to times of prosperity and wealth before the Civil War. Bullets from the guns of Yankee soldiers are embedded still in the walls of the White family's old homestead (or what is left of it).

A deep belief in and firm adherence to Christian Evangelical thought shaped Gene Sr.'s ideas of life. His formal education ended with grammar school, but his fundamentalist background molded his beliefs and guided his behavior. Gene Sr. read the Bible as the Word of God; predictably, he didn't believe in dancing, smoking, drinking whiskey or playing cards. A man of very strong opinions, he was intolerant of those whose beliefs differed from his own. Interestingly, he never expressed animosity towards Blacks, Jews or other specific racial or ethnic groups; his intolerance was limited to ideas and practices that deviated from his simple, Bible-based religion.

His social activities, too, were defined by his beliefs. He routinely went to church, attended the meetings of the Board of Stewards and the Wednesday evening prayer sessions. His religious beliefs and activities provided a structure that shaped family life in the Stead household, and thumbed its lifelong imprint onto young Gene Stead's own ideas. Dr. Stead himself never developed a strong religious belief, but his early lessons on the value of structure to a person, an organization, or a system were ever visible in the later stages of his own life.

In sharp contrast to her husband, Emily White Stead came from a family whose relative wealth allowed her to attend Girl's High School in Atlanta. As a result, education was always important to her, and she read a great deal, both the classics and contemporary periodicals. Because of her influence, the Stead children always had books to read and to read without censorship. Gene Sr. didn't always approve of the books his children read, but his protests were

3

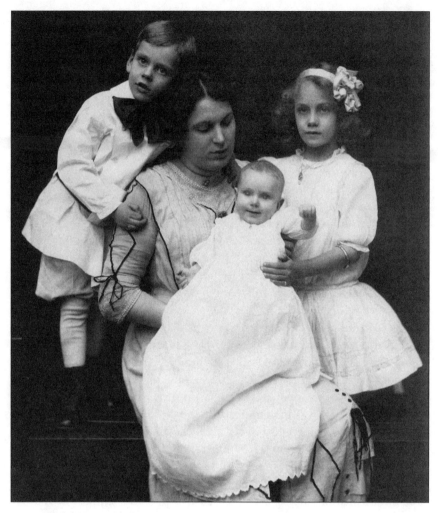

Eugene Stead Jr., at age 5 in 1913 with his mother, Emily White Stead, and sisters Emily (in mother's lap) and Mary Cleo.

barely audible above his wife's enthusiastic and unflagging support of learning. Emily Stead used her unobtrusive influence as wife and mother to balance her husband's doctrinaire rigidity. From his mother, young Gene learned a passion for reading and the infinite value of education.

Most of her life centered around the home, but when some activity or cause captured her attention, Emily Stead would devote whatever free time she had to it. She was an articulate woman, able to express herself very well, and so, although generally a quiet person, she would campaign hard for issues about which she felt strongly, such as replacing a congressman she didn't like. Her involvement with such activities was quite limited, but she was persistent once she got going. Watching his mother's tactics in such matters made Gene aware of the effectiveness of her methods. It was how, in fact, he learned the "dripping-water-wears-away-rocks" approach that he later made his own in dealing with medicine and medical administration.

Eugene A. Stead Sr. was a traveling salesman who reportedly could sell nearly anything. As a teenager and young adult, he sold lamps, worked as a carpenter, and held a variety of odd jobs. By the time his children arrived, he was the distributor of a patent liquid headache remedy named Capudine, which literally means "head pain." He then went to work with his older brother who had been to pharmacy school and was a licensed druggist. In those days it was possible to study pharmacy and achieve formal accreditation without going to school, so Gene Sr. studied in the back room of the drugstore and eventually became licensed. It was then not unusual for even distinguished professionals to have attended a proprietary school, of which there were many. For example, the noted physiologist of the day, Dr. Morris Fisher, studied independently in order to become certified as a medical practitioner. Later, when Gene Stead enrolled at Emory, he met an old doctor there named Carl Aven who outdid Morris Fisher in his creative approach to accreditation: Dr. Aven was reputed to have formed his own medical school, graduated by himself as a class of one, and then closed the school! In the context of the time, Gene Sr.'s back-room studying was neither an extreme or singular phenomenon.

Knowledge of pharmacy made Gene Stead Sr. an effective salesman. He could go into a drugstore, inventory its stock, determine the pattern of sales, and formulate a reasonable sales presentation. When druggists bought from him in quantity, they always received a discount, and the more they bought, the better the discount. He traveled the rural routes and urban avenues of Georgia and surrounding states, visiting all the druggists in his travels. As a licensed druggist himself, when he was in Georgia, he had the advantage of being able to help pharmacists with their work. Unlike today when customers pick pre-packaged medications off a shelf, pharmacists then had to compound their own preparations. If, as sometimes happened, the druggist were busy, Gene Sr. would step behind the counter and help fill prescriptions.

Because he was honest and hard working, Gene Stead was well liked by his customers. They knew that when he gave them information about a product, it was correct to the best of his ability. He maintained an active reputation by attending pharmacists' conventions and keeping in touch with his business associates, which also gave him political leverage in the drugstore industry. In keeping with his beliefs, however, Stead never drank, which was rare among pharmacists, who in those days were fairly riotous. Within the confines of his religious and moral tolerance he was a good negotiator and, indeed, found that sobriety often worked to his advantage, leading him to tremendous influence in Georgia pharmaceutical politics, and bringing honors from the Georgia Pharmacy Association.

In spite of his active career in drug sales, Gene Sr. never did earn much money, and the Stead family was poorer than most Georgians, who in general were quite poor. Emily Stead kept the home and cared for the children, which was considered her job and her contribution to the household, but this meant there was only one income. As a result, Gene Sr. had to creatively expand his earnings whenever possible. Being a traveling salesman meant working only one job, so Stead arranged with his employers to supplement his income during the summer. Once Gene Jr. had reached adolescence, his father took him along on his business trips and the two would camp by the road, cooking their own meals for about three months each year. The company paid the elder Stead a stipend for lodgings and meals for himself and his son; since their expenses never exceeded the stipend, Gene Sr. would retain the difference. For the most part, young Gene enjoyed his time alone with his father. In spite of the older man's strict religious beliefs, they had fun on the road and saw a different side of life; they were even freed from church attendance. To entertain themselves, the two sometimes flipped knives, threw an axe at a tree, or played other games. The closest they came to religious activity was a game in which the two would work their way through the alphabet quoting a biblical verse for each letter. Gene Jr. always enjoyed reaching "J," for which he handily had at his disposal the shortest verse in the Bible, and which he took much joy in reciting: "Jesus wept."

One troubling aspect of being on the road, however, was that the younger man became the older's confidant, a role he would rather have avoided. Hearing the concerns of the adult world made the boy grow up fast, and he became aware of things with that might otherwise have escaped him. For instance, his father confided his worries about how he would pay for the children's college education; problems of one sort or another were always part of their discussions. To further complicate matters, when his father went off alone and young Gene remained at home, his mother would confide in him. From an early age Gene was keenly aware of the problems that arose from having five children and relatively little money. And although his parents never indicated that they thought life would have been easier with fewer children, it was not difficult for the boy to surmise that it would have.

Gene Jr. was the only one of the Stead children to accompany his father on his sales routes, and when he went along he worked beside his father distributing advertisements and samples, for which the company paid him directly.

With the first money Gene earned, he bought a bicycle for his younger brother Bill, with whom, despite the ten years difference in their ages, he always enjoyed a close relationship. He bought his brother this rather extravagant gift without bothering to ask his mother for permission, because he knew she disapproved of bicycles.

Dr. William Stead:

> Two things bring tears to my eyes when I talk about Gene. Mother told me about the first, and I'm sure he doesn't remember it. After I was born at home in 1919, Mother heard a soft sobbing one afternoon. When she turned, she saw Gene in the shadows quietly crying. Mother, of course, thought, "Here comes trouble," and she asked Gene what was bothering him. He said, "I'm just happy to have a brother." And, honestly, Gene treated me that way. He's been a damn good brother all through my life.
>
> When I was 8 and Gene was 18, he had a job sweeping the floor at the local Buick repair shop. He spent the first money he ever earned to buy me a bike because he hadn't had one. I remember it not because I was told about it, but because it was firmly planted in my memory as a wonderful gesture.
>
> I have a profound love for Gene, and admiration for him, and for the most part I thought he could do no wrong. The only time I was embarrassed by Gene was when we were quite young. Gene, and a friend and I were camping. We had to go into town once a week to get provisions, and so we'd go on Saturday morning when all the farmers were in town. One Saturday Gene wore an old sweatshirt over his bathing suit. That's common enough now. The shirt came down just low enough that you could not tell that he had on a bathing suit; you simply couldn't see it. He had these very long legs hanging from beneath his sweatshirt, and our friend advised him to put on some pants. He didn't pay any attention to this suggestion though, and as we walked from the store to the drug store, people turned to stare at him. When we went to the post office, there were 6 or 8 people in a circle talking. Gene walked over to the counter and bought his stamps, and as the people crowded together you could tell they were looking at him and talking about him. One little boy snuck into the middle of the circle and hid behind his father's pants legs, pulling them apart enough to peer out at this apparition. Soon a policeman came up and told Gene to get in the car and cover himself up. Gene didn't know what he was talking about because he knew he was

clothed, but nobody else did. We had to finish the shopping without Gene who had to sit in the car in the shade of a tree. I thought he could have used a little shyness that day.

As boys, we liked to camp. Dad and Gene had bought a little piece of property on a mountain near Clayton, Georgia, where they camped for many years. But when Gene got to the point where he could drive a car, we began to camp on Lake Rabun, which is down the hill. We would camp at a place that was about a mile or a mile and a half by canoe, and couldn't be reached by road at all. We'd swim in the lake and go over to the mountain stream and cool off. We were there one day, happily camping with our little canoe, when our parents arrived. They had written us a postcard and we hadn't answered it. They insisted that we drive with them to Highlands, North Carolina, which was one of mother's favorite places. On the way, the automobile boiled over from going up so many hills. We had to stop on the road and go down to a creek and get some water, but first we had to let the radiator cool for fear of breaking the block if we didn't. So we were sitting around waiting for the car to cool, and Gene was sullen. He'd been dragged out of his camping place and we were stuck on the road and there wasn't going to be any fun. The sky was socked in with clouds and so on, so Gene was ticked off. He pulled out the Saturday Evening Post and read it. He was not sociable. Mother often said that this was the time she learned that her son wasn't perfect.

It was an advantage in college to have a brother ahead of me who could point out the road signs. Yet he wasn't a father; Gene wasn't of a different generation; he was still studying in school just as I was, although several years ahead. But the norm was studying, the norm wasn't goofing off, because that's the way all the members of the family were.

Gene Stead and his father made their sales travels in an antique touring car with running boards. His father would hire three other boys in each town they visited to work with young Gene distributing samples. Gene Jr. competed hard and took great pride in his ability to deliver more samples than any other boy he met. The boys would stand on the running boards of the car, jumping on and off to deliver samples or replenish their supplies. Young Gene became proficient at taking just enough samples in the bag he carried with him for about two blocks worth of houses. It was strategic on his part, because if the bag were too heavy, he would be weighed down and unable to move quickly; too light and he would lose time running back to the car for more supplies. On entering a neighborhood, the car would slow down and the boys would jump off and run from house to house. A bag full of samples was great protection against dogs, too, because "when a dog would jump up, I'd pull the bag up in front of me like a shield. I'd often go to areas the other boys avoided because of their fear of dogs." This strategy, of course, produced monetary rewards.

Driving with his father through streets lined with mill houses and row after row of outdoor privies exposed young Gene to a great variety of rural and urban poverty. They sold products mostly to the poor people clustered in cities or towns. The mass-produced headache remedies cost little to make and, as a result, the selling price was low. In order to make money, Gene Stead Sr. had to sell a lot of Capudine, and he was helped by the fact that in densely popu-lated poor neighborhoods his sales pitch could reach more people in less time. And, fortunately, poor folks bought as much as the rich. The Steads, of course, were poor themselves, but because their lives were structured, their poverty never went any deeper than the bottom of their pockets. The love and discipline of their home life were not related to income; the quality of their lives was not connected to father's earnings. Mother was at home to look after the children, and provide for their emotional and physical needs.

By watching his father, young Gene was able to see the power of direct com-munication. On a number of occasions over the years Gene Stead Sr. went, unavoidably, deeply in debt. The first time occurred when Gene Jr. was five years old and quite ill, as was his sister. The heavy medical expenses made it difficult for Gene Sr. to meet all the costs of raising a family. As soon as he re-alized this financial plight, he contacted his creditors, explaining the situation to them and proposing a plan for repaying them. Watching his father deal forthrightly with these difficulties underscored for young Gene the value of open and honest communication. The first time his father found himself in financial straits was not the last, but he dealt on each occasion as he had the first, and remained in good standing with his creditors as a result. To the watching boy, his father seemed fearless, able to face anything. Over the years, these repeated lessons led Gene Stead to realize that many of the world's prob-lems arose from people's lack of communication about their problems and the potential solutions.

Dr. Stead:

> My father never showed signs of fear toward the kinds of things of
> which I've been afraid. He stood up for whatever he thought was
> right, and was not intimidated by a lack of formal education. By con-
> trast, I was afraid of the dark, worried about money and whether I
> could earn a living, and was afraid to speak in public. But my father

was never afraid of those things. My sister Emily once swam out into water that was over her head in a lake in northern Georgia, and she wasn't able to get back on her own. My father didn't know how to swim, but he somehow got out to help her, but once he reached her, he couldn't swim her in. Because the water was not terribly deep, he was able to bring her in by holding his breath and walking underwater along the lake bottom, pushing her along as he went. When he could no longer hold his breath, he surfaced long enough to refill his lungs before lowering his weight again and walking her into shallow water. Later when I was in high school I taught him to float and then to do a side-stroke in the Atlanta City Park.

If my father did have fears, they ran on a different level, and were integrated with his views on morality and religion. We lived Decatur, which was about seven miles from Five Points, the center of Atlanta. Like my father, many of the people in Decatur were suspicious of their city neighbors whose lives were different from their own. And they were afraid of the young people being contaminated by the people of Atlanta. So in order to prevent any possible interplay between the two communities, the people of Decatur had their holidays on Sunday and Monday. We went to school Tuesday through Saturday and attended church on Sunday. Then on Monday, when the Atlanta children were back in school, we were free to roam about. It worked to keep us separate and protect us from the big bad city people—as those Atlantans were perceived to be.

Emily and Gene Sr. early settled their differences about how their children were to be raised. A child could not go around one parent and get permission to do something from the other; both parents gave the same answer, and that made an impression. As befitted a structured home, dinner was on the table each night, and after dinner the children knew that they were expected to help clear the dishes. Each day, too, the blessing was said at their house, and at night before the children went to sleep either their father or mother heard their prayers. In that way, a set of values was formed within the Stead family, values that provided a structure for life. So the poverty Gene Stead knew as a boy was of a different kind than that found in the broken homes of today where love is elusive and discipline unknown. When one or both parents are absent or preoccupied, it's difficult for children to have their basic needs satisfied. Too often there's just not enough time for meaningful contact between the parent and child.

The Stead children sometimes thought that five offspring was too many, but their parents didn't seem to think so. They never indicated that they didn't want all of their children. Problems arose later between the parents and their daughters, but in those early years all the children felt welcome and well loved.

The people young Gene saw as he traveled from door to door had a very different kind of home life, and suffered from a more integral kind of poverty. They were destitute on a level more personal than material. Their houses were filled with a prevailing sense of disorder and, as was obvious to the eye of the discerning observer, lacked any tangible form of discipline. Through the cracks of doors held slightly ajar, Gene Jr. could glimpse the chaotic lives of people within. Babies lay unattended on the floor, crying for their mothers, who themselves wore the mask of bitter distraction, in homes of permanent confusion and filth. As if to underscore the disturbing quality of those lives, the neighborhoods were suffused by the offensive smell of dishwater routinely thrown out back doors onto the clay earth where it sat and baked in the Georgia sun. The disorder of those lives was as unappealing as the fetid, fermenting mud—a pungent recollection that Gene Stead could conjure up at will.

These experiences impressed young Gene Stead with the fact that you could survive without much money, but you did need order. Having accompanied with his father in visiting hundreds of mill houses in South Carolina, Alabama and Georgia, he realized that to have some measure of order it was necessary to forego immediate gratification and think beyond the pleasures of the day. These early observations were later incorporated into his philosophy and discipline as a physician—with the added proviso that each day must, in itself, provide its own satisfactions and rewards.

Rules and a sense of order were the basis of life in the Stead house. The children were respected by their parents, and because (or in spite) of the strict rules for their behavior, the children were respectful of their parents wishes, as well. Gene, in particular, was not a rebellious youth. He disagreed with his father's religious beliefs, but did not argue for his own ideas. He understood that his father's convictions were genuine and a part of his everyday life, and he respected that. Religion was never an issue between them.

Being at home with their mother most of the year while his father traveled, Gene and his siblings were expected to help with chores around the house. When his father was home, there were projects of greater proportion. Together Gene and his father built a cow barn with a loft, and a garage. A plot of land owned by the Steads was cultivated in summer and planted with corn, lettuce, black-eyed peas, beans and other vegetables. Gene Sr. took great pride in his work, whether on the road selling medicines or at home engaged in tasks he had created for himself. He instilled in his son a sense of pride and satisfaction in a job well done.

Dr. Stead:

> Father always did things better than anyone else I knew, even though
> he had held low paying jobs most of his life. He believed in individ-
> ualism and was very anti-union. He believed in hard work and
> thought that he would do a better job than someone else because he
> would work harder. And he felt that he should be paid for what he
> did. The general union notion of a whole class of jobs in which
> everybody was paid the same seemed to him to be ridiculous. Con-
> sidering that he never went far in the economic world, I found his
> perspective remarkable, and I applied that lesson later on when I
> paid my faculty different amounts of money, even though their ti-
> tles might be the same.

Both Stead parents took pride in their children's intellectual achievements and
were interested in their school performance. Their mother read often to the
children, leading Gene to a deep love for books and an insatiable appetite for
reading. He read whatever was available. A neighbor loaned him a complete
set of Horatio Alger books and he read them all. During the summers of his
youth, he often read six or seven books a week. One year at school he was
asked to turn in a list of all the books he had read over the summer. The
teacher skeptically reviewed the extensive list Gene handed in, and warned
him that there would be a few questions about the books he had listed. Gene
proudly agreed to answer any questions the teacher might have, knowing, of
course, he had read them all. Engrossed in the pages of a book, the rest of the
world grew dim as he gave himself over to the power of the written word. He
would forget to eat and barely managed, if others approached him with a
question, to rise to a level of consciousness that would satisfy their brief demands on his attention. When absorbed in something in which he was interested, such as the Horatio Alger stories, nothing else mattered.

Because of a marvelous memory, Gene Jr. did well in school, and most
years, was the outstanding male student in his class. In some ways, though,
he was an indifferent student. Being unusually shy, he avoided speaking in
public, and during recitation periods, if asked a question, would pretend that
he didn't know the answer. He was saved by his ability to do extremely well
on written exams, and so what amounted to a social handicap did not ad-
versely affect his grades.

Outside of the context of his family, there was little praise for intellectual at-
tainment. Decatur offered virtually no culture at that time, and the limits of
achievement were narrowly defined. The school system, a product of lower
middle-class southern society, was certainly not very good, and provided little

challenge for students of superior capability. In an attempt to expand the limited academic offerings, Gene's mother organized the "A-Pin Club" for outstanding students. She also asked the principal to recognize students' scholastic performance by offering an elective in college algebra to the highest achievers.

One curious story illustrates Emily Stead's enthusiasm for education. Without knowing anyone there, she supported Emory University long before her children were of college age. Living nearby, she was able to watch the school being built, and once it was complete, she attended all of the undergraduate commencement exercises as a spectator. Her greatest satisfaction came much later when her son Gene became Dean of the Medical School at Emory and handed out the medical diplomas. She was very proud and, though the ceremony was held every nine months and Dr. Stead himself grew somewhat tired of it, his mother never did.

Dr. Stead:

> I had a head start from the beginning. My sister Emily was a very bright girl and we spent a lot of time together when I was small. When I was six years old and it was time for me to enter grammar school, Emily, who then was eight, enrolled me in the second grade. She explained to the teacher that she had taught me everything I needed to know about first grade. Decatur at the time had just converted from a school without formal grades to a graded school that differentiated students, but the school was still fairly informal, so I saved a full year. I was an October child who normally would have had to wait another year to enroll. But the system was fairly loose and nobody said very much about it. Later on I had another break that saved me a year of high school, and so I was just a month short of sixteen when I went to college.

Gene Stead was a quiet child with few friends, who played mostly by himself. This was due, at least in part, to health problems. Because of an episode of bronchopneumonia when he was young, he was considered sickly; after school, he would return home to fly a kite, build a dam or read a book. Concerned about the effect of activity on her son's health, Mrs. Stead consulted Dr. James Paullin, the family's physician (and later an important influence on Gene's adult life). Dr. Paullin asked how Gene was doing in school, and his mother admitted that attendance had little effect on his grades. And so it was decided that the boy be allowed to decide whether or not he was feeling up to school.

Many of those days at home were spent in the big field beside his house chasing butterflies, exploring the underside of rocks, and just enjoying the freedom conferred on him by Dr. Paullin and his mother. Because his absences from school were sanctioned by adults, they weren't considered hooky, but he didn't have to be very ill to stay home and from time to time exploited his license to do so. Life continued to be structured for Gene Stead, but he had a great deal of freedom within that structure. He used that liberty to explore his inner and outer worlds, separate as they were from the regimen of the other children.

Growing up, the five Stead children spent much of their time in the living room with their parents. As a result, Gene learned to study amidst great noise and confusion. Someone might be playing the radio or the piano while others were working; consequently, Gene learned to do two things at once. Although impossible for most people, he could write a theme for a term paper and carry on a conversation at the same time. Later in college, he tried to talk with his neighbors while writing an examination, but it was looked on very unfavorably by his teachers, who were not impressed when he told them he had always done so at home! Nor did his fellow students appreciate such demonstrations of how he could beat the system.

Southern schools were segregated during Gene's childhood. The Steads had black help in the house, but the Stead children had little other exposure to black people. Jacob Simm, a man of about 60, and his wife, a tall, angular woman who took in wash, were the only black people with whom Gene had close contact. Mr. Simm did odd jobs for the Steads when Gene was a young boy; he was a very strong and upright man who was paid by the hour for his work and he called young Gene "Sir," something the boy never thought twice about. Jacob's presence was more of necessity than a luxury since there were so many chores to do around the house and Gene Sr. was away on business so much of the time. Emily Stead's brother, who ran a meat distributing businessan, had given her an enormous cow named Bessie. One of Jacob's regular jobs was to milk Bessie and he was unusually good at this, able to make her milk last a long time between calves. It was expected that the Stead children would work alongside Jacob, which they did, but when it came to Bessie, she was too big for anyone but Jacob to handle. When that cow turned its enormous head to shrug a fly, it would pick Gene up and toss him around. So the children worked at other chores, and in the summer, when Jacob was out plowing the field, Gene Sr. was there working along side of him.

There was never a discussion of civil rights in the Stead house; they just accepted things as they were. Gene was personally unaware of the prejudice of the society around him because habitual behaviors were so ingrained they were not identified as wrong or malevolent. Only many years later, when he came across a book about the seeds of tragedy being sown between whites and blacks and the need to resolve the situation before a terrible harvest was reaped, was he able to see the evil inherent in a system he previously had taken for granted.

CHAPTER 2

RIDING HIGH ON GOOD MEMORY — THE COLLEGE YEARS

When I examine myself and my methods of thought, I come close to the conclusion that the gift of fantasy has meant more to me than my talent for absorbing positive knowledge.

Albert Einstein

Of the fifty graduates in Gene's high school class, only five went on to college. Gene was one of them. No one in his family knew anything about college courses because no one before had been to college, but there never was a question about whether the children would go. Emory University, which was about two and one-half miles from the Stead house, offered a scholarship to the male graduate of the local high school who had the highest scholastic average. When Gene won the award, the decision to go to Emory was more or less made.

Surprisingly for someone who was to become a great educator, Gene Stead's method for studying was to cram. He would wait until near the time of the final exam, then absorb a semester's worth of material with several days of intense study. This method is generally frowned upon by professional educators, but Stead found some advantages in cramming. He understood that in order to successfully pass an examination with little preparation, the material had first to be organized in a structured way so that it could be learned. The admitted disadvantage to his method was that a week after the examination he could recall none of the information. Having been assigned to the unretentive ranks of short-term memory, the information was never assimilated in a form that would allow future recall. Still, because he was very good at written exams, Gene Stead invariably made grades of 98 or 100. In fact, it became his stock-in-trade to go into a final exam with an 88 average, then score 100, giving him an 'A' in the course. Nothing to it for Gene.

When Gene was a college freshman in 1924, his sister Emily became engaged to a young man who was a biology laboratory instructor at Emory. He suggested to the 16-year-old Gene that he take biology, which was known as a difficult course and hence not very popular with freshmen. If he did well in Freshman Biology, it was likely that Gene could obtain a laboratory assistantship in his sophomore year. Unbeknownst to the freshmen who were busy dodging biology, the laboratory assistantship was the most attractive one on campus. The Professor of Biology, a man named Rhoades (and predictably referred to as "Dusty"), was independently wealthy and doubled the normal stipend for the laboratory position, making it a choice assignment. The prospect of a lucrative assistantship, coupled with the challenge of the course, piqued Gene's interest. Ironically, Gene would never have taken biology had it not been for the lure of the job; he didn't have a clue as to what biology was all about.

Dr. Rhoades turned out to be the teacher who had the greatest influence on Gene during his undergraduate years. A reflective man, Rhoades was known among the students for a saying that captured Gene Stead's ear: "Life is the succession of generations, with heaven on earth as its goal." Eventually Gene was appointed to the laboratory assistantship, where his job was to look after the protozoa that Dr. Rhoades cultivated. The older man never did any real investigative work, but he was fascinated by protozoa and liked to look at them.

Stead's first and only triumph during his laboratory assistantship came while he was working with a flagellate called *Heteronema acus*, a protozoon that fed on *Euglena gracilis*, a tiny one-celled organism. Gene learned to coat a microscope slide with egg white so that the organisms would adhere to it, then flood the slide with a fixative solution like osmic acid, and stain it. The stain highlighted the digestion process of *Heteronema*, which Gene and his teacher then examined under a microscope. They made camera lucida drawings of their observations, and both teacher and student reveled in the simple tasks that were a threshold to the larger, more complex world of science.

As an undergraduate student at Emory, Gene Stead made a few friends, but generally spent his time alone, much of it in the laboratory, although it was hard for him to account for exactly where all the time went. Because he lived so close to Emory, it was easy for Gene to get back and forth. Often he would work until 10:00 or 11:00 PM. then walk home; Saturdays and Sundays, too, were devoted to the biology lab. The job didn't require the long hours he put in, but to Gene it hardly seemed like working at all. Time simply evaporated as he was drawn deeper and deeper into the new world that Biology was opening up. However, it is not clear that he would have chosen medicine as a career solely because of his new-found interest in biology. Actually, his decision to enter medical school was not even a matter of serendipity—it was a fluke decision resulting from a conversation with some friends. Most young people say they to want to become doctors because of exposure to role-models or life experiences; Gene Stead's logic was rather different.

Dr. Stead:

> I became interested in medicine for two reasons: I had to do something after I graduated, and I was drawn to the challenge of medical school. Towards the end of my junior year, I became involved in an argument with some of the people I played chess with and who were already in medical school. They pointed out how difficult it was. I had never found anything very difficult at school, so I laughed and bragged that I could easily get very good grades if I went. I had never declared myself pre-med or given it any prior thought. However, not knowing what else to do, I made up my mind to go to medical school if I could get the money. I didn't go to medical school for altruistic reasons or to save lives. I went for the intellectual challenge and the career. It was no more profound than that. By 1928, when I graduated from college, the boll weevil had already hit Georgia and everyone was poor. I thought that medical school would be a safer haven than simply graduating and trying to eke out a living, and I thought that it was one thing I could do for which my family would continue to give me support. Although my father grew up with a limited education, he was determined that his children would go to school and turn in a good performance or else they would go back to work.
>
> My mother had great respect for the medical profession and liked the idea of my becoming a doctor. My father, on the other hand, was perturbed by biology. He was smart enough to know that if the theory of evolution really was correct, the fundamentalist interpretation of the Bible would have to go. He was annoyed when, as an undergraduate, I took the assistantship in biology, but he had to yield to the reality of economics. Biology was the best chance I had to make money and so this didn't lead to any arguments. I never tried to talk my father out of his beliefs; I simply didn't discuss issues I knew would make him uncomfortable. He had taken good care of us and I respected him, despite the fact that he had little educational advantage.
>
> Having decided late in my college career to go to medical school, I had to make up some requirements. This meant taking more subjects at one time than the school allowed. By going to summer school, I was able to complete the full course in half of the usual time. Before

the authorities caught up with what I had done, namely, maneuvering an end-run around them, I completed the work. When they discovered my strategy, they informed me that it couldn't be done. I argued that it could because I had already done it. However, by taking the summer courses I missed out on an opportunity to do research at Woods Hole Laboratory on Cape Cod during my last summer in college. I had earned a student scholarship to go, but wasn't able to take advantage of it; and I always regretted that lost educational opportunity which was so highly prized among biology students.

CHAPTER 3

MEDICAL SCHOOL AND
Two INTERNSHIPS

Social graces and medical skills are not always related.

E. A. Stead Jr.

Gene Stead was 20 years old in the fall of 1928 when he entered Emory Medical School. As it turned out, it was for him an oasis in the terrible economic drought known as the Great Depression, which affected the South even before it dried up the rest of the country. The boll weevil had wiped out the cotton crop, making money and the things that it bought very scarce. There were even fewer economic opportunities in the South than had been the case just a few years earlier, when Stead had graduated from high school. There was no question as to where he would go to medical school; without funds, Emory was the only available option. He borrowed money from the Atlanta Rotary Club Scholarship Fund, which he was expected to repay, and did, though he was granted a deferment until after he had finished his education.

As a medical student, Gene spent time away from school to prove to his friends that he didn't have to spend as many hours learning and studying as the other students. He continued to cram and continued to make superior grades. However, his methods proved dangerous to any fellow classmates who tried to imitate him. His dissection partner in anatomy, for example, was a very bright young man whom he had known as an undergraduate. Unfortunately, he tried to mimic Gene Stead's work habits and flunked out of medical school!

When his partner flunked out, Stead teamed up with student named English McGeachy, the son of a Decatur minister. In the middle of the year, they and several other students became curious about what would happen if they connected a sensory nerve of a dog directly to its motor nerve, bypassing the essential connections in spinal cord and brain. The idea is about as naive as hooking up the carburetor of a car directly to the drive shaft, bypassing the motor. Furthermore, although naïve, it was technically difficult to do. Stead engineered the logistics of the project, including borrowing instruments from the operating room. For four weeks they worked on the project, attempting to suture the nerves together. Although they found it an exciting, original project, they learned little beyond how technically complex such a procedure was. And because they didn't have any way of giving post-operative care to or preventing infection in the dog, it survived only a few days after the experiment was abandoned. For students eager to be involved in the practice of medicine, the experiment was a real opportunity to probe the possibilities of investigation, regardless of the naiveté of the undertaking. At that time, students saw very few patients during the early years of medical school, in part because Emory University Hospital was a community hospital and not a teaching hospital; the teaching was centered in downtown Atlanta at the Grady Hospital, miles away from the Emory campus, where the first two years of study were spent.

There were three outstanding internists in Atlanta at the time; by far the most prominent was Dr. James Edgar Paullin, a Johns Hopkins graduate and distinguished physician who later became President of both the American Medical Association and the American College of Physicians. He was known for having identified Brill's disease (scrub typhus), not previously known to occur in Georgia. An excellent physician, he was the Stead family doctor when Gene and his younger sister, Cleo, suffered from bronchopneumonia as children. Because he had seen Gene as a patient, Dr. Paullin recognized Stead in the halls of Grady Hospital, where Gene trained clinically during his later years of medical school.

Dr. Stead:

> Dr. Paullin was the first person to teach me that if you were really good at something, you could get paid for it. He charged more than the other internists in Atlanta, and he justified his fees by the fact that he had the medical experience of working at Grady Hospital. When I went down to his office to see him, I was very aware that the place was run well. He had an orderly office and there were one or two young doctors working with him who stayed with him for a few years. In those days he had his own x-ray equipment and was well-to-do by our standards.

Dr. Paullin was quite accomplished, in contrast to the Chair of the Medical Department at Grady Hospital, who was rather ineffectual. The Chairman's extensive travel schedule meant that he spent a good deal of time away from the hospital. His experience as a student convinced Stead that staying at the hospital was the single most important element of a chairman's success, far surpassing intellectual brilliance.

As everywhere in the South at that time, Grady Hospital was segregated by race. The "Black" and "White" Grady Hospitals sat across the street from each other, but they were run as separate hospitals with separate administrations. In his third year of medical school, Stead was assigned to the ward at Black Grady Hospital where Dr. Paullin was in charge of the patients, and Stead the medical student lived at Grady Hospital just as he had lived in the biology building as an undergraduate. Dr. Paullin made rounds at Grady every Tuesday morning, and on Wednesdays he went to Emory to give a Clinical Pathologic Conference (CPC).

The medical services of Black and White Grady each comprised two large wards, one male and one female; each ward had forty beds arranged along the walls and center of a dimly lit square room. One of the first patients Stead treated was an elderly black man with fine white hair whose major complaint was diarrhea, but whose diagnosis was not clear to the fledgling doctor. The patient had a fine tremor of his hands and fingers, and had lost weight despite a big appetite. Stead wrote up his findings the night of admission, but the diagnosis eluded him. The next morning, while riding into the hospital on the streetcar with his classmate and friend English McGeachy, the two discussed the case. McGeachy asked what the laboratory work showed and Stead said that there were a large number of lymphocytes in the blood, but that the other tests were normal. McGeachy, who had just been reading about the causes of lymphocytosis, said that hyperthyroidism was one of them. The signs and symptoms were absolutely classical for thyrotoxicosis; a light went on, and Stead was able to put it all together. "Oh my God," Stead said, realizing that he had been overlooking the obvious. Abnormalities of the blood cells seemed like a funny way to arrive at the diagnosis of hyperthyroidism, but the significance of solving the dilemma by discussing the case with a colleague made a deep impression, which Stead never forgot.

At the hospital, Stead recounted the patient's case to an intern named Hugh Wood, whose competence and knowledge as a doctor impressed Stead. Dr. Wood was young, but Stead admired the way he handled patients and students. In time, Stead discovered that Wood worked in Dr. Paullin's office. Until that time, Stead's vision had been limited to the Atlanta horizon and getting through Emory Medical School, but as he tagged along with Dr. Wood, he asked about his background and his training. When he learned that Dr. Wood had interned at Peter Bent Brigham Hospital in Boston, Stead decided that was where he, too, wanted to go. To help him, Dr. Wood later wrote a recommendation for his young proselyte.

Medical students at the Grady were given a great deal of responsibility in caring for patients with life-threatening diseases. Gene Stead had always been extremely shy in social interactions, but he never felt alarmed or apprehensive about going to see patients. From the beginning, he was confident that he could do something for them. If a man had diarrhea, for example, at the very least, he could help him get to the bathroom. The fact that he could do little things for patients while he was learning, gave him a sense of usefulness. And because the hospital was short of help, whatever the students did was appreciated by the patients. Despite this, Stead's uneasiness around other people led his medical school classmates to the opinion that he would not be a successful doctor. As it turned out, meeting people socially and caring for them professionally were two separate issues. Gene Stead knew early what his classmates later learned: that social graces and medical skills are not always related.

As a medical student, Stead was aware of what little research was going on at Grady. Dr. Carter Smith used an electrocardiograph (ECG) machine to measure the electrical activity of the heart, in particular the cardiac rhythm of people who were dying. It was the first piece of clinical research Gene Stead ever saw, and he was intrigued by the fact that more patients died from cardiac standstill than from abnormally rapid or irregular cardiac rhythms. When Stead learned that Dr. Smith also had trained at the Peter Bent Brigham Hospital, he was interested in learning more about him, but his reserve hindered him from approaching the older man.

Junior students at the Grady were assigned to work on Tuesday morning, but Stead decided that it would be more useful to attend Dr. Paullin's 10 AM Tuesday conferences with the residents. At these meetings, Paullin carried out a very thorough history and physical on a "difficult patient," reviewed any relevant laboratory data and discussed the basic science that lay behind a particular illness. Stead, eager to be involved and not at all reserved about what he knew, spoke up enthusiastically whenever he knew the answer to a question that had stumped the residents. This embarrassed the residents but pleased Dr. Paullin, and caught his attention.

Dr. Paullin was later very helpful to Stead. As a member of the Association of American Physicians, Paullin knew academic physicians around the country, and he had a position of influence in the medical community at large. He was a personal friend of Henry A. Christian, Chairman of the Department of Medicine at Peter Bent Brigham Hospital, and when Gene applied for an internship there, Dr. Paullin strongly supported his application.

As a medical student, Gene Stead had a lot of obstetrical experience, and delivered more babies than most Professors of Obstetrics. Like the other students, he lived at Grady Hospital, and so was ready to deliver babies whenever they arrived. Dr. McCord, an obstetrician, was the only person other than the Dean who was paid to work full-time at Grady Hospital. McCord was interested in eclampsia, a potentially serious form of hypertension and kidney disease that occurs during pregnancy. He gave his students a list of instructions on how to care for patients suffering from eclampsia; on the bottom of that list he had written, "If you're in doubt, call me." The fact that he always responded when summoned left a lasting impression on Gene Stead.

Stead was one of the few Emory Medical students who excelled in Neurology because it depended on a knowledge of neuroanatomy, a subject he found fascinating. Psychiatry, on the other hand, was another matter. Practical instruction in psychiatry was not available at the Grady Hospitals. As a result, the course consisted of a few lectures at Grady Hospital and case work at the Federal Penitentiary. The lectures presumed a theoretical background in Psychiatry, and Stead was hard put to understand them. It was the one clinical course he didn't like. At the penitentiary, he found it difficult to determine whether the convict patients were lying or telling the truth (a difficult task even for experienced psychiatrists); as a result, he didn't know how to treat them and didn't like them. He also found it unnerving to enter the prison grounds with its big walls and armed guards. In all, it was a haunting experience that later moved him to enquire further into the field of psychiatry and to find out how it could be useful to patients.

Pediatrics, which consisted mostly of classroom lectures, came to life during Christmas of Stead's senior year. Signing on as a student-intern to replace house officers who were on Christmas vacation, he worked on the pediatric ward in the evening. This gave him his first chance to perform a pericardial tap, inserting a long, hollow needle to drain fluid from the sac around the heart. You learn fast when you are faced with responsibility.

Everything seemed to be going quite well as Gene Stead finished his final year of medical school and prepared to visit the Brigham Hospital to take the examination for internship. He enrolled in a lecture course in urology, and managed to make his usual "A", but he didn't attend the lectures, which piqued the instructor no end. As the semester came to a close, the teacher told Stead that he was going to give him an "F" because he had not attended the lectures. Stead went to see the Dean who reassured him by saying, "Gene, why don't you and I just not worry about this." Recording of the grade was delayed, and this saved his chances at obtaining a Brigham internship, which surely would have been compromised by an "F" on his record.

The interview at the Brigham was the occasion of Stead's first trip away from Georgia. The travel expenses and the additional costs of the trip meant some economic hardship for the Stead family. Before the visit, Stead bought the eight-volume medical encyclopedia edited by Dr. Christian and Sir James Mackenzie. The faculty at Emory would never have assigned such advanced reading to a medical student, and his classmates thought Gene peculiar for undertaking challenges that were not required. But, motivated to learn more than the courses at Emory could provide, he read not only Henry Christian's books but Dr. Paul Dudley White's *Diseases of the Heart* as well. He knew he wanted to be prepared for his examination when he got to Boston.

Young Dr. Stead was accepted into the Peter Bent Brigham Hospital program, and eventually spent seven years in Boston. After one internship and several months of fellowship, he undertook a second year of internship (in surgery), had 18 months of residency in Cincinnati, and returned to Boston for a research fellowship. Considering that most postgraduate training in the 1930s lasted only one year, the amount of time he spent in a white suit was quite remarkable, but he was young and he loved the work. In fact, clinical work as an intern was less demanding than what he had seen as a student at Grady, so he had no difficulty adjusting to being a full-fledged doctor. Doctors at Grady Hospital practiced rough and ready medicine, treating a lot of emergency cases but almost never seeing patients with illnesses that weren't life threatening. At the Brigham, by contrast, his first three months as an intern were spent as a virtual lab technician, making measurements of blood chemistry values for ward patients.

The medical service at the Peter Bent Brigham Hospital appointed three new interns every four months. Stead was the only one of the three in his group who knew how to interpret an electrocardiogram. The ECG apparatus used at the Brigham was, in fact, more primitive than the one at Emory, and was used only to identify disorders of heart rhythm or to diagnose simple myocardial infarctions. Because of his extensive hands-on training gained at Grady, Stead was quickly recognized and touted for his accomplishments. That was when he recognized that giving honor to learning is what makes a faculty.

Going to the Brigham expanded his contacts with people. Sitting in the library, he couldn't help but feel a sense of awe over the fact that he had daily contact with people whose names he read in the journals before him: Samuel Levine, Joseph Aub, Henry Christian, Merrill Sosman, Fuller Albright—all great men of American medicine. It pleased him greatly to be even a small part of such a group of productive people. It was one of the reasons he wanted to go to the Brigham to begin with.

Fifty percent of the graduating class at Emory Medical School went straight into practice without even an internship, and 80% of the remainder entered practice after a year of internship. Because most of his Emory classmates went so quickly into practice, Stead's parents were a little bewildered by his seemingly unending education. His mother was supportive, however, even though she didn't understand the reasons for so many additional years of education. But her son was training at one of the Harvard hospitals and anything connected with Harvard had to be good. After several years of internship without a foreseeable end in sight, even his mother found it difficult to explain to inquisitive friends exactly why her son needed so many additional years of training. "I guess Gene's just a slow learner," she told a neighbor one day for lack of a better reason. "You know, your mother might be right," teased Soma Weiss, Stead's boss at the time.

Dr. William Stead:

> Dr. English McGeachy, Gene's classmate at Emory, came back to Decatur and was already in practice by the time Gene had just begun his second internship. At the Brigham, each internship lasted 16 months, so altogether he was an intern for 32 months. In the meantime, McGeachy's practice became solidly established. Then more of Gene's classmates came back to Decatur to practice, with no sign of Gene's return in sight. The parents of other classmates and our neighbors were always asking when Gene was going to come back. His "internship" went on and on and on. Although there was a lot of support by our parents, they did have a tough time explaining to the neighbors exactly what Gene was doing for a living.

Stead's parents visited him only once in Boston. They drove from Georgia to Massachusetts only to find that the demands on their son's time were so great that he had energy for nothing but sleep during his time off. Years later, when Stead visited his own children who were interning, he found they followed the same time-honored tradition. Nevertheless, his parents were extremely proud of him. His father, the pharmacist, had considerable respect for his son, the doctor. He didn't always believe what doctors said, but he did respect them. The fact that young Gene was interning at the Brigham Hospital (and would later join the Harvard faculty) was a considerable source of pride for his mother.

Dr. William Stead:

> Dad died of tuberculosis at the age of 83, and when we traced it back, it appeared likely that he had been infected by his father, who died of it when Dad was 15. Dad had a flare-up of the disease in 1902 when he was 27 years old. Nobody told him that he had tuberculosis, but they did tell him to sell his drug store, where he worked 12 to 15 hours a day, and to live and work outdoors. So he became a traveling salesman. He died in 1957, having been in the Milledgeville State Hospital in Georgia on two separate occasions. All the x-rays showed was a little streaking in the right upper lobe of his lung. When he died three years later, he had tuberculosis of his kidney and lung. Looking back, it was apparent that he'd had trouble in both places for

many years. As a result of my father's illness, I became interested in chest disease and tuberculosis.

Just as at Grady, the staff at the Peter Bent Brigham Hospital were largely part-time employees. The only full-time person at the Brigham was Dr. Henry Christian, the Chief. Dr. Christian's medical background was in pathology, so he trusted mainly what he could learn from studying microscope slides of diseased tissue. He knew a great deal more than Gene Stead, but Stead knew that he could readily learn that kind of medicine. Dr. Joseph Aub made a greater impression on Stead because he asked questions the answers to which were not found in books, questions that Stead had never thought about. Having seen so much clinical medicine at Grady, Stead was already a good bedside doctor, but Aub introduced his younger colleague to things that were totally new. Aub had done some important work related to lead poisoning and to overactivity of the parathyroid glands (which affects calcium balance and causes bone and kidney disease). When he talked about these subjects, he touched on things that Stead had never before encountered.

Given a choice as to which teaching rotation he would take, Stead elected to work under Dr. Aub. The other possibility was Dr. Sam Levine, a fine bedside doctor and brilliant cardiologist, whose knowledge of physical examination made him more popular with the residents than Aub. Levine always had "pearls" of clinical information to share—subtle and helpful diagnostic clues not found in standard textbooks. But Stead was intrigued by Aub's way of thinking, and traded off as many rotations as he could in order to work with him. The admiration was obviously mutual, because for many years thereafter Dr. Aub fostered Stead's career by providing recommendations and nominations to key medical societies.

Following his internship in Medicine in 1933, Stead undertook eight months of laboratory fellowship with Dr. Christian. The Chairman had an allotment of fellowship money, which allowed him to provide young doctors the opportunity to conduct research under his supervision. Having no other prospects at the time, the fellowship allowed Stead to keep learning. He had no real notion of how a laboratory worked, but the fellowship gave him an opportunity to look around and determine what he wanted to do thereafter. He was able to live with the medical students in Vanderbilt Hall, the quadrangular residence hall on the Harvard Medical School campus. In the lab, he studied how mercurial diuretics helped patients suffering from edema to eliminate excess fluid. The question was whether diuretics changed the way kidneys excreted water or whether they somehow moved fluid from the edematous tissues into the bloodstream to be excreted by the kidney. It seems a fairly simple problem now, but at the time there was little knowledge about how diuretics worked.

Dr. Stead:

> There seemed to be two approaches to the problem: an easy one, and the one we took. Our first assignment was to make dogs edematous, or swollen with excessive fluid, which turned out not to be simple. We read books describing how plasma was removed from a dog and the protein-rich plasma replaced with water. We got pretty good at doing this, but our dogs didn't get edematous. After several months, we hadn't made any progress, until one night when the animal assistant came in and asked what we were trying to do. He said, "That isn't so difficult. All you have to do is put a tube into the stomach of the dogs at night and give them 1000 cc's of salt water." It worked, of course. Reading the literature didn't help because they failed to say that you had to administer salt solution and not just water. When you really want to find out how something is done, you have to go to the laboratory.

> By measuring the blood protein and hematocrit levels in these dogs we could tell how the fluid was being eliminated. If the fluid moved into the bloodstream from the tissues, the protein concentration would be diluted; on the other hand, if the blood protein content remained constant, we would know that the diuretics were working directly on the kidneys. However, it was a cumbersome technique and the methodology was very slow.

> Of course, the simpler way would have been to determine whether a minimal amount of the mercurial diuretic injected directly into the renal artery caused diuresis. That would have answered the question more directly. Nevertheless, I learned how important a good instrument shop is, since we had to fashion our own experimental tools. I began to see a little bit about the nature of research and we did publish a paper on our findings.

After an initial discussion with Dr. Christian about the fellowship, Stead spoke to him again, to confirm his desire to participate. At the second meeting, Stead discovered that he and Dr. Christian had different recollections about the proposed stipend. Stead thought it would be $1,000, but Christian remembered $800. It was an awkward position. The amount of money was important because it was to fund the medical education of Stead's brother, Bill. Mustering his courage, Stead went again to see Dr. Christian; as it turned out, the older man was very gracious, saying, "I certainly mean to pay you exactly what we agreed, but my memory is still that we agreed on $800." Because it had been an oral agreement, it was simply a matter of one man's word against the other's.

Stead persisted, sure that he hadn't made a mistake, and knowing how his brother was depending on the money that he would receive. Christian finally said, "It appears to me that the matter is much more important to you than it is to me, and therefore you are more likely to have remembered it correctly."

Dr. Stead:

> I had always been very close with Bill, and I was glad to give him the money. I didn't need very much because I didn't smoke or drink, and I lived at the hospital. Bill benefited not only from my being frugal, but also from my educational experience. I was able to help him plan his summers and to tell him which teachers to see. He had the advantage of having somebody personally interested in him, and he received much more direction over the years than I did. Consequently, he took much more chemistry, math and physics than I did.

Dr. William Stead:

> One of the advantages I had in college was that I had somebody ahead of me who could point out the road signs, but was still close enough to me in age to be considered part of my generation. Gene was studying in school, just as I was, and he was a good role model because he worked so hard.

Stead's extensive experience at Emory meant that knew a lot about caring for sick people, but he was extremely shy and had great trouble speaking in public. Whenever he was called on to speak, he would develop incapacitating shakes and tremors. He had managed, for the most part, to avoid such occasions, but at the Brigham, circumstances conspired against him and he was forced to confront his fear.

Dr. Stead:

> During my surgical internship, which I took after completing my medical internship and fellowship, I saw a patient in the emergency room who had injured his hand. My diagnosis was that the patient had a small linear fracture of a metacarpal bone. However, the x-ray report came back the next day saying: "Normal wrist." So I wrote a little note on the chart saying, "As usual, the X-ray Department made a mistake," and didn't think anything more about it. But the Medical Record Librarian knew that this wasn't an appropriate notation to have on the chart. She took it to Dr. Merrill Sosman, the Professor of Radiology, and after looking at the x-ray, he explained to me that

what I was looking at on the x-ray was a nutrient artery, not a fracture. Christian had always said that Sosman wasn't a great radiologist, and that the other doctors didn't believe anything he said; in fact, if Sosman said the patient had one thing then the patient must really have the opposite. So I said, "Let's put the bright lights on that x-ray and look at it again." Bony details show up better on very bright illumination and sure enough, there was the fracture. He was very nice about it, however, and we developed a closeness.

One day Dr. Sosman told me he was going to help me learn to speak in public. He explained that he had quite a lot of experience in this realm, and at the time was going around to the County Medical Societies making presentations at medical conferences. He invited me to go with him, saying he would have me present a patient to the audience each time and, no matter how bad I was, he would save me. He assured me nobody would remember, and he always picked up the presentation in such a way that nobody ever knew how bad I was. Although presenting the patient was a grueling experience, I enjoyed it overall. I enjoyed the car ride with Dr. Sosman, and I appreciated the fact that he always did what he said he'd do; he came in and saved me whenever I needed it. With Dr. Sosman's help, I made a start on overcoming my fear of public speaking. Much later when we had "Sunday School" presentations at Emory and Duke, and the residents were asked to present a conference for an hour before all of their colleagues, I always helped them out. If we were getting near the end of the hour and the resident wasn't doing too well, I'd rescue him in the last five or eight minutes so that nobody ever knew the worst that this person could do. I'd come in and say, "You've carried the ball long enough in this conference, let me try to summarize what you've said." Then I'd say what the resident hadn't quite been able to say. I was able to rescue the resident because I had once been rescued.

I still get nervous for the first 30 to 60 seconds at a presentation. It is a very common problem, but I had it in a severe form. When I was growing up I would walk around the block rather than face my professors. It took me until I was about half way through medical school to get over this. As a by-product of these experiences, I was always sympathetic to shy people. I think that the milk of human kindness will go a long way towards helping students feel more comfortable, but you can't cure others of this problem because it's not your problem, it's their problem. A young doctor once came in for an oral examination and exhibited all the signs of anxiety. I got him to sit down and I asked him to tell me about anxiety and what happens to you when you're very anxious. He finally got through the exam and when he realized he himself had a clinical disorder, it put him at ease, and he had an opportunity to get his head together. He's never forgotten this because he reminded me of it many years later.

Dr. Stead himself later developed a training career path for young doctors, but in the 1930s no such path existed. Most doctors went into general practice after a year of internship or perhaps took another year of residency to specialize in internal medicine. Stead had no long-term plans other than to follow those things that interested him. Having completed an enjoyable medical internship and an eight-month research fellowship, he followed his nose back across the street to the Peter Bent Brigham Hospital where he became an intern in surgery. Internship can be a grueling experience and rare is the person who takes more than one. But, in terms of learning about people, the clinic was better than the laboratory. Stead knew enough medicine to make a real contribution to the surgical service, but he lacked the highly developed dexterity necessary to be a surgeon. Still, he thought he would have a good time caring for patients who had been operated on by the surgeons, and this turned out to be true. Stead was unique among the surgical interns because he had no true interest in becoming a surgeon. However, he did remove a few appendices and repair a few hernias, and he became very good friends with Dr. Hartwell Harrison, the urologic surgeon who later performed the first kidney transplant.

Dr. Stead:

> I was quite tentative in the operating room, and found that it was easy to make mistakes. Whereas I was never uncomfortable in medical decision-making, I was uncomfortable in the use of my hands. However, I've been glad that I had the surgery experience, if for no reason other than to discover how tired you get after working all night. Surgeons stay up all night with an emergency and then have to be in the operating room again at 8:00 in the morning. Knowing this, I've never gone to see a surgical patient in consultation just to be smart, or left a lot of orders for the surgeon to carry out. If something needed to be done, I did it myself. Consequently, I related well to my surgical colleagues over the years.

Dr. Stead's introduction to the surgical staff at the Brigham, however, involved a controversy that was vintage "early" Stead. While he was still a medical intern, a 25-year-old man was admitted to his service. The patient appeared basically strong, but very ill with a high fever. On examination, Stead found that he had fluid in his chest; when this was partially drained with a needle, it had the foul smell of anaerobic bacterial infection. Stead took the fluid to one of the surgeons saying, "This stuff doesn't smell good; we ought to drain his chest surgically." Because it was too late in the day to operate, the surgeons planned to put a big hollow tube in his chest to drain off the fluid first thing in the morning. Unaware of how dangerous the situation was (the infection ruptured into the patient's bronchus and flooded the lung), Stead went for dinner. When he later returned to the ward, the patient was unconscious and having trouble breathing. Stead quickly maneuvered the patient so that his head was hanging down over the edge of the bed so that the pus could run out of the young man's mouth. The patient gradually regained consciousness, and Stead stayed beside him all night, holding him on his side so that he could oxygenate one lung. The next day, Stead stopped by the operating room to see how the patient was doing. He found the patient was lying on his back on the table, turning blue. The surgical staff had positioned the patient in such a way that his good lung was being flooded and he couldn't breathe. In a rage of fury, Stead picked the man up in his arms and carried him back to the ward. Determined not to take the patient back to the operating room, Stead then had to figure out how to keep the patient alive.

Dr. Stead:

> I didn't have the right instruments or equipment with which to drain him. Fortunately, I was friendly with one of the Senior Assistant surgical residents who was somewhat independent; I told him I needed to drain my patient, but didn't want to take him back to the operating room. He figured out how to perform a closed chest drainage procedure on the ward. With his help, I got my patient through the day fairly well, with a tube draining into an underwater bottle to provide suction. He began to look better, but as the night wore on I had more and more trouble keeping the tube open because the patient tended to lie on his side and twist or kink the tube so that it stopped draining. Finally, I decided that I needed the tube to go directly down, and the easiest solution was to put it straight through the mattress. I made an incision in the mattress and ran the tube from his chest down through the hole in the mattress, and it worked fine. Of course, we had to keep the patient still, but he was quite cooperative, and I continued to stay with him.
>
> The next day, the Nursing Supervisor discovered what I had done and, without ever talking to me about it, reported me to Dr. Christ-

ian, claiming that I had ruined her mattress. Dr. Christian said that he thought it was a unique situation. He was a gentleman about it and told me if I ever had an unusual situation like it again or had a complaint, I should go to him directly. In fact, the reason I got a surgical internship so easily was that the Chief of Surgery got wind of the whole story and thought it was pretty amazing. He'd heard that I had taken the patient out of the operating room, but he never said anything about it to me until I went to apply for an internship. When he interviewed me for this very competitive position, he said he knew about my credentials and would be glad to have me.

Aside from learning about the seriousness of anaerobic bacterial infections of the chest, I learned some other interesting lessons from that patient. He had come in big, strong and robust, but his illness lasted for quite a while. After he had been in the hospital about two months, I approached him with a needle, and he began to cringe. He was a good example of how illness can traumatize a person, and cause them to react in ways they might not when they're well.

CHAPTER 4

Unpopular in Cincinnati

No one can give authority, it must be taken.

E. A. Stead Jr.

In December 1935, after finishing his surgical internship, Stead went back to the laboratory at Harvard Medical School, working on dogs. It was extremely smelly work and the odor tended to cling. After work one day, he decided to shower in the intern's quarters at the Peter Bent Brigham Hospital, across the street from the Medical School. As he was taking a hot and steamy shower, somebody came in and got into the adjacent stall. The other person, a little taller even than Stead, looked over the partition and asked who he was and what he was working on. He said he was Gene Stead from Atlanta, but that he didn't really know exactly what he was doing. He was three years out of medical school and still didn't know what his next step was going to be.

The fellow bather turned out to be Dr. Tom Spies from Cincinnati. After talking for a while, Spies said that Dr. M. A. Blankenhorn, the recently appointed Chief of Medicine at Cincinnati General Hospital, didn't like the candidate who was slated to become Chief Resident from the current housestaff, and had sent Spies to Boston to find another Chief Resident. Cincinnati had developed a residency program that lasted for five or six years, but Blankenhorn wanted to shake things up by bringing in a Chief Resident from outside the system. Gene said that, given his unstructured background, he wouldn't be very popular in a structured medical service like Cincinnati's. Furthermore, he had no money and couldn't afford to move from Boston to Cincinnati. Spies persisted and arranged for Stead to have breakfast with Dr. Hartwell Harrison the next morning. Harrison was just starting his illustrious career in urology, and he and Tom Spies had both known Blankenhorn at Western Missouri where he had been a most popular medical professor before moving to Cincinnati.

Dr. Stead:

> We discussed the possibility of my going to Cincinnati, and I reiterated my reservations. But before the breakfast was over Hartwell told

me he had a "rich uncle" who liked to do things for people and would happily loan me the money. So if I wanted to go to Cincinnati, I shouldn't worry about the money. That was an offer I couldn't refuse.

Tom Spies had never worked at the Brigham. The day Gene ran into him he was merely visiting a friend at Harvard. By sheer happenstance they both took a bath at the Brigham at the same time on the same day. Stead never would have thought about Cincinnati if it hadn't been for that shower after work in the dog lab. So often do career opportunities turn on just such serendipity.

In January, 1936, Dr. Stead started work as an Assistant Resident at the Cincinnati General Hospital, knowing that he would become Chief Resident in July. Amongst the rest of the resident staff, however, "I was not very popular for the simple reason that those people who had been there before would have liked the old system to continue. They would have preferred that one of their own people become Chief Resident."

Cincinnati General had the same type of patients as Grady, but was much larger. It was a great learning experience because it demonstrated the relationship between acute illness and poverty, and put on display the advanced disease of patients who often arrived at the hospital in terminal condition. But it also had all the problems of large city hospitals: no full laboratory or x-ray units, and none of the ancillary facilities taken for granted at private institutions. As Assistant Resident, Gene Stead took to the medical service with the anticipation that on July 1 he would make a great many changes. And so he did.

Dr. Stead:

> As Chief Resident, I was in charge when the Chairman was away. And no one could gainsay me without going to see Dr. Blankenhorn. Slowly I learned that authority can't be given, but it can be taken. I ran the medical service in a very high-handed fashion, and I'm not entirely proud of the way I ran it. But nobody argued with me. I wouldn't let any patient be transferred to or from the Medical Service unless I saw the patient personally. I took a great deal of responsibility for teaching students, and supervised their lab work and their medical work. I was interested in these things and it seemed like a practical way to run a service. I really lived in the hospital and enjoyed my residency at Cincinnati. Dr. Blankenhorn later signed a photograph of himself to me and it reads "To Gene Stead, a Chief Resident in every sense of the word."
>
> In those days, you wouldn't be admitted to the hospital unless you signed an autopsy permit in case something happened and you died.

I must say that in return for the somewhat autocratic way in which we ran the hospital, we really took exceptional care of the patients. We were in the hospital at all times, and gave the patients the very best of our knowledge about how to care for sick people. If a nurse wasn't there, we carried the bedpan to the patient. In a sense, we were making a bargain with the patient and it seemed fair to us at the time. As I say, it's not a time I'm particularly proud of, but it shows how we used poor people to learn medicine in that day.

One of the problems at the Cincinnati General Hospital was that it had a rotating internship. Rotating internships have a theoretical advantage over straight internships in that the interns spend time in medicine, surgery, obstetrics, and pediatrics in the anticipation that, after those varied internship experiences, they will select a specialty area for residency training. But rotating internships have some serious drawbacks. One loomed so large that Gene Stead thought it called for drastic action. Around Christmas time, when the interns were notified of their July 1 residency appointments, they tended to lose interest in those rotations that lay outside their chosen field. As a result, the Medical Service was difficult to operate over the Christmas holidays.

Dr. Stead:

I solved the problem by identifying interns who had a real interest in a career in Internal Medicine, then arranged for them to swap rotations with colleagues who had less interest. In this way, we got the desirable ones to spend a longer time in medicine, and the others were not a concern of mine. I persuaded the interns to agree to swap by employing a very simple method. I had to sign the interns' evaluations, verifying that they had completed the medical portion of their internship successfully. I simply told the people whom I didn't want on the service that I wasn't going to sign their certificates. I suggested they go somewhere else to study medicine as an intern because, if they didn't, they would end up getting no credit from me for taking the medicine rotation.

I wanted to be involved in all the major decisions on the Medical Service, but Dr. Blankenhorn could not give me that authority, which I obviously could give myself. Fortunately I had a good group of senior and junior medical residents; and my personal system of selective rotation supplied me with good interns.

Unlike the Grady Hospital, Cincinnati had full-time staff, but their numbers were limited. Dr. Blankenhorn was full-time, but also did a fair amount of private practice, earning perhaps half of his income from private patient fees. There was a full-time gastroenterologist named Schiff, who became very well known, but all the other doctors were part-time. Tom Spies was there doing nutrition work, but he was frequently absent because he conducted a lot of his work in Birmingham, Alabama.

Dr. Stead:

> The Emergency Room was very active and I found it highly produc-tive to my learning and to the patients' welfare if I wandered through there at all times of day and night. Some of the staff were a little skep-tical about my methods, however, because the service had previously been oriented toward practical medicine with the anticipation that its young doctors would go into practice after they finished training. We brought a much more clinical research oriented approach to it. The teaching emphasis had been based on what was known about medi-cine; I simply shifted that emphasis to what was *not known* about medicine. Nearly all the teaching was done with the patients in the room, and that made it uncomfortable for some people.

> I personally desegregated the Medical Service of the Cincinnati General Hospital, which was segregated when I arrived. The adult service was divided into units for men and women and then further divided into black and white. As a result, we always had unused beds in some sections and a dearth of space in others, and very sick peo-ple who needed to be taken care of. I didn't like the idea that there were special areas restricted to the use of one particular group, and so I set out to change as much as I could. I didn't ask for permission. I simply ordered the change based on expediency for patient care. I did not change the preference system; there were always more black patients on the old black wards, and more white patients on the old white wards, but I managed to effect a 10% or 15% mix because we never rejected a patient on the basis of color. The reaction to the in-tegration of patients was varied; some of the housestaff thought the solution was very sensible and some resented it. For me, one of the virtues of the system was that unless Dr. Blankenhorn was on the ward, my word ruled. Our new arrangement increased the work of the housestaff because they couldn't count on having any empty beds, but I must say I didn't really worry about what the staff thought. I was having a great time.

> The force of culture is very strong and can make it difficult to see the needs of a particular group when you've grown up in a place that

has become indifferent to those needs. In the South, many indignities were put upon blacks because white people never knew they were indignities. The Cincinnati General Hospital had a ward of approximately fifty beds, which was entirely a black male ward when I arrived there, and there was about a 35% mortality rate from lobar pneumonia on that ward. There was only one nurse on duty at night, and it seemed to me that it would be very hard for the nurse to give any kind of comfort to that many sick and dying patients. I went to the Hospital Superintendent and told him that the situation was intolerable, and I threatened to go public with details about the ward unless there was a change. Under duress, he agreed to give me a second nurse at night. However, the second nurse had been trained at the General Hospital and was used to the existing practices and attitudes from having been a student on that ward, so her presence accomplished nothing. When I walked through the ward in the evenings I saw that there were two nurses sitting down instead of only one. I had to go back to administration and tell them that I had not succeeded in improving patient services, and that I could not justify the additional nurse. People's attitudes toward what had once been the serving class hadn't changed much. A lot of time had passed, but we hadn't yet gotten over letting old habits dominate our behavior. If somebody stopped and asked those nurses what they were doing and why they were doing it, it would become clear that they had no bad intent. But it was not possible to effect much change because the nursing department at the General had a very strong hierarchy and they really didn't appreciate my change, simply because it had always been done the other way.

During that year as Chief Resident, I had a number of informal meetings with and taught a number of nurses, so I learned a great deal about communicating with people who had different formal educational backgrounds. Consequently, I have always felt some debt to the Cincinnati nurses, both graduate and undergraduate, who put up with me in my learning time. I practiced my speaking skills and worked on overcoming nervousness in front of an audience of strangers. By that time, I had gotten to where I could speak loud enough to be heard, but it took me some time to figure out what was useful information to impart to the nurses, given what they were going to be doing in their careers, and what wasn't useful information. I had more trouble sorting out the material to be presented than I had actually presenting it.

Dr. Stead had a central role in the vitamin scandal, as it was called in Cincinnati. In the spring of 1937 or '38, members of the housestaff at Cincinnati General Hospital developed a rash accompanied by gastrointestinal problems; Gene checked into the poor diet provided to the hospital staff and discovered that the residents were all deficient in the B vitamin, niacin. They had contracted pellagra from eating the hospital food! This became front-page news in the Cincinnati Enquirer. Dr. Stead was the one who made the diagnosis and it's ironic because he was first recruited by Tom Spies, a nutrition expert who was a Professor of Medicine at Cincinatti.

Of course, Stead's influence at the hospital was limited to the medical wards, and on those wards he reigned, but in other arenas he ran up against very strong, organized structures, which he had no way to change. He didn't pay the salaries of those people, they weren't responsible to him, and they would still be at the General after he had moved on. Like civil servants in Washington dealing with a new president, they would outlast him. He didn't make any progress with nursing, or with the laboratory or x-ray services. The food was bad, and remained bad. The only thing that he really affected was the care of the patients, and the attitudes and work habits of doctors who were on the medical service. It was a sharply circumscribed influence.

Dr. Stead:

> Having enjoyed a positive learning experience and the time I spent in Cincinnati, I was never sure in my own mind why I was able to leave so easily. In a sense, I went to Cincinnati a boy and came out a man. I didn't know I could be a leader until I went to the General, but after that experience, I knew that quality was something I possessed. I was still socially pretty inept and ill at ease despite the help of Dr. Sosman, and was always concerned about my interactions with people. I somehow never felt that I had anything important to say and therefore avoided conversation because it seemed to me that I was imposing on another person. I was peculiar and felt myself to be so. Yet somehow, I believed in the field of medicine and I wanted to be cured of my shyness, so I was willing to do whatever it took to make that happen. But I was kind of a queer mixture. I was clearly domineering when I ran the General, and I didn't take "No" for an answer. In nearly all other relationships I was as timid as could be.
>
> The few times I did get involved socially with people at Cincinnati General, I was just as ill at ease as ever. The housestaff, of course, picked up on this and called me "Professor" from the time I got there. Interestingly enough, I never worried about it; I guess I thought that

someday, maybe I would be a professor. But I didn't find much resistance to my methods. Only one or two residents remained from the old guard, because Dr. Blankenhorn and I had weeded out at least 80% of the former residents. The group that I had were largely Stead people from the beginning.

In Cincinnati, Gene was fortunate to meet Dr. Morton Hamburger, a very urbane and cultured young resident at the General. His uncle had been a distinguished member of the medical faculty at Johns Hopkins for many years. Hamburger was Jewish and had benefited from his family's cultural background, which led to an interest in music, an area unfamiliar to Gene. In fact, Hamburger's whole orientation and interests tended toward things that were totally foreign to Gene. Hamburger introduced him to Gilbert and Sullivan, to fine foods (he had never before eaten cheese!), and widened Stead's horizons with a variety of new experiences.

Stead had always been a careful student of history but, given our tendency to mythologize American history, he had no real sense of what was true and what was not. Hamburger gave him Beard's *American Civilization*, a book that is still in Stead's possession. The book opened up for Stead a whole new way of looking at particular points of historical time, and made him realize how unimportant most of the history he had learned really was. In addition, Hamburger was widely read in the medical literature. "Under Morton Hamburger's auspices, I saw my first patient with periarteritis, a serious blood vessel disorder, and my first case of a dissecting aneurysm, both of which are difficult diagnoses to make during life, and both of which he had already diagnosed. He was a senior resident and two years later he was Chief Resident. He remained in Cincinnati and became involved with infectious disease."

Dr. Eugene Ferris was a graduate of the University of Virginia who had a two-year internship at Boston City Hospital as a research fellow with Soma Weiss, then came to Cincinnati General as a full-time Assistant Professor of Medicine. Spies, Ferris and Schiff were the three full-time faculty members under Dr. Blankenhorn. Gene Stead became friendly with Ferris because of the Boston connection and because of Ferris's interest in research. During the last six months of his residency, Stead spent one afternoon each week in the laboratory with Ferris. Among the instruments used by Ferris was a double manometer that allowed him to measure pressures in blood vessels. Stead became interested in measuring venous pressure in patients with various clinical conditions, so he got himself a little tray and carried the apparatus to the wards. In patients with obstruction to blood flow in the chest (such as from tumors compressing the great veins) the manometers were a useful way to show that the flow of blood was obstructed. Naturally, Stead also interested the residents in the use of this technique.

Dr. Ferris used a plethysmograph to measure blood volume in the hand, and a kymograph to record dynamic changes in volume on smoked drums. A change in circumstances like cooling or heating the hand caused major changes in blood flow, as did diseases that affected the blood vessels of the arm. Plethysmographs and smoked drums were primitive but classical measuring instruments found at the time in all physiology departments. They had been around for a long time, but using them to study blood flow in sick people was new; it was Stead's first try at clinical research. He had no real notion of what to do, but since Gene Ferris was often not there, Gene Stead was on his own. He would go to the ward and find a patient on whom to make simple observations of venous pressure. And, importantly, he reported his findings.

This seemingly casual experience played an important role in his professional life. Midway through his year as Chief Resident, Dr. Ferris invited Soma Weiss to spend five days at Cincinnati General Hospital as Visiting Professor. Stead and Weiss spent a good deal of time together, mostly seeing patients. Weiss was interested in many things and the General had a large number of patients with different diseases. Weiss and his colleagues in Boston had just finished work on alcoholics who developed the nutritional deficiency disease called beriberi, and Weiss had described patients with what was called carotid sinus syncope (a curious condition in which pressure on an overly sensitive carotid sinus in the neck causes fainting).

Dr. Stead:

> One particular patient I saw with Dr. Weiss piqued my curiosity. It was a lady with rheumatic heart disease that had led to mitral stenosis and auricular fibrillation. I had been struck by the fact that some patients with mitral stenosis had a heart sound, heard through the stethoscope, that came after the second sound, after the "dub" in "lub-dub" as you listen to the heart. The extra sound was significantly louder than the normal second heart sound and was striking when it happened. It occasionally occurred in patients with mitral stenosis and fibrillation who had all the typical x-ray findings in the heart and lungs that are expected in mitral stenosis but who really had little or none of the classical murmur that is the tell-tale sign of mitral valve narrowing. As it turned out, this sound was later to be known as the "opening snap" of the mitral valve, and if I'd been a little brighter, I would have realized this right away. I pointed this sound out to Soma as an interesting finding, indicating that there had been very little or

no research work done on this. The sound was so striking that it initiated my interest in mitral stenosis.

As Dr. Stead wrote in a 1955 letter to Dr. Blankenhorn:

> What a flood of memories comes to me as I begin this letter! I came to your service as an immature uncertain assistant resident and I left it 18 months later as a confident doctor. The sense of being at home in medicine which grew into me on your service has lasted throughout the years.
>
> I remember many small things that you have long since forgotten: the man with the chronic emphysema and contracted chest who I thought had atelectasis from bronchial obstruction—you asked for a needle and out came the pus; the first sympathectomy performed on a desperately ill patient with hypertension; a patient apparently recovering from pneumococcal pneumonia in whom you heard the early diastolic "whiff" indicating the development of bacterial endocarditis.
>
> I have never forgotten the support that you gave to your resident. He was free to run the service and to try out his own ideas. For me it was a year of great growth in my relationship to other people. For the first time, I began to understand how to work with other people and to get them to help me.

CHAPTER 5

RETURN TO MECCA

Many people like to fish and play golf. I like to work with my head.

E. A. Stead Jr.

Dr. Stead:

When Soma Weiss was getting ready to return to Boston after his visit in Cincinnati, he asked me to come to the Thorndike Laboratory the following year. But I told him that there were certain considerations involved in my decision: I was still paying off my medical school debt, and was determined to pay my brother's tuition at Emory, so I would need to have $1,500 a year. I had been paid $1,000 as Chief Resident at Cincinnati. Dr. Weiss replied that they had never paid a Fellow $1,500 and he couldn't swing that. I really didn't know any other place that I would want to go for clinical training. My experience over the past 18 months had been pretty rich and I thought that when the academic year ended in July, I would take a one-month vacation and then go into practice in Atlanta. I told him if he returned and found that by any chance there was a little more money, I would be able to join him at the Thorndike. At that time I didn't want to go into research on a full-time basis, because I really didn't know what it was. On the other hand, I knew I was a competent clinician and wouldn't have any trouble handling patients because, as it turned out, my shyness was never a limitation with them. I also liked the Atlanta area, so returning there to practice seemed to be a sensible decision.

In May I got a wire from Dr. Weiss saying that he had found the money. I was convinced that Dr. Weiss was one of the few people I'd learn much more clinical medicine from. The Thorndike possessed a certain standing in the medical world and I appreciated the fact that it would open up doors that I might or might not be able to walk through.

Stead returned to Boston (the Mecca of American Medicine) in 1937 at the lowest academic rank of Assistant in Medicine. It was an important career de-

cision because he had been offered a number of other choices, including staying on at the Cincinnati General Hospital. Dr. Blankenhorn thought that the
Thorndike was a good idea, but also suggested the Rockefeller Institute—an
outstanding research institution, but not one that interested Stead who, for a
number of years, had wondered whether he was suited for a research career.
He was confident in his ability to take care of people, but uncertain about
work in a laboratory. The American Heart Association offered to make him a
career investigator, but he never saw himself as primarily a researcher.

Dr. Stead:

> I knew I could be some kind of an educator, some kind of a doctor,
> but I had no desire to go into research full-time. I was never certain
> that, over an indefinite period of time, I could continue to produce
> and contribute new knowledge, as you need to do in research. I did
> think I could remain competitive in teaching and caring for pa-
> tients—the things that I liked—for as long as I lived, but I didn't
> think that by the time I got to be 50 years old, I could compete with
> young people in the research game. I really wasn't very well trained
> as a scientist, and that was a gap in my education. When I got beyond
> high school I didn't know what I was going to do and so, as a result
> of not taking preparatory courses, my education in the physical sci-
> ences was limited. I also knew there were some areas in which my
> limitations weren't obvious, at least not to me. I didn't want to be in
> a position where my performance was only satisfactory; if I couldn't
> be really outstanding, I wasn't interested. My judgment was quite
> right. When I went to college, I really didn't know what I should
> learn. Over time I discovered that I could ask penetrating questions,
> which, in the end, even I couldn't find the answers to. That made me
> useful to some researchers but would be a limitation on my own abil-
> ity to conduct research. If I had been better trained, I might have
> made the wrong decision and decided to go into research.

After finishing as Chief Resident in Cincinnati, Stead knew that he could teach
and that he could encourage younger people to reach a level of research productivity that wouldn't occur without him in the picture. He interacted well
with physician-researchers like Jack Myers, John Hickam, and others, but he
never took credit for a project on which he didn't actually work (his name
doesn't appear on a single one of Myers's many important papers). Curiously,
at the time of decision about post-Cincinnati life, he could have been lured to
Atlanta by an offer of $2,000 from the Grady Hospital because he knew he

could be helpful there. As things were to happen, there would be time enough for that later.

Stead began work in Dr. Weiss' lab on July 1, but he arrived a few days early to get acquainted with his new surroundings. Weiss, Associate Director at the Thorndike, was on one of his regular trips to Europe, so on Stead's first day at work, he went to see Dr. George Minot, the famous hematologist who had won the Nobel Prize for discovering the cure of pernicious anemia, and was then Chief of the Medical Service at the Boston City Hospital. Stead reasoned that, since he was being paid enough to be a Chief Resident but his only assigned task was to turn off the hospital lights at night, he should make himself available to Dr. Minot, should his services be needed.

Besides Stead, Dr. Weiss had one other fellow, Dr. Charles Kunkel (who would later become Stead's Chief of Neurology at Duke). On June 30, just before the official start at the Thorndike, Kunkel accidentally hit Stead in the face during a squash game. Gene had the gash over one eye sewn up by an intern but had a tremendous bruise around the injured eye and was left with a noticeable scar. He was still able to explore on his own the next day, and discovered that he not only had a laboratory to work in, but a technician as well. He introduced himself to Sophie, and asked who had been there before. She said his predecessor had been a man named Wilkins, so Stead asked what Dr. Wilkins would be doing if he were still there. She explained that he and Dr. Weiss were investigating ways to make people faint so they could study the physiology of fainting. Subjects would stand perfectly still, like soldiers at attention, until they felt faint, presumably because insufficient blood was being pumped to the brain, then the investigators would see if they could alleviate the faintness with a new drug called epinephrine. In the course of this process, they would monitor the pulse and blood pressure.

"They have a thing called a plethysmograph to record measurements with," Sophie said, and Stead told her he'd heard of that. "They set the plethysmograph on the subject while he's lying flat and make some measurements and then stand him up and put the plethysmograph up on the x-ray stand. Your duty is to lift the plethysmograph when the patient rises into a standing position so I can make some more measurements. When the patient is ready to faint—however long it takes—you lie him down and lower the plethysmograph."

It seemed straightforward enough, but clearly they needed a subject. Sophie told him to go up on the ward and find a patient who was scheduled for a hernia operation and tell him that in preparation for the operation it would be important to do some special studies. Once the patient was in the lab, he would be rigged to the plethysmograph, stood up while measurements were made, put back down, given some epinephrine, stood up again and the process repeated. Before Dr. Weiss was back from his trip, Stead had finished a number of studies and written his first paper. Such were the rough and ready clinical research mores of the day.

Dr. Weiss had a secretary, Marion, whom he shared with Dr. William Castle, perhaps the most famous of the great Boston City hematologists. Marion had excellent editing skills, so Stead took the paper to her and said, "I'm a lonesome boy in a great big city and I've got this paper and I need somebody to read it."

Dr. Stead:

> Well, she read it and she told me it was the worst paper she ever saw, told me to take it back and read it over and find out what I had done wrong. Further, she threatened that if I dared hand it back to her with the same mistakes she'd never help me again. I thought that sounded fair to me, so I read it over and made some changes and Marion typed it for me. Then I took it in to Dr. Castle, saying, "Marion thought this was the worst paper she ever read. Would you be willing to read it in Dr. Weiss' absence?" I think it is typical of Dr. Castle's character that he was comfortable reading a paper that was not in his field. He made some very helpful, straightforward and simple suggestions, which I incorporated. When Dr. Weiss returned, he was satisfied with it. After some debate, I persuaded him to put his name on it because I felt strongly that having his name on the first two papers I published would lend them stature, and it had started as his project. We submitted it to the Journal of Clinical Investigation and it was published six weeks later.

Stead had actually met Dr. Castle several years earlier. During the last four or five months of his Brigham internship, Stead had served as resident on the Infectious Disease Service at Boston City Hospital. One day he was consulting on a patient who had a urinary tract infection. The senior medical resident met him and they sat on the steps right inside the doors of the hospital while the resident told him about the patient. When he was through, Stead told him that he didn't think the information held together, and that the story probably wouldn't check out when he saw the patient. For good measure, he didn't think very much of the way the resident was planning to handle the patient. The resident responded that he thought they were going to do all right because Dr. Castle had stopped by to see the patient and had agreed with the plans. Never having met him, Stead said, "I don't care who Dr. Castle is, or what he thinks, because he's wrong." About this time, they noticed someone standing behind them on the steps; they turned around and the gentleman said, "I'm Dr. Castle and I'm interested in this discussion." Stead later recalled: "Of course I was tremendously embarrassed. But that remark was characteristic of Dr. Castle. He was never paralyzed by what he didn't know. He had enough confidence to always say, 'I don't know that' or, 'We'll try to get the information.'" In Stead's eyes, Dr. Castle was the most original thinker at the Thorndike.

Dr. Stead:

> I think this had to do with the fact that he was unencumbered by information that he didn't need to use at the time. This impressed me to such an extent that I began to watch for this among my residents and students. Over the years we did have a large number of fairly compulsive learners, and I observed that truly compulsive people, who have to know the latest about everything, are really not original thinkers. They don't have time to be because they are completely submerged in the process of learning other people's thoughts and ideas. At the same time, you do need clay and straw in order to build bricks; if you don't have sufficient materials to work with, in this case knowledge, you also can't be creative. But the ability to say "I don't know" is terribly important, and it was very characteristic of Dr. Castle not to be encumbered by things he didn't know at the time. The freshness with which he looked at problems was delightful.

During his time at the Thorndike, Stead lived in room 606, a number famous in medicine because it had been assigned by Paul Ehrlich to the first successful anti-syphilis drug, Salvarsan. As a result, Stead had no difficulty remembering where he lived. The Thorndike Lab, on the other hand, had a troubled relationship with Boston City Hospital, whose administration didn't understand the reason for a research hospital on their campus. The administrators were irritated if they saw the lights burning all night at the Thorndike, so every evening Stead walked through the entire building, solemnly turning off all the lights. Years later he learned that at the same time that he was saving money at the Thorndike, Hollis Edens (a future President of Duke University) was turning out lights at Emory University.

Dr. Lowell Rantz, later the Professor of Medicine at Stanford, worked in a laboratory across from Stead. One day, Dr. Weiss asked Stead to substitute for him on rounds and Gene invited Lowell to join in. Stead always involved anyone who was present in the discussion on rounds; he believed that no one should stand around and not take part. So whoever was in attendance on rounds was invited (or provoked) to participate, and there was always electricity in the air. On this day a well-dressed gentleman turned up, asking where Dr. Weiss was making rounds. They told him that they were making rounds in Weiss's place, and asked him to come along. As the discussion turned toward the unknown aspects of medicine, they incorporated their guest and quizzed him a little. "He was extraordinarily well informed, though we didn't know who he was. He stayed with us the whole two hours and thanked us when he left. I remarked to Lowell about the depth of his knowledge. When I later met Soma in the hall he told me he was having lunch with a visitor from Columbia University and invited me to join them. When I got there, Dr. Weiss's guest turned out to be the gentleman who had participated in rounds with us earlier—Dr. Robert Loeb, Chairman of the Department of Medicine at Columbia, and author of a famous textbook of medicine. He really was a very nice man. He had a very wide range of knowledge." No wonder about this: Dr. Loeb was probably the most famous doctor outside of Boston. Curiously, they did not introduce themselves when they first met, but were to have many contacts in the future.

Soma Weiss was a most dynamic individual. He came by the lab each morning and invariably asked, "What's new?" Every day Stead set up an experiment so that they would learn something new, no matter how small, that they could talk about. They did no experiments on Sundays, Christmas or Thanksgiving, but on every other day of the year there was a set of new observations and measurements to discuss. Before leaving in the evening, Dr. Weiss stopped by and asked again what was new. In a very few minutes he would know what they were doing in the lab and why. The questions got harder to answer, but these were exciting interactions for the young scholars.

Despite his close interactions with those doing the work, Soma Weiss didn't carry out experiments himself because he was involved with so many other things. Only once did Stead see him at work with his own hands. They wanted to get blood from a patient's internal jugular vein above the point where the facial vein entered. Stead had never done this before and didn't want to mess up the experiment, so Weiss came in and made the venipunctures. "He was quite apt with his hands, much more so than I am; I'm not very apt, which is why I could never be a surgeon."

Stead spent two years at the Thorndike. When Soma Weiss was then called to chair the Department of Medicine at the Peter Bent Brigham Hospital, it was clear that he was going to take somebody working on blood circulation to the Brigham with him. There were two candidates: Stead and his predecessor at the Thorndike, Wilkins. "I'd have to say in all honesty that Bob

Wilkins was a more imaginative researcher than I turned out to be. He had excellent training and had a much more sophisticated background than I had. But I had one advantage over him; I was simply further along into my clinical training." Two other lucky breaks contributed to Stead's eventual appointment at the Brigham. Each week Dr. Weiss held a CPC (clinico-pathological conference) during which the chart notes of all of the attending doctors were read aloud, after which the pathologist demonstrated the autopsy findings. Early on Stead figured out that whoever saw the patient last would probably have the best notes. That doctor would benefit from everyone else's thoughts as well as from the terminal observations, which sometimes were important (for example, in cases of bacterial endocarditis it is sometimes difficult to culture bacteria from the blood until close to the end of life). So even elusive diagnoses can become evident near the end. Stead arranged that the senior intern running the wards would keep him informed of all difficult diagnostic problems likely to end up in the autopsy room. Stead would examine the patient and the chart near the end, and add his own notes. As a result, his were the best. One of the people who helped him most was Lewis Thomas, a senior medical student at the time, who later became President of Memorial Hospital in New York and noted author of the most graceful essays about medicine and biology.

Stead was also fortunate to know Dick Ebert, an intern who became an important figure in medicine. They saw a number of patients together and Ebert was familiar with Stead's work in the laboratory. It was clear to Ebert that Stead was destined for a career in academic medicine because he knew so many things that other people didn't, so he said to Weiss: "I hope that Dr. Stead is going with you to the Brigham; if he does I want to work in his laboratory." (Stead says this kind of thing is "luck"; Disraeli said, "We make our fortunes, and we call them fate.") In any case, Stead went with Weiss and Wilkins didn't, but "Bob did extremely well with his career, and we have remained friends over the years. I have no real notion as to whether he even wanted the job at the Brigham, but it would have seemed perfectly reasonable if Soma had taken him. There weren't a whole lot of other candidates in those days."

The year before Weiss was appointed Chief at the Brigham, Stead was offered the position of Chief Resident there with Dr. Christian, who was in his last year. At the time it was not known that Dr. Weiss would succeed him. From across town at the Thorndike, Stead was very pleased to be offered the position. He remembered how impressed he had been with the Chief Resident he met when he first came to the Brigham as an intern and "I was really just a boy from Georgia." Dr. Christian and Stead carried on some negotiation about the position, but Stead was still supporting his brother in medical school. Dr. Christian proposed that Stead's transfer from the Thorndike to the Brigham would result in his brother Bill's transfer to Harvard Medical School, thus alleviating the financial problem. "I went back to Soma to discuss this offer, and he was perfectly honest with me. He said, 'Don't sign up with the old Chief, wait and sign up with the new Chief,' who, of course, turned out to be Soma although he could not have been sure about that when he gave me this piece of advice."

CHAPTER 6

YOUNG FACULTY—
EARLY LESSONS

People don't choose their careers; they are engulfed by them.

John Dos Passos

The medical experiences in Boston made Gene Stead come to life. He couldn't know it then, but he and his young colleagues were destined to shape the future of clinical medicine in America. They did so through clinical research that illuminated normal and diseased physiology. Soma Weiss was particularly interested in the nervous system, especially the reflexes of the autonomic nervous system, because so many things were amenable to experimental measurement. At that time, a young psychiatrist named John Romano was working at the Thorndike, and Romano, like Weiss, thought that the brain was the determinant of behavior. Because there was a good deal of interchange between the medicine and psychiatry services at the time, Weiss got to know Romano and appreciate his abilities. Consequently, when he moved to the Brigham, in addition to Charles Janeway in Infectious Disease, Gene Stead in Cardiology and Jack Gibson in Isotopes, Weiss appointed Romano to Psychiatry and Neurology at the Brigham Hospital. Between 1939 and 1942 Stead spent a lot of time with John Romano. Together with Charles Janeway, they started a small private practice clinic at the Peter Bent Brigham Hospital.

Dr. Stead:

> They gave us a little office in which to see patients, and I discovered that Romano was very helpful in taking care of a variety of patients whom I didn't know what the heck to do with. They didn't have heart failure, their kidneys worked, they weren't bleeding and so on, but they felt chronically unwell. I had now gotten to the point of appreciating someone who had the background that Romano had in psychiatry. He could be a very useful ally. By that time I had realized that professional physicians should be able to take care of a variety of

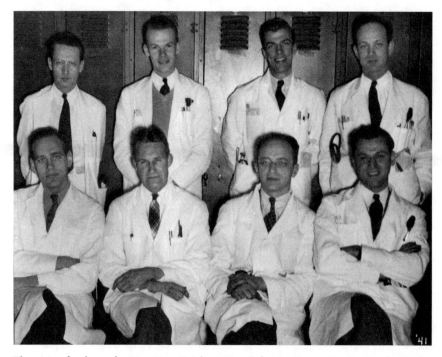

The young faculty at the Peter Bent Brigham Hospital, 1941 Front: Eugene Stead, Charles Janeway, Soma Weiss, John Romano Rear: Residents Jack Myers, Jim Warren, Louis Hempleman, Max Michael.

partly incapacitated people who weren't psychotic, and in whom the usual kinds of tests of mental faculties were likely to be normal. Doctors like Romano could do that. In turn, I was useful to him because I had ways of measuring things in the laboratory that John didn't know about. So I helped him to write his first papers that had anything to do with science.

Together, Romano and Stead wrote a paper on electroencephalographic (EEG or brain wave) changes in a woman who, it was thought, had an overactive carotid-sinus reflex, which caused her to faint. In this rare condition pressure on the carotid sinus in the neck slows the heart rate enough to induce fainting. One classic case described by Soma Weiss involved a businessman who often fainted while riding on the train going to New York City, but never on the return trip home. The mystery was solved when it was learned that his tight collar pressed on his overly sensitive carotid sinus only when he turned his head to the right to look out the window at the Hudson River on the way into New York. On the way home, he turned to the left, and had no trouble.

In studying their patient, Romano and Stead collaborated with a man named Gibbs, who did most of the early EEG engineering. Unfortunately, he used a mechanical way of reading EEGs that was not accurate, but Stead did not realize it. The paper they wrote using the faulty data was published in the *New England Journal. of Medicine*.

Dr. Stead:

> We only found out later that what we were thinking was brain wave activity induced by the carotid-sinus, was an artifact built into Gibbs' new machine, and had nothing whatever to do with the physiology of the carotid sinus. It's the only paper I've written in which the data were incorrect. George Engel, who was interested in vascular reflexes, read our paper and detected the artifact. At the time he was an intern at Mt. Sinai Hospital, but was visiting the Brigham for the summer. While he was in Boston he tracked us down, saying, "I want to see the people who wrote this paper. It's a very bad paper and no one should write papers like that." After he had thoroughly berated us, John and I said, "Well, we think you're pretty smart, and although you don't think we're so smart, we're smart enough to offer you a job." So he joined up with John Romano just as the war was coming along. I went to Emory as a Professor of Medicine, and John moved to Cincinnati as Professor of Psychiatry, taking George Engel with him. Of course, George later became very famous in Psychosomatic Medicine. I knew George had a twin brother (Frank Engel) who also was involved in medicine, and so I kept an eye open for him and he did figure in my career a little later.

Dr. Weiss gave his three young faculty members as much leeway as he could, as long as they all went about their business, making ward rounds, attending conferences, teaching. Whenever Weiss was away, one of the three was in charge of the service. As Stead recalls, "We did nearly all of our teaching on the ward, and I would have to say that we were on top of the heap. We were always available to the Housestaff and students."

Dick Ebert and Gene Stead were good at getting permission for autopsies on patients who had been treated by the Housestaff. If a patient died and the Housestaff couldn't get permission for autopsy, Stead or Ebert would go to the family's home and most often got permission from the family.

Dr. Stead:

> I remember one famous Brigham patient with hemosiderosis, a condition in which tissues such as the liver and kidneys become iron-

loaded after many blood transfusions for anemia. The housestaff was very interested in why she had been so anemic in the first place. We had done many studies on this patient to no avail, and Max Michael, the intern in charge of the patient, hadn't been able to get the permission for the autopsy. I went out and got the autopsy permission and afterwards, I joined Saturday morning Grand Rounds. The group was just coming out of one of the wards when Dick and I came along; Max was talking to Soma. We said we'd just come from getting the autopsy permit from the patient's family and Soma said, "That's pretty good, how did you manage it?" To Max's consternation, I replied, "We just went down and asked for the autopsy. You've got to teach your Housestaff how to do this." But that's the way it was at rounds; they tried to ace us and we tried to ace them.

It was fortunate for me that we all had a good time together. We rarely went out socially because we were simply too busy, but in the hospital setting we enjoyed being together. The people closest to me, were Jim Warren, Paul Beeson, Jack Myers and John Hickam. Otherwise my relationships really centered on professional activities, which were very rewarding for me, and I assume they were rewarding to other people. Somehow they didn't seem to be friendships in the traditional sense of the word, although I may be wrong. I don't know if I've ever really had any close friends in the usual sense. Clearly I've had people who I liked very much, and I've done a lot of things for a lot of people, but in the sense that most people have friends—there aren't many people who became heavily involved in Evelyn's and my life outside of our professional activities. Maybe I really don't know what a friend is. Obviously it has different meanings for different people.

Dr. Jack Myers:

I first met Gene Stead at the Peter Bent Brigham Hospital in 1939. He had been working under Soma Weiss at the Boston City Hospital; when Weiss was appointed the Hersey Professor of Physic to succeed Henry Christian, he brought three bright young men with him: Gene Stead, Charlie Janeway and John Romano. All of then became professors and Department Chairman. I was an Assistant Resident in Medicine at the time, and I suppose that when Gene came in he was called an Assistant Professor.

There were four assistant residents in medicine at the Brigham, and we admired all three of those young faculty members. The residents beside myself were Dick Ebert, who went on to become the Chairman of Medicine at Minnesota, Gus Dammin, who became Professor of Pathology at Harvard, and Franklin Paddock, who came up from Columbia and went into practice out in the Berkshires of Massachusetts. We were a tight-knit group, but Dick Ebert formed a closer bond with Gene Stead than the other three of us. In fact, after he completed his assistant residency, he took a fellowship under Stead at the Brigham. But a small group like ours meant we had close personal contact with everybody on the faculty.

I became Chief Resident in late 1940, a little over a year after Gene came. Paul Beeson had been Chief Resident, but he had a Canadian background, and became quite exercised about World War II. When Harvard University formed a Harvard Red Cross Hospital Unit to go to the relief of Great Britain, Paul went to England with that group, and I became Chief Resident. That meant even closer contact with the faculty than I had as an assistant resident.

Dr. Weiss had a teaching philosophy, and I know Gene shared this. In fact, he may have picked up a good deal of it from Weiss. The idea was that young people learn medicine by doing medicine, not by passive information transfer. So all of our students—and there were some very bright ones at Harvard, of course—actually joined the team. Bob Glaser, who later became head of the Kaiser Family Foundation in California is a good example. We made him a clerk in the Harvard Medical School curriculum; he was a member of the team and learned from all of us.

Every Friday morning Soma held Grand Rounds at the Brigham, and they were truly Grand Rounds then. The team assembled and went from ward to ward, and bed to bed, and we saw as many patients as we could see. The last Grand Rounds that Soma made included a lady who had a ruptured congenital cerebral aneurysm and died. A week or so later, he suffered the same fate and also died.

About that time, we got orders for the Fifth General Hospital to go on active duty, so I had to get a uniform. I inquired around Boston, but uniforms were scarce because everybody was being taken into the army. I was advised that the best deal at that time was at Brooks Brothers. So I went downtown and walked into Brooks Brothers, and the salesman said, "You're Dr. Myers, aren't you?" I said, "Yes, how do you know?" He said, "My wife was in the Brigham Hospital a couple of weeks ago and died of a ruptured aneurysm in her head." It was a remarkable coincidence.

Dick Ebert, and I joined the Harvard Fifth General Hospital. It was headed by the famous elder statesman of surgery, Harvey Cushing, and it was the first American general hospital to go overseas. Dick was married and so when the troop train was leaving Boston one Saturday morning in January of 1942, he went down with his wife. I had a call from Gene and Evelyn Stead a day or so before to say that they would like to take me down to the troop train. I was unmarried then, and instead of wandering down by myself, they accompanied me to South Station, which meant a great deal to me.

Two issues warrant clarification. The first has to do with the clinicians who worked with Dr. Soma Weiss in Boston, and later helped bring American medicine to a pre-eminent position. The second concerns Dr. Stead's highly favorable attitude towards experts in behavioral medicine, which was not yet a generally recognized field. This attitude shaped his care for patients, and his teaching of young doctors. And it began with Dr. John Romano.

Dr. John Romano:

Gene Stead and I met in September of 1938 at the Boston City Hospital. He was working with Soma Weiss, and I was a Rockefeller Fellow on the Neurology Service. On Tuesday evenings, Dr. Weiss would make rounds, starting on the Neurology Service and extending through the whole hospital, seeing interesting patients. It was always a great teaching experience. Everyone in the whole hospital, which had housestaff not only from Harvard but also from Tufts and Boston University, got to know Dr. Weiss. I met Stead on one of these occasions and we became friends.

On September 1, 1939 Charles Janeway, Eugene Stead and I moved to the Brigham to be part of Weiss's Department of Medicine. I remember the date because it was the day Hitler bombed Warsaw. Soma Weiss met with the three of us that day along with Samuel A. Levine, James P. O'Hare, William Murphy, Marshall Fulton and a few others of the Grand Old Guard faculty at the Brigham. Soma said, "Gentlemen, these are my three young men and I hope you will give them the opportunity to earn your respect." I'll never forget that day because they brought me on rounds and, since I was a psychiatrist and therefore the most vulnerable, they presented a medical patient to me. She was a very beautiful young woman who, they told me, had a rare disorder called periarteritis nodosa, involving the median nerve in the right arm and causing weakness of the fingers. But I noticed that somebody had done a very bad venipuncture, and there was a huge bruise over the antecubital fossa, so I doubted that periarteritis nodosa had caused the median nerve injury. I was right. She had compression from the blood around the median nerve. After that they decided Romano wasn't so bad, for a psychiatrist. I even knew where the median nerve was!

Stead and I worked together for a number of years, beginning at the Boston City Hospital. We worked on problems relating to blood volume, the physiology of fainting and other matters, and together with the Brigham housestaff, we published a number of joint papers. Our work together led to Stead's Three Laws of Fainting: 1) Never use a dog if you can find a house officer; 2) Bleed them until they faint; and 3) Do it again! We had great fun with these pioneering studies, and Janeway, Stead, and I were sort of the three seniors of a very young group.

When we were doing blood volume studies I was a subject as well as an investigator. One time I had tourniquets on two legs and one arm to pool my blood and lower my blood volume. I was lying recumbent, and when Stead and the others looked down at me, I was white and sweaty. Ebert said, "Jesus Christ, Romano, you're fainting, you don't look good." And I said, "What do you mean I don't look good? Who's doing this to me?" When the tourniquets were released and the blood came back into my legs and arm I had a pain like never before. It was a visceral pain, like a testicular pain—very, very painful. We used a tilt table in order to position the research subject (me) and later on we inserted a balloon in my rectum or in my stomach to record pressures. This was the life of science in those days.

Vigilance was one of Stead's great characteristics. He had a tremendous capacity for single-mindedness, for paying attention to what he was doing. I've seen him sit at the desk in our combined office, writing a paper while all kinds of hubbub were going on around him. He was undisturbed by it all. People could be in the midst of a loud argument and he wouldn't lift up his head from the paper. Those powers of concentration were set in childhood.

Gene was really interested in patients. It wasn't a show; it was quite genuine. I remember one patient, a woman with alcoholic cirrhosis of the liver. She was very distraught, and had been abandoned by everybody. Gene was attentive to her and listened to her. He was genuinely interested in what he could do to relieve her pain and distress. I was impressed by how genuine he was. There was no artifice about him.

He was interested in the world of persons as well as the world of things. He had a genuine relationship to his patients and I admired that.

At Grand Rounds, we were entertained by Soma's slips of the tongue. For example, he would say, 'That fellow he's neither fish nor fry." One day Eliot Joslin, who founded the famous diabetic program that bears his name, asked, "Soma have you read this yet?" and Soma answered, "Yes, not yet." Another time, when a Grand Rounds was rather tedious and going on and on, he turned to Dick Ebert and said, "Dr. Ebert, do you have to say something?" instead of "Do you have something to say?" Evelyn Selby, who became Gene's wife, was Soma's secretary. Sometimes Soma would walk by Evelyn's desk and say "Miss Selby are you under snow?' instead of "Are you snowed under?" He had a Hungarian accent and Lewis Thomas who, as a student, worked with at the City Hospital used to say, "There are two great men at the City: Houston Merritt (a famous neurologist) and Soma Weiss. I'm getting suspicious of Soma Weiss, however, because his accent is getting worse."

Soma was a lovable fellow and he lent himself to fun. But he had very high standards, too. One time at a morning conference I reported that one of the residents thought that more attention was paid to medical students than to housestaff. Soma got very mad and wanted me to name the resident. I said I wouldn't do so because I had been told in confidence. Beeson and Stead backed me up on that. Soma was mad at me for a while, but then he got over it.

Then Soma died tragically of a rupture of the anterior communicating artery in the brain, with subdural, subarachnoid, and intracerebral bleeding. Charlie Janeway and I took care of him at his house, and when he died, my wife and I had all of the housestaff over. I think we bought some beer and spent the whole night long, like an old-fashioned Irish wake, talking about Soma and laughing about all of his slips of the tongue and jokes and stories and it was a time of sadness, but also of joy.

After Soma's death, Stead ran the hospital from April through June or July. He then went to Emory as Professor of Medicine, and later on, Dean. That was just about the time I went to Cincinnati as a Professor in Psychiatry. Stead wanted me to go to Emory and he courted me awhile, so to speak. I went to Atlanta and spent a few days outlining a prospectus because they had no Department of Psychiatry to speak of, and I pointed out the need for a hospital, the need for a program for teaching medical students and for research. Gene then embarked on a program to seduce me to Atlanta. He made elaborate arrangements for my visit. I met the head of Coca-Cola, the head of Georgia Power, the mayor and the city council, as well as Margaret Mitchell, the author of *Gone With the Wind*. She entertained my wife and me at the Piedmont Driving Club, a very fastidious, snobbish club. When we met her she was wearing one of those Queen Mary hats; she was a very nice woman and told us how imposters were taking over and forging her autograph on books. Everybody wanted me to come there, but I turned down the offer because I was involved in all kinds of war research in Cincinnati and building the Psychiatry Department there, and didn't think I should leave. Stead was disappointed, but he understood and I helped him. I went back and forth to Atlanta a couple of times to give some lectures and had a delightful time with all of my old friends there who had joined Gene in Atlanta.

Dr. William Stead:

When he was one year old, our nephew John came to live in my parents' home because my sister's husband was ill. At age 5 John developed primary tuberculosis, and Gene had to explain to him that he had to stay on the bed, though not necessarily in it, for six months. This was a hard thing to do. John Romano had shown Gene his technique for getting children to understand this illness, and so Gene approached it as John Romano would have. Gene told young John all about his illness, and what he needed to do in order to get well. Then Gene asked John to repeat what Gene had told him. John said, "It's just like you said." So Gene realized he had to approach it a little differently. He took a sofa pillow and squashed in one corner and made it look like a hat and set it on another pillow and said, "John, let's pretend that's a friend of yours. Now I want you to tell him what I just told you." When John couldn't do it, Gene sat down and said, "John, I want you to listen because I want you to tell your friend about this." So Gene repeated his instructions about having to be quiet in order to get better, and afterwards John recounted it beautifully. Then Gene said, "Now, John, who is that friend?" And John said, "Well, it's a pillow, what do you think?" Gene said, "No John, that's really you." And then the light dawned and John went to bed for 6 months and he really did recover.

Dr. Romano:

Gene insisted on high standards. Anything that was shabby or shoddy he drew attention to immediately. I remember times when he pointed out that the student could have done better. Also, he was frank enough when he made a mistake. One time he used a wrong decimal place in an experiment we were doing together. He said, "I never forgave me for that." But I did.

Gene contributed significantly to American medicine, not only through his investigative work, but also in the role that he played. Today the generalist in medicine is an endangered species. Before, people like Stead and Jim Warren and John Hickam and all the rest were comfortable making rounds on all patients, no matter what disease they had. Today teachers who stray one or two standard deviations away from a molecule that they're studying are lost. They get anxious and scared and angry. Very few young doctors now are generalists. They all have vertical skills in a very narrow area. Gene was a model for the generalist physician.

Dr. Stead:

John Romano was the real scholar among us. Oh, the rest of us all read books, but Romano was a scholar. He made tremendous contributions to the development of the medical school in Rochester."

CHAPTER 7

COURTSHIP

[Evelyn] has been the dominant force in keeping our family together.

E. A. Stead Jr.

While Gene was still at the Thorndike, he met his wife to be, Evelyn Selby. After graduating from Mt. Holyoke College, she applied for a job as secretary to Dr. Soma Weiss at the Brigham. There were two applicants for the position, which was one of the most desirable at the hospital. One candidate was a skilled secretary from a well-to-do family, but Dr. Weiss selected Evelyn because she was supporting her mother, and needed the job. He correctly surmised that she'd stay with him because she had to work for a living.

Gene and Evelyn met in the hall when she came by the Thorndike for an interview before Dr. Weiss had begun at the Brigham; Gene went to the Brigham in September, and they were married the following spring. Dr. Stead had one earlier serious love affair. While he was a surgical intern at the Brigham, he met a "young lady I was very fond of; she was very attractive, but she wanted to get married and I wanted to go on and be a resident before taking on that kind of responsibility. We were engaged through the time I was in Cincinnati, but then it became clear that I was going back to the Thorndike and there would not be any extra money for us to live on. Of course, I wasn't drawing any big debts compared to today's standards, but when Evelyn began to think seriously about marrying, I was paying for Bill's education and Evelyn was paying back her college debts. When we did get married, we devised a common budget and we made out very well. We had flowers on the table every night and ate steak regularly."

Gene and Evelyn came from quite different backgrounds. Evelyn was an only child, her mother had divorced very early, and she had been raised largely by her maternal grandparents, who were the dominant force in her life. Unfortunately, her mother was there but not really in charge of Evelyn because they were living in the grandparents' home. In those days divorce was frowned on, and Evelyn's grandmother was ashamed of her daughter. "Evelyn never really derived any fun out from her relationship with her mother. I think Evelyn looked on her as a failure as well." Evelyn's grandparents had eight children but Evelyn's mother was the only one who had lived. Her grandfather was proud of Evelyn because of her success in school, and she was given whatever she wanted, until her grandfather became ill and lost all of his money. So Evelyn had to support herself after her first year in college, and for many years thereafter, had to support her mother.

Gene's parents did not meet Evelyn until after the wedding. One of his sisters got married at the same time and much closer to Georgia, so Gene Sr. and Emily attended their daughter's wedding. Gene felt no need to ask his parents for permission to get married, since he had been away from home for so many years.

Dr. Stead:

> Fortunately, Evelyn and my mother became very close friends. My mother had long before decided that I ought to be married, so there was no question about that. My father liked Evelyn too; he thought I was grown up enough to be making my way in the world. On the other hand, I was very lucky because I got along well with her mother. We were married at the Weiss home and it was lovely. Because it was some holiday we had Sunday and Monday off, and went to a little inn near Boston, I think in Andover. When Evelyn packed she locked both of the suitcases and then lost the keys. I spent the first part of our honeymoon wandering about searching for a key or someone who could open the suitcases without breaking their locks. But we finally found the keys and were able to open the bags.

The newlyweds adjusted easily to living with one another. Evelyn knew how Gene lived and knew his obligations, including that of working at night. Evelyn never complained about his schedule. Because of her experience earning a living, Evelyn knew the value of a dollar. She took pride in her own work and Gene, in turn, took pride in the fact that whatever she did, she did well. "I think she felt the same way about me. If we had been different people, quite obviously different things would have happened. But Evelyn has always been totally supportive. I think she figured out fairly early that if she was going to work for somebody, she probably wasn't going to have a major career role, so if she was going to work, she might as well work within the family. She has been the dominant force in keeping our family together."

Evelyn Stead:

> I arrived in Boston on September 1, 1939, to begin work as Dr. Weiss's secretary. With him Dr. Weiss brought Gene, John Romano

and Charlie Janeway, (who later became head of the Children's Hospital in Boston), and that was when Gene and I really got to know one another. Gene, Paul Conlin and Mike Mickeljohn shared a house in Brookline on what they called Pill Hill. Their landlady was a very peculiar woman, who came to dinner in a long dress and she had proper help to serve meals and whatnot, but she also took in boarders. She struck a deal with Gene, Paul and Mike that, if one of them didn't come to dinner, the others could bring one guest free. It was a long time before I met Mike because I ate Mike's dinners. The first time Gene asked me out, we went there for dinner and after dinner he said, "You know, I forgot I had a date to play chess tonight," and so he had to take me home and go play his chess game.

Gene, Mike Mickeljohn and I took German lessons together at the Berlitz School. Our instructor was a German lawyer who had only been in this country for three weeks. He had a terrible time with us because we all sounded different: I was from New England, Gene was from Georgia, and Mike was from Scotland. He couldn't understand us, we couldn't understand him, and I'm afraid he didn't last at the Berlitz School. One night, coming home from Berlitz, we came out of the subway at the Fenway stop, and we'd had a blizzard and had to walk. I lived near the Medical School, and Gene and Mike got me there, but then they still had to walk to Brookline. We didn't even know how hard it had snowed until we came out of that subway station and found nothing was moving above ground.

Our courtship lasted less than a year; we were engaged in April and married in June of 1940; I was 25 and Gene was 31, to be 32 in the fall. I paid the last of my college debt just before we were married. We had a very small wedding—I think there were fourteen of us including the minister and the Weiss family. Jean Davis, Gene's secretary, played the piano.

Gene used to have a nervous little laugh, and I think I was aware of his nervousness. I didn't think I was all that sophisticated, but he certainly felt that I was. I'd been working for a woman at Mt. Holyoke who was writing a book about Elizabeth Barrett Browning's family, and in connection with my job, I'd been to the New York Public Library. For some reason this impressed Gene. When I worked at Mt. Holyoke I had to close my apartment in June and reopen it in September every year because in the summer I went away to work. When I moved to Boston I remember saying, "Well, at least I won't have to pack up in June," but I was wrong, I did have to pack up in June.

Dr. Stead:

We were married in 1940 and Nancy, our daughter and first child, was born about four years after that. Then we had Lucy fairly soon afterwards; Bill, the youngest of the three, was born in 1948.

I think the two best pieces of advice to give a young person starting out in the academic world are to be careful not to travel too much, and to live simply and within your means. We were very fortunate that Evelyn and I never had a disagreement about money. From the very beginning we were aware that material things were useful, but that they could not be the reason for living. We always saved and had independent savings accounts. Evelyn's a better mathematician than I am, but she wasn't interested when I tried to persuade her to look into stocks and investments. So essentially, I've done the investing, trying to increase our capital. On the other hand, Evelyn keeps very accurate accounts of where the money goes, and so, with the exception of the investments, she spends the money. We've always had a joint checking account.

Now I've always employed Evelyn for her services. When I was a young man, the laws were such that if I had died, certain things in Evelyn's name would cause tax problems unless she could prove that she'd had a hand in earning them. I had an interest in showing that she had earned part of our savings over the years, so I'd sent her a check every month. The laws have since changed, and they're much more fair to women. But when I left the VA as a Distinguished Professor, I had to sign a piece of paper stating that my wife and I agreed on how the pension would be divided. There never was a question in our minds.

CHAPTER 8

THE 'CHIEF' IN ATLANTA

In the fields of observation, chance favors the prepared mind.
Louis Pasteur

Dr. Stead's invitation to chair the Department of Medicine at Emory was influenced by people he had known as a student. Dean Oppenheimer and Dr. James Paullin, his former teacher and mentor, both favored his return to alma mater, but the dominant voice in convincing Emory of Stead's desirability was that of Dr. Arthur Merrill.

Already a prominent Atlanta physician, and teaching at Emory, Merrill had been a student in the class behind Stead's at Emory. In fact, Stead had coached Merrill in biology when Merrill was a junior student. Stead charged $5 an hour to tutor selected students, usually B+ students who wanted to move to an A. The two continued their acquaintance in medical school and later at Cincinnati when Dr. Stead was Chief Resident there. Merrill was impressed with Stead and stayed abreast of his career as it took shape. He knew something of Stead's special interest in cardiovascular disease and was convinced that Emory would benefit by his unique professionalism. Of course, Merrill had to persuade his colleagues that Stead was a wise choice because his reputation was not yet well established beyond Boston. However, Dr. Merrill was a leader among Atlanta's private practitioners, and his persistent recommendations led his colleagues to offer Stead the Chair of Medicine at a salary of $6,000 per year. Gene was 32 years old at the time, and had spent seven of the ten years after graduation in a white suit. Stead responded, "If I come to Emory for $6,000, I will clearly have to do other things than run the Department of Medicine in order to create extra income. And I don't really think that's what you need. You'll have to pay me $8,000 or I'll stay in Boston."

Dr. Stead:

> My friends and professional colleagues at Harvard advised strongly against accepting the Emory offer. They said that the outlook for weak private schools was dim, and that even with money, I could

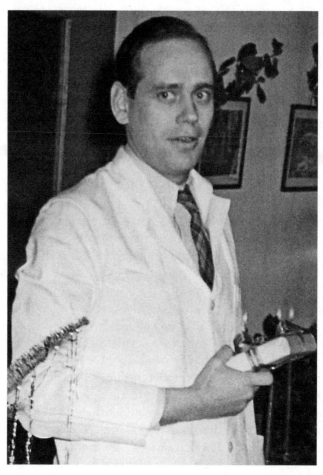

Eugene Stead at a Christmas party at Emory in 1945 or 1946, shortly before he departed for Duke in 1947.

never attract a distinguished faculty. The one exception was my Chief, Soma Weiss. He said one should go where one was needed, and that it was time to determine whether I could move from being a man of promise to a man of achievement. If I were better suited for practice than for academia, the sooner I found this out the better.

By summer of 1941, Stead had joined the Harvard Hospital Unit as an Army Captain. While he was in negotiation with Emory, the Brigham contingent was called overseas (the first medical unit called to active service during World War II); if Stead did not go to Emory, he was likely to be sent to Europe. And even if he did take the job at Emory, there was no guarantee that he would not be called to serve. With the War adding to the ante, the stakes of negotiations climbed higher for both parties. Emory needed some staff members who were protected from the draft, and it needed someone who could encourage the growth of its Department of Medicine. According to Dr. Merrill, Gene Stead was that person. It is remarkable that Emory would even consider appointing a 32-year-old junior faculty member from Harvard, consider making him full Professor and Chairman of Medicine, but this was, in part, a reflection of the respect for Boston medicine, as well as the candidate himself. Emory finally agreed to a salary of $8,000, if Dr. Stead could be exempted from army service. But since all of his friends were being called to serve, and seeing no reason why he should be an exception, Stead decided that he would not actively campaign to be exempted. Furthermore, if he came to Atlanta, he would not actively oppose leaving Emory if called into service, but he agreed not to volunteer.

The prospect of war with all its uncertainties made the early 1940s an emotionally difficult time for all young men. Emory obtained Stead's release from the Army, but as he prepared to leave Boston for Atlanta, many of his friends were going overseas. Dick Ebert and Jack Myers joined the Harvard Fifth General Hospital, and left Boston in January of 1942. With Soma Weiss's death and the outbreak of the war, life had taken them on an unexpected detour.

When Stead's junior associates at the Brigham—Jim Warren, John Hickam and Eddie Miller—learned of his decision to accept Emory's offer, they cornered him in the lab one afternoon. "We're going with you," they announced as they surrounded him. Not knowing what resources would be available to him or what positions might be available, Stead had never considered asking any of his friends to join him. At best, he could offer them positions paying only $400 or $500 annually; at worst, nothing at all. And since Emory had nowhere near the reputation of the more prestigious schools of the Northeast, it was a risky venture. Dr. Stead told them so. "Well, we're not here to ask you if it's alright," they asserted, "we came by to tell you that we'll see you in Atlanta on July 1."

Dr. James Warren:

> I was a research fellow when Soma died and the bottom fell out of the blood volume project I had been working on. So at the end of January, 1942, soon after Pearl Harbor, all the young people who thought they were draft-eligible tried to get into the Harvard Red Cross Hospital Unit. I did, too. There was a great deal of uncertainty at the Brigham because we didn't know who the new chief would be, and

this caused a lot of apprehension. The pull of Dr. Stead in Atlanta was so great that it seemed like a very natural decision to make. John Hickam would be Chief Resident, and I would be a special fellow on a war-time cardiovascular project. I liked Boston and the Brigham, but the challenge of Atlanta seemed much more exciting.

In May of 1942, Gene Stead set out for the familiar territory of the South, returning to the place that had started him in medicine. When he arrived in his old hometown of Decatur, he seemed much the same as when he'd left, with the exceptions of a newly acquired wife and a job. Evelyn had never been further south than Philadelphia, and she looked forward to experiencing first-hand the South she'd only read about in books or heard about from Gene. She was excited about meeting her new husband's family and exploring the geography of her new life, but her sense of adventure was tempered by the prevailing threat of the war. Being far away from home and the people and places familiar to her, she worried that Gene might be called to active duty. Those fears were soon realized. Shortly after they arrived, the young Chief was summoned to appear before the several faculty members who made up Emory's Procurement and Assignment Committee. On the appointed day, the committee sat at a long, metal folding table that might have been borrowed from the cafeteria. "Sit down," said the Chairman as Stead entered the room. Several minutes of silence passed as each committee member reviewed the docket before them. The Chairman finally spoke, "Where did you get your degree?" he asked Stead, all the while scanning the sheet he held in his hand. "You know I was educated here, at Emory," Stead replied, noting the uncomfortably hard seat beneath him. The committee huddled at the center of the table, whispering. Then rising out of the deliberation, the Chairman shook his head regretfully. "I'm sorry, Gene, it's nothing personal, but we simply can't justify keeping you out of the army. We're going to recommend that you be called to active duty as soon as possible." "That's fine," Dr. Stead replied and rose to leave. He had reservations about going to war, but staying home when everybody else was going presented a conflict of its own. Stead was determined not to resist the decision made by his peers.

When Dr. Paullin heard that Gene had been recommended for conscription, he knew the impact that decision would have on the medical school. Before Stead's appointment there had been virtually no full-time staff at Grady Hospital. As a result, the medical and surgical services, and the teaching program were seriously hampered. Now that the Department of Medicine had a chance to overcome this hurdle, Paullin was determined not to allow a step backward. Using his influence as a member of the Draft Appeals Board, Paullin worked hard to thwart the Committee's decision. Three days before

Stead was scheduled to leave, papers came in from Washington officially excusing him. Evelyn and Dr. Paullin heaved sighs of relief.

Dr. Stead:

> I was called to active duty about four or five different times. Each quarter I'd appear before the Procurement and Assignment Committee and they'd assure me that they thought I was doing a good job, and that they didn't mean anything personal by it, but they couldn't justify keeping me at home. You see, back in 1932 when I was a senior student, there were no paid members of the Department of Medicine, and the men on the committee had been my teachers. They asked me how I had gotten along, and whether I was a competent doctor. I answered in the affirmative. "Who taught you?" I replied, "You did." "Then why can't we teach the current students? Why do we need you?" I responded, "That is a question that you will have to decide." They decided the question quickly and processed my papers for immediate active duty. The next day James Edgar Paullin, who for many years had served as Chairman of Medicine without pay, took the train to Washington to appeal the decision. My orders would be revoked. I never actually left Atlanta during World War II.
>
> The committee members and I remained good friends, but they never conceded the fact that a research-oriented, full-time teacher, living in Grady Hospital, could inspire students to see beyond the immediate needs of good medical practice. The members of the committee and I remained good friends because I didn't take their attitude personally.

Stead always had the facility of separating professional from personal differences; one didn't spill over into the other. Recall that Grady Hospital was still divided into separate Black and White facilities located across the street from one another. Each had a separate administration. Dr. Stead went down to Emory believing that he would be Chief of both hospitals. Black Grady had been run almost totally by the housestaff, and through his powers of persuasion Dr. Stead quickly assumed control of that facility. However, because there was a more established line of command at the White Grady, it took more time and political persuasion for him to become Chief there.

At the Cincinnati General, Stead had learned that authority could be taken but not given; he applied this principle at Grady Hospital. He was there 18 hours a day whereas the nominal Chiefs of Service never spent more than a single hour a day in the hospital, so it did not require a struggle for him to assert his authority. Whenever there were problems with patients or resources, Stead was there, and his ability to find answers was soon recognized. Furthermore, he would be able to rely on his Boston colleagues for support when they arrived. In keeping with his philosophy that the world belongs to those who work harder, he got up early each morning and went to bed late each night; eighteen months after he arrived, the chiefs of both Gradys resigned and he was appointed Chief of Black and White Grady Hospital.

A lack of full-time senior staff meant that the hospitals were run, for the most part, by housestaff, even though care was the nominal responsibility of the professional staff of Emory Medical School. It was immediately obvious to Dr. Stead that Grady Hospital would benefit from the kind of discipline and commitment he was accustomed to. On his first tour of the medical wards, Stead found an Assistant Resident seated at a nursing station, his feet up on the desk, a cigar in his mouth, and his shirt unbuttoned to the waist. A lethal combination! The lack of professionalism and seriousness conveyed by the resident's posture gave Stead an opportunity to both assert his authority and establish, unquestionably, the standards he expected of the staff. He quickly arranged for the resident to be out of Grady Hospital and enrolled in the ranks of the army. Shortly after that episode, shirts and ties appeared on all the wards, as did a more professional and sober attitude. After he had a chance to survey the entire group of house officers he had inherited, Dr. Stead notified the army to expect several more soldier-doctors. He had no hesitation in weeding out those he thought would be of little value to his program. "They wanted to stay," he observed, "but everybody knew that life was uncertain at that time."

Before Soma Weiss died, Stead had had little exposure to medical administration. He thought, naively, that hospitals functioned because of what doctors did. The role of Acting Chief of Medicine at the Brigham gave him insight into the complexities of budgeting and administrative organization that were to be a significant part of his new responsibility. Drawing on these lessons from Boston, Stead was able to assess the needs of Emory's Department of Medicine, and to formulate plans for building the department and establishing the policies and procedures by which it would operate.

He had general goals for a department of medicine that would provide a foundation for his educational program. In order to accomplish his goals, it would be necessary for him to "stay at home" until the department was on a sure footing. This was (and still is) an unusual decision; most department chairmen travel frequently to Washington to serve on governmental advisory committees or to other medical schools where they function as visiting professors and lecturers. But Stead avoided the national scene and did not involve himself in outside committee work, lectures or conferences. He was sometimes criticized by his colleagues for an apparent lack of interest or involvement in outside activities, but he believed in his plan and systematically set about implementing it. Knowing that he needed a firm base of operations before moving on, he rejected any criticism of his actions. After establishing a secure base, he could later move into the broader medical world, but he intended to work outwards, moving always from a base of excellence in his own department.

Because of the war, Stead's Boston recruits did not all come immediately to Atlanta. This meant a manpower gap between the time Dr. Stead assumed his position and the arrival of his colleagues. Further complicating his life in 1942 was the task of hiring interns who would not be summoned off to war; Stead had to find people who either were ineligible for the draft or had fulfilled their military obligation. Jim Warren was temporarily protected by his contract study of the use of concentrated human serum albumin, which the military was interested in developing for injured troops. He arrived within a week after Stead, but John Hickam, who was to be the Chief Resident, became ill and wasn't able to start for some months. So Warren assumed the job of Chief Resident until Hickam's health improved.

Dr. James Warren:

> Before we arrived, the housestaff literally ran Grady Hospital. Most of the clinical teaching was done by volunteer faculty from the community. There was practically no full-time faculty, and no one knew what it was to have a well-staffed hospital. When we got to Emory, we were very short-handed. Gene started from nothing, but we did pretty well.

Paul Beeson, who had been at the Brigham with Stead, and had served with the Red Cross Hospital in England in 1941, was scheduled to return to the States in 1942. When he learned of Beeson's imminent return, Stead, who had accepted the position but not yet moved to Emory, offered his former colleague a job in Atlanta. The story of the recruitment of Dr. Beeson, who was later to become one of this country's medical leaders, tells a great deal about Beeson, Weiss and Stead.

Dr. Stead:

> Soma Weiss, David Barr of Cornell, and I were all negotiating with Paul Beeson who had satisfied his military responsibilities by spending two years in England with the Harvard Red Cross Unit. He was the prize academic candidate of the year because anyone else with his health and achievement would be called to active duty. Weiss made

the first offer—an assistant professorship with an annual income of $3,000. At the same time, in December 1941, Weiss wrote to Beeson at the Harvard Hospital Unit in Salisbury England:

Dear Paul: You have received or will soon receive a letter from Gene Stead about simultaneously with this letter of mine. You well know how much I am interested in your future progress, and therefore I thought that I would like to write you about how I feel about Gene's undertaking. Emory University School of Medicine has always been an important center in the South, but I am certain that with the recent development there in surgery and now in medicine and with the future plans, it will become one of the most important centers in the South. You know Gene's ability, so I don't have to add anything on that point. He is taking several younger men from the Brigham in the capacity of assistant residents. The clinical material and opportunities there will be very great. I am also confident that the various foundations will see the significance of Atlanta as a medical center, not only in undergraduate but also in graduate education, and it is my sincere belief that they will support worthwhile undertakings. The understanding and treatment of infectious diseases have been particularly neglected in the South, and therefore if you decide to go to Emory, you will be certain of a good opportunity to develop yourself clinically. I also believe that if you do good work, you will have no difficulty in getting other even more important positions if that is your ambition. I don't want to influence you, because the decision is up to you, but I thought these lines might be helpful....

Dr. Stead:

Soma Weiss was a good prophet. As you know, all of his predictions came true! Weiss died on January 29, 1942 before his arrangements with Beeson were completed, and in the administrative confusion surrounding his death the offer to Beeson lapsed. I offered Paul the rank of associate professor and a salary of $4,000. Meanwhile David Barr had decided to establish an infectious disease unit at New York Hospital, and asked Beeson to be its Director. I gave Paul a deadline for my offer and to my great joy he accepted. Shortly thereafter Barr made a definitive offer and upped the salary to $5,000. Beeson regretted his acceptance of my Emory offer, but being a gentleman as well as a scholar he came to Emory. After four and a half years he succeeded me as Chairman.

Barr, with space on his hands, approached Walsh McDermott who was deferred from service because of tuberculosis. He said that Walsh could take the position offered Beeson. If he was successful, he could stay on at Cornell, and if unsuccessful, he would have delayed going into practice by only 12 months. McDermott stayed on and became one of the most distinguished members of the Cornell faculty. In time Beeson and McDermott collaborated as editors of five editions of the Cecil Textbook of Medicine. When they learned many years later that they had been candidates for the same job, they laughed about it because instead of being warm friends, they might have become hated rivals.

In the meantime, staff shortage was weighing heavily on Dr. Stead, who already was working 18 hours a day seven days a week. He rode the streetcar from his home in Decatur to the hospital in the early morning and back again each night. One day, entering the ambulatory clinic after rounds at 9:00, Stead realized that he would have to single-handedly treat the 150 patients who would pass through the clinic that day. With luck, he would be done before midnight. As he steeled himself for the long day ahead of him, Dr. Eddie Miller reported for assignment. After exchanging greetings, Miller took off his coat, and the two men went to work and didn't stop until the last patient had been seen around six o'clock that evening. A long day, but better than some.

Shortly after their arrival in Atlanta, the Steads' first child, Nancy, was born, and so on top of all his other responsibilities he added fatherhood. But it didn't slow him down. He spent time with her in the late evenings after the day's work at the hospital was done. Despite his long hours, he could only do one job at a time. Even with Drs. Miller and Warren, who worked the same long hours as Stead, the responsibilities exceeded the capacity of his small staff. The demands on time were distributed among teaching, medical and administrative duties, and he needed to have as many assistants as he could recruit. It was then that he wrote to Beeson and told him he would have to receive his reply within a week's time.

Short staffing on every level meant that senior staff had to take on even the most routine tasks, like pushing patients in wheelchairs or providing bedpans when necessary. Stead hadn't realized how badly the war would deplete the ranks of housestaff, so he wasn't prepared to answer the question of how Grady Hospital was going to operate. Without people like Miller, Beeson, and Hickam, Grady Hospital would not have functioned at all. Stead needed more staff, but none were available, so he decided on a simple expedient: he conscripted medical students. Choosing the best senior students, he abbreviated their training and put them to work as interns. As an added incentive, he pointed out that the army would be waiting for anyone who didn't get his work done. After several weeks of careful supervision and instruction on the ward, Stead could find no difference between the performance of interns who had been taken prematurely from their textbooks and those who had completed the prescribed course of study. As a result, he concluded that, through a series of demonstrations and questions, he could teach nearly any bright student how to take care of a patient. Students didn't need medical school in order to perform as doctors. Not many medical educators believed that was possible then or now.

Dr. Stead:

> Interestingly, there wasn't one who failed the test. People with less than half the normal amount of clinical instruction did as well as other interns when they were properly supervised on the wards. And so, obviously the body of knowledge provided by more schooling wasn't necessary to becoming a good intern. I decided that medical school had to have a purpose other than just making competent doctors because, based on my experiment, you didn't need medical school for that.
>
> One of the purposes of education is to broaden the range of brain cells that you are able to use. If you want to develop the best brains, you have to take the time to develop an intellectual framework. There is a big difference between a neural network that has a wide range of applicability, and a neural network that is tightly patterned. I think you need both to function effectively. I couldn't possibly practice medicine without having a tight neural network of repetitive behavior and knowledge. That would be ridiculous. It would take so long to see a patient that I would never get through. One needs an ordered system for taking a history and doing a physical examination on a patient; you can't re-invent the process every time you examine the head or the chest. On the other hand, I wouldn't want to spend a whole day performing the same repetitive task.
>
> Despite what I learned from my "experiment" during the war, I've never really been a believer in short education, and I would hate to see medical education shortened to the point where one didn't have many experiences out of which to select a future discipline. When I conscripted students for intern positions, I did think that the students lost out on a great deal of education, because many experiences which they didn't need in order to become technically competent were simply cut out. They missed a lot of experiences and a lot of fun. If you pursue learning in a way that makes the day more interesting, you can really enjoy yourself. Consequently I've never really been a believer in "short" education.

Medical educators idealize the process of medical education. We honestly tend to kid ourselves. Content is irrelevant to the learning process. The basic science faculty believes that certain habits make a good chemist. In fact, one could do a great deal of chemistry without having those habits, but there is a large part of professional training that can only be learned through repetition. A surgeon learns how to tie off arteries that are bleeding by performing the act over and over again. There is very little material in pre-clinical or basic science work, however, that medical students have to learn to the habit level. If they have studied well, the students will have learned a new language of science and what can be accomplished by the successful practice of that science. But they can learn that whether or not the subject matter has direct relevance to being a doctor. Professional skills don't depend on the mastery of such subjects. A student should know what a biochemist does, and should track three or four exciting innovators in biochemistry, and get to know the practices common to the field prior to choosing a profession in which they will rely on those habits and practices. They don't need to know the work habits until they're ready to select a career. It's faulty reasoning to assume that the language of science is necessary to perform the tasks associated with the medical profession. I've always been amused by the large fees cardiologists earn for interpreting ECGs. One can read ECGs as patterns without even knowing the medical terminology; nearly any bright high school teacher can learn to read ECGs simply because distinct patterns are known to occur in specific heart conditions. It's like a mathematical formula. One pattern reveals a posterior myocardial infarction, and another pattern indicates atrial fibrillation. You don't have to know what atrial fibrillation is to identify the pattern, in fact you don't even have to know that it reflects the activity of a heart or where the heart is! It's just matching patterns and words.

All schools had personnel shortages during the war, but Grady was particularly hard-hit because it began with fewer interns and residents than most other hospitals with comparable patient loads. Because they lost so many of their resident staff to the army, everybody pitched in and performed whatever tasks needed to be done for the patients. The young doctors and the entire staff knew that what they were doing was important. And this knowledge, coupled with the awareness that others had been called to war in their place, inspired them to work selflessly, fighting for life on the medical front. However, war was not the only motivating factor. Stead's commitment to hard work and excellence, and his zeal for medical education provided the young doctors at Grady with a spirit of excitement about medicine and how to look at the problems of sick people.

Dr. Albert Heyman:

> Before Dr. Stead arrived, Grady Hospital was pretty much like New York's Bellevue Hospital—or any large city hospital in which the housestaff were kings—because we did everything that needed to be done. We saw a tremendous variety of diseases and, for the most part, were on our own, except for very complicated cases. At that time, typhus fever, malaria and diphtheria—diseases that had long gone out of prevalence in the civilized community—were still common in Atlanta, and most cases were treated by interns and residents like me. Obviously, attending staff people made rounds, and the teaching staff taught students, but education at Grady was quite primitive. Many of the faculty were part-time people, who spent most of their time in their private practices; with very few exceptions, there was no full-time staff. But within a very short time after Dr. Stead's arrival, things had turned over completely. Grady went from being an interesting place to being a first-class teaching hospital. More important even than the sudden appearance of a teaching program, we had enthusiasm and a new and refreshing orientation. House officers at Grady were fascinated by the exotic diseases that they saw, but now, for the first time, we had somebody to explain and to teach us about those diseases. And it was not just Dr. Stead, but the faculty he brought with him who made it obvious that everything was changing, and all for the better.
>
> The new faculty brought research fellows with them and they, too, increased the enthusiasm of the housestaff and students tremendously. The full-time staff had offices in the building, so we could clearly see that we now had teachers who were interested in the patients and interested in teaching. Instead of having offices downtown or at Emory University on the other side of town, Grady's doctors now had offices in the hospital. Those for Drs. Stead and Beeson were on a corridor in the hospital's basement, and they were the least pretentious things one could think of—very small and with one tiny window each. When it rained hard, the floors flooded and Stead and Beeson would have to mop up their offices. If you happened to be in the basement at the time, you were expected to pitch in and help.
>
> Because there had been no full-time staff to speak of, no objections were raised to the changes that were taking place. You see, Dr.

Stead arrived just six months after the bombing of Pearl Harbor. Most house officers were preoccupied with whether they would be drafted, so they weren't in any position to resent all the new work. Going into the service was an alternative, and a number of those who rebelled at the workload did go.

In our day-to-day activities, we were expected to know everything about a case. It was assumed that we had read the textbook, and knew all the symptoms; we were expected to perform at our very best. It was also important that our case-management be correct, but I never heard any nasty remarks about what we did or didn't do. We were just expected to perform. I don't remember anybody being torn apart at rounds, although that might occur at morning report, which was another thing. Every morning we had to report our admissions from the preceding day. We had to be sure we covered all the bases, and recorded the case material because Dr. Stead was sure to ask. He was almost psychic in knowing what hadn't been done.

Our work took on new meaning under the informed guidance of Stead and his insightful colleagues. Before they came, we were seeing patients with hundreds of different kinds of diseases and we were learning, within the existing limitations, the best ways to treat them. For example, when I was seeing patients with typhus every day, I treated them as effectively as I could in those days before antibiotics were available. Well, when Paul Beeson realized the invaluable source of case material we had available, he gave Dr. Eddie Miller the job of writing an article on typhus fever; the fifty or one hundred Grady cases he cited became the basis for a seminar on endemic typhus fever. So we realized that experts like Drs. Beeson and Miler could tell us about the diseases we were treating, and we had the opportunity to work on cases that were going to be part of a medical report. For the first time we appreciated the scientific aspect of what we were doing daily. This made us keep good records as well as take good care of the patients— we didn't want to say that this patient died, or that we didn't know what happened in another case because it was going to be in a report.

When I later went to the Massachusetts General Hospital to learn neurology, I was impressed with the spirit of the housestaff there. Their attitude seemed to say "This is Mass General, and Mass General and Harvard expect a high level of achievement." So they worked hard to uphold the Mass General tradition. Well, hell, nobody had ever said, "This is Grady Hospital at Emory University." Grady and Emory had no tradition. We worked hard for another reason: because

Dr. Stead and his staff expected us to and because we were learning and enjoying the challenge.

At that time, Stead's regimen had each resident on duty every day and night of the week except for one weekday night off each week and one weekend day and night off every other week. In addition, we had ward rounds and the famous "Sunday School" of specialty rounds. Of course, our "weekends off" weren't really off because we were expected to be there on Saturdays, but we didn't know any better then. For all of this we were paid five dollars a month. Not much, but more than the better internships paid in Boston and New York—and we were given Grady Hospital food which was raised at the county prison camps. We ate mostly vegetables like okra, rutabaga and collard greens, and everything was served with a large plate of gravy loaded with bacon fat.

I found it quite distressing whenever I learned that Dr. Stead had come by my ward while I was out getting a haircut or going to the dentist. I was never reprimanded for being off the ward, but I learned to postpone those activities in case he might stop by. When he did wander through the wards he'd ask "What have you got that's interesting?" and there was an awesomeness in that experience. It wasn't so much that we wanted to please Stead as we wanted to be up to scratch. Before he came to Emory, we might slip out in the afternoon to play tennis or go downtown and shop. Suddenly we were expected to be at the hospital. The whole atmosphere had changed. We were responsible for our ward and we were expected to be there. Of course the other side of responsibility was that we could always talk with Dr. Stead or Dr. Beeson or any of the others. They were always helpful and interested, and they always tried to teach us something. So if we felt inadequate in the face of this drastic change, their readiness to help us made up for it.

Among his innovations at Grady, Stead introduced "Morning Report." At eight o'clock each morning, the residents reported on all patients who had been admitted to the ward during the previous 24 hours. And woe unto any doctor who was a minute late; that meant that the entire group might sit in silence for the full 30 minutes. This conference helped the Chief detect any problems on the wards, and decide where energy needed to be directed. It also let him identify the very sick patients whom he needed to see immediately. Perhaps the most noticeable change introduced by Stead was that he installed his offices in the hospital basement. For the first time ever, housestaff had full-time senior staff available to help with difficult cases or to provide guidance and support. And not least, Stead instituted his unique form of Grand Rounds, held on Sunday mornings and known familiarly as "Sunday School." Sunday School convened in a makeshift auditorium in another basement room. Stead and his senior staff used these meetings to discuss interesting cases or important medical topics; because it was so scintillating, Sunday School attracted a large audience of doctors from the community as well as from the Emory and Grady staff. Sunday School provided doctors with the latest in medical science from the best and brightest, and they came like flies to honey.

Dr. James Warren:

> Sunday School, the major intellectual exercise of the week, was pretty heavily attended by community doctors and those affiliated with various military establishments. Gene Stead, Paul Beeson, John Hickam and a few others, including me, put on all the presentations. It was good for my medical education because I studied and presented talks on topics that I would otherwise never have thought of talking about at Grand Rounds.

Having been at the Thorndike and the Brigham, Stead understood that, in order to fulfill its real potential, any institution needed an active research program to attract attention and establish a national reputation. However, purchasing restrictions brought about by the war and the limited Grady budget slowed the process of getting established. In order to start, Stead needed funds beyond what Emory could provide. In addition, Dr. Stead couldn't run Grady Hospital with its many very sick patients unless some senior staff members were granted military deferments. By constricting services and pushing his residents, he was able to stretch his staff, but it was clear that he needed to keep his senior staff members if the hospital was going to continue to function. Stead had the brilliant idea of protecting his faculty by having them perform research that was of vital importance to the military and for which they would be deferred from military service. Stead could see two such options: one was the study of shock and its possible prevention, because this was a major battlefield problem, and the other was the development of rapid treatment systems. Perhaps they could do both.

In the early 1940s, the Public Health Service became very interested in rapid treatment centers, and was willing to offer deferments to those working in this area. One such area concerned the treatment of syphilis, a widespread problem that brought many patients to Grady (over 50% of Atlanta's civilian population had a positive serology test for syphilis, and Grady was considered the syphilitic aneurysm center of the world). Albert Heyman, then a first year Resident in Medicine, talked to Dr. Stead about working on syphilis. Having seen a large number of syphilis cases, Heyman was especially well acquainted with the nervous system effects of the disease, and so Stead agreed that he should pursue this avenue. Heyman, who had been at Grady when Stead arrived, had earned Stead's respect as a serious young doctor; he was one of the few residents who survived the new Chief's social Darwinism, which culled weak performers. But the other side of Stead's hard edge was his commitment to staff who were dedicated and hard-working. He would help these young doctors take their careers in new and exciting directions. He had a unique ability to see opportunities for research in what appeared to others as routine practice.

Dr. Albert Heyman:

> Dr. Stead had a keen awareness of the overall significance of the cases we were seeing at Grady. At one point he asked me to write a paper on syphilitic meningitis. The clinical manifestations of this aspect of syphilis weren't described in textbooks because nobody had seen enough cases. Well, I had seen a dozen or more, and Dr. Stead realized this was significant because he knew there was no literature on it. He asked me to write a paper, which I did.
>
> Atlanta had a major problem with venereal disease, and the Public Health Service wanted to get venereal disease under control. The City Council donated some money, and the City Health Department asked Grady Hospital to work with them because so many of the venereal disease cases were seen there. Dr. Stead told me that he thought this was an opportunity to do something important and asked me if I'd like to learn about infectious and venereal disease. He offered to send me to Johns Hopkins or anywhere I wanted to go, so I visited Hopkins, Bellevue, the University of Pennsylvania, the University of Michigan and other places known for achievement in this field.
>
> The City Council and the Health Department donated $18,000 to build a clinic with a waiting room, examining room, and offices. I was put on the State payroll, and suddenly went from earning $60 a year to earning $3,000. I thought this was massive riches, so much so that when I could hire only one nurse on the clinic budget, I used part of my salary to hire another nurse (something my wife never let me forget!). We had a public health nurse and a patient nurse who helped with syringes.
>
> I don't really recall specifically how Dr. Stead introduced the idea to me, but I remember that he called me into his office and told me that he thought this was an opportunity. The fact that I'd be working mostly with him and Paul Beeson did sound like a good idea. I

enrolled in the Public Health Service, which kept me out of the army, although I assume Stead had the prerogative of saying, "The people I select are needed here for civilian service."

I never did figure out how Dr. Stead knew that venereal disease was an area that I'd be interested in. I think that he just saw a job and the need for a person to do the job. At first I had no special interest and in fact I said, "Why would I want to go into venereal disease? I'm going to have a miserable group of patients." When my family heard I was going into venereal disease they weren't exuberant. They were proud of me, of course, but they didn't tell many of their friends, and the few they did tell said, "What? Is that the best Albert can do?" Most people thought that only the dregs of humanity contracted venereal diseases. But, like anything else, the more you know about a subject, the more interesting it is. Syphilis gave me a marvelous opportunity for me to expand my scientific horizons and advance my academic career. It let me write a great many important papers.

Drs. Stead and Warren debated getting involved in the rapid treatment of syphilis. It was a pervasive disease that demanded attention, but was difficult to treat. Penicillin was not yet available and the standard treatments involved toxic arsenical drugs. If the patient made it through the therapy, then the drugs might cure the syphilis, but rapid treatment was full of complications such as severe skin reactions, limb pain and severe abdominal pain, and even paralysis.

While they were debating the question of syphilis, Dr. Alfred Blaylock, a friend of Dr. Stead's and an expert on the subject of blood volume, brought another research opportunity to Stead's attention. The government was interested in using blood substitute products like dextran to treat shock. They wanted treatments that could be used on the battlefield by medical corpsmen tending soldiers wounded during combat.

Colorimeters had just been introduced to measure blood hemoglobin concentration, but few people knew how to measure blood volume. This was an important question because very rapid loss of blood, such as from trauma, lowers blood volume dramatically even though hemoglobin concentration can remain normal for hours. The only way to estimate the amount of blood lost (and needing to be replaced) was to measure the volume of blood remaining, and there was no way to do this at the time.

Dr. Jim Warren:

One fine day I was working away at the lab when a high-level delegation visited. Dr. Alfred Blaylock from Johns Hopkins and Dr. Joe

Wern from Cleveland asked Gene to establish a cardiac catheterization program at Grady, jokingly saying it resembled a battlefield more
than any other place in the U.S.A. They wanted the program pat-
terned after the one at Bellevue Hospital run by Drs. Andre Cournand and Dickinson W. Richards. Gene wasn't interested. He knew
that measuring cardiac output wasn't going to help him take care of
our patients, and he really turned his back on the idea. I wasn't in the
room and I can't tell you exactly what happened, but in effect, they
went away without an acceptance.

I was still young, and militarily vulnerable, but the draft board considered me essential because Emory medical school didn't have any faculty in Atlanta. Still, everybody was going to war, and I was not above
trying to pick a good spot to go to. Earlier, when I was at the Brigham,
Dr. Robert Loeb had been the visiting Professor of Medicine there, and
he stayed in a room right next to the Assistant Resident's room that I
used. He sort of depended on me to guide him around and I got to
know him that way. Later he became the person most involved in making research assignments for the military. Since our albumin project
was coming to an end and Dr. Stead didn't want to pick up the catheter
project, I said, "I think I'll go up to New York." Dr. Loeb invited me to
come up and talk. Well, I just walked in his office and he said, "What's
the matter down there at Emory? Here's the most exciting project I
know of, and Dr. Stead turned it down." And I said, "Well, I wasn't in
the room. I heard he'd turned it down, but I don't know just what went
on." He asked me how long I was going to be in New York and I said a
couple of days and he pulled out a little pad of paper and said, "I want
you to go downtown to Bellevue Hospital and look up Dr. Cournand."
He gave me the names of two or three other people to see at 1st Avenue
and 24th Street, so I called one of the people he mentioned and went
down there the next day. I watched them insert a catheter into the heart
of the victim of a subway accident. I got tremendously excited about
it. This was, of course, the first time I'd ever seen this done. I told Dr.
Loeb I would like to do something like this as wartime research if I possibly could. He said, "I want you to go back to Atlanta and tell Dr. Stead
that you think this is the thing to do." Well, I did do that, and I must
have carried the day in the sense that he agreed to go up and look. Less
than a month after that I was back in New York as a special resident at
Bellevue Hospital, and I was right there when the shock work went on.
I spent something like three months at Bellevue with Drs. Cournand
and Richards, who later won the Nobel Prize for their work.

After I went back to Emory, we found a nurse, and set up the first catheter lab there. We got a contract from the Office of Scientific Research and Development, and the whole thing went ahead. We never talked much about why Dr. Stead changed his mind, but he quickly and enthusiastically did. The positive point of the story is that he wasn't afraid to change his mind; he didn't have to do any back stepping or anything like that.

There is a wonderful story about Dr. Stead's first grant. He wrote the application rather blindly, especially in trying to estimate the cost of conducting the study. Because of his inexperience and a raging wartime inflation, he was quite far off in his estimation, and submitted a figure that would cover only about one-tenth of the actual costs (a mistake he would never make again). The government accepted the proposal, but fortunately made an accounting error of one decimal place and awarded a grant for $50,000 rather than the requested $5,000. And that turned out to be just enough money to cover costs of the project.

It soon became obvious to the local medical community that Grady Hospital was conducting research that required financial resources well beyond the budget allocated by Emory. With the inception of the research program Stead had at least achieved local recognition. The national scene, however, would require more than a display of resources; it would require results.

Stead and Warren were quite certain that solutions of albumin and dextran would work as blood substitutes. Given intravenously to expand blood volume, either could substitute for plasma, which was in short supply and had a limited shelf-life; either could be used under battlefield conditions to allow wounded soldiers to be transported to a hospital. Blood substitutes could save many thousands of lives. In order to conduct the research, all that was needed were patients who had suffered massive blood loss. As it turned out, Atlanta was a hotbed of Saturday night stabbings. Many a drunken brawl ended with victims torn and bleeding from knife and ice pick wounds. In one year alone there were 365 stab wounds into the chest.

Stead and Warren would go into work early on Saturday mornings and work through the night, but even at Grady, the staff could never predict just when they would have patients whose blood loss was sufficient to produce shock and thereby make them suitable subjects for the study. So every Friday, Saturday and Sunday, a team of doctors was available and ready to work around the clock, waiting for victims of major trauma in whom they could study blood circulation during shock. One night a young black man was admitted with multiple superficial stab wounds. He had been attacked with an ice pick, and was wearing badly slashed and blood-stained pajamas when he entered the emergency room. The staff set to work, pulling off his pajamas, and infusing plasma. Jim Warren, playing the role of major domo, looked to see if the patient would be a suitable subject for their shock study. As it turned out, he needed extensive superficial suturing, but had no penetrating wounds of the chest or any major loss of blood. Dr. Warren, having completed his survey, turned the patient over to a resident. "We're through with our studies, you can admit him now." "Admit him?" the resident retorted, "He's fine, he's been sutured and can go home." Dr. Warren had been so engrossed in making measurements that he hadn't noticed that the cuts had all been sutured. The patient, wrapped in a sheet because his pajamas were gone, was released and, having nothing else to wear, trudged to the door wrapped in the sheet. A nearby nurse protested as the man walked out, but he didn't turn around or let on that he'd heard her. He walked off into the darkness, presumably to find his attacker and even the score. These were rough and terrible times in large inner-city emergency rooms, not much different from today.

In terms of scientific progress, the shock-study group was most productive on nights when only a few patients were available. Waiting for the next emergency, they discussed congestive heart failure and how they should study it at Grady. It was a simple next step to begin an actual study. They continued to work on their first priority, shock patients, but the large number of patients with congestive heart failure put at their disposal a ready supply of subjects.

Dr. Stead:

> We always had patients at Grady Hospital with heart failure, so when we weren't engaged in the blood substitute business, which was very erratic, we were studying a whole variety of patients with heart failure. We were going to spend the night at the hospital, so we might as well be productive. We were already interested in heart failure, and all the tools were the same—the nurses, the needles and us.
>
> In retrospect, we discovered what should have been fairly obvious: there were tremendous similarities between the abnormal physiology of shock and that of congestive heart failure; the circulatory dynamics in each were nearly identical. In both circumstances, the heart was unable to provide the brain, kidneys or liver with the amount of blood they needed, and they were deprived of oxygen and nutrients as a result. The body compensated for the deficit of blood with a series of responses, the upshot of which was that the patient became sick. The one difference, of course, was the fact that in heart failure, the venous system is full of blood and in shock it is empty. It's like a car engine shutting down because the carburetor is clogged with grit as opposed

to shutting down because the gas tank is empty. The causes are different, but the end results are the same. In heart failure either the valves were too tight to permit adequate blood flow or the heart muscle was weak, or both conditions existed. By contrast, the heart muscle is usually normal in hemorrhagic shock, but the heart can't supply blood that it doesn't have to pump, and the effect on the organs is the same. In shock, because the heart muscle is still working, there is time to fill the system with fluid—blood substitutes in our case. Fluid congestion does not occur in shock as it does in heart failure unless fluid is given to the patient intravenously. But if salt solution is administered intravenously at a rapid rate, it will leak out of the capillaries nearly as quickly as it is put in and flood the system because the salt solution lacks protein or a protein-like substance to keep the fluid in the vessels. The kidneys then shut down and the system becomes waterlogged. Shock is a fairly acute condition and if you don't do something about it rapidly, the patient will die most of the time.

The body has time to make compensatory changes in heart failure and so, although the heart is no longer able to provide the normal supply of blood to the organs, the vital organs receive proportionately more than their share, keeping the body alive. And this process of compensation can endure over a long period of time.

As it turned out, Warren and Stead picked up where Stead's earlier studies with Dick Ebert in Boston had left off. They studied the relationship between extracellular fluid pressure and blood volume in dogs. They used plasmapheresis to reduce the blood protein concentration, and found that the blood volume was quite low. Then they tied off the ureters so the kidneys couldn't excrete water, and gave the dogs massive amounts of saline fluids until the blood volume and fluid equilibrium returned to normal. It took a tremendous amount of fluid to restore the equilibrium, because most of the fluid leaked out of the blood vessels into the tissues; by the time they were done, they had given the dog about half its body weight in extracellular fluid.

Next they studied the weight increase that sometimes occurred in patients with congestive heart failure. They knew that some patients developed heart failure while carrying out normal daily activities, but when those people were put at bed rest and the work of the heart reduced, the heart failure would subside. But they were interested in a more stable group of patients, those who exhibited chronic heart failure whether they were active or at rest. Patients in this category might have a rapid and irregular heart beat called atrial fibrillation, or tight mitral stenosis in which the opening through the mitral valve has been narrowed by rheumatic fever, or other forms of heart disease. Such patients were easy to identify because they sat up in bed puffing for air. They couldn't lie flat because fluid would collect in their lungs and prevent them from breathing. Heart failure of this type can be controlled by medications and salt-restricted diets, but in the early 1940s a great deal remained unknown about heart failure. In the course of their studies, Stead and his team helped to unlock the key to the nature of heart failure.

Dr. Stead:

> We took a couple of patients who were always in heart failure, even when resting, and followed their plasma protein levels by repeatedly measuring protein concentration as the congestion subsided. We then measured the pattern in which congestion recurred as their tissues re-swelled. When we took this information back to our lab, we determined that these people were all in a state of excess renin production; this made their kidneys reabsorb salt and water instead of excreting it in the urine, as a normal person would do. As we continued to observe these patients, it became clear that weight gain and the onset of visible edema appeared before there was any increase in heart congestion or venous pressure. So we established that salt and water accumulated in such patients before the heart actually failed and before there was a rise in venous pressure, a tell-tale sign of a failing heart. We could measure the venous pressure by inserting a needle attached to a measuring device (called a manometer) into an arm vein that connected with the right atrium of the heart. The pressure in the vein gave us an accurate indication of the pressure within the heart. We had already figured out that when the ventricle of the heart failed to pump its normal share of blood, the blood dammed up behind it, forming something like a lake. This, in turn, caused edema. Then, when a patient drank and ate excessive amounts of salt and water, the blood volume expanded and fluid leaked into tissues like the lungs, causing severe shortness of breath, particularly when the patient was flat in bed, a condition known as paroxysmal nocturnal dyspnea. Without an excessive intake of salt and water, heart failure patients did much better.
>
> We knew, of course, that the only blood available to dam up behind the right ventricle was that normally pumped out by the left ventricle. From personal experience, I knew that a lake doesn't form by just damming up a river, but from water that collects when it rains up in the hills. If it rains long enough, you get a big lake. So blood damming up behind the right ventricle didn't seem likely to be the

sole cause of edema; there had to be some "rain in the hills" for a person to swell to the degree we were seeing in these patients. And very simply, it seemed that the most likely cause of the excess fluid was what a person ate and drank. Since we already knew that the body is quite able to get rid of distilled water, but much less able to eliminate salty water, our guess was that the intake of salt plus water was too high. And we arrived at an extraordinarily simple thesis: the amount of water in a lake or in a biological system depends on two or three variables: the amount of water you put in, the potential for evaporation in an open system like a lake, and the drainage system. If you altered any of these (changed the amount of rain, or opened up a clogged drainage system) the amount of accumulated water would change.

For many years people had believed that the generalized increase in venous pressure in patients with heart failure was due to a reduction in output by the heart. As our research proceeded, however, it became obvious that all the things we associated with congestion occurred when the fluid volume became great enough. We arrived at the conclusion that the water and salt which people drank and ate, like the rain in the hills and that the clogged drainage system, had to reflect the kidneys not working properly. And, of course, this turned out to be true. Understanding how all of this fit together led to entirely different ways to treat heart failure, including the use of low salt diets and diuretic drugs, which increase the excretion of salt and water by the kidneys.

Stead's group at Grady was one of the first to demonstrate a scientific basis for the efficacy of salt restriction. The less salt in the diet, the less the kidney would reabsorb water, which was the principal component of edema. Their studies demonstrated practical things that could be done to help patients in heart failure. They learned very early on that lack of adherence to a diet program rather than lack of understanding of how to properly prepare food was the chief obstacle to effectively putting this knowledge to work in the clinic. They studied fluid in legs or arms with drainage problems from prior surgery or disorders of the lymphatic or venous systems. They learned that localized pools of fluid, which sometimes occur in unusual places like the upper rather than the lower lobes of the lungs, often were the result of a prior injury to that specific part. Once again they learned that fluid accumulation had to do with both inadequate drainage and the amount of salt and water contained in the body.

Dr. Stead's work on heart failure was paid for out of the research contract to study shock. If they hadn't studied heart failure, the group would have wasted a lot of time waiting for suitable shock patients to arrive. As it turned out, Stead's group was able to satisfy the requirements of the contract by producing excellent results. In addition, they learned a lot about heart failure of all types. Working with patients suffering from pericardial tamponade (where the accumulation of fluid within the sac surrounding the heart prevents filling of the heart with blood), they discovered that they could relieve the tamponade by inserting a needle into the pericardial sac and extracting the fluid. They studied the effects of anemia on cardiac output. It was a brilliantly productive period, and it that opened up whole new areas of research, as well as answering very specific questions about the treatment of disease.

Dr. Stead:

> We got up early in the morning and worked late into the night. We never took ourselves too seriously, and we thoroughly enjoyed what we were doing. Our notebooks showed that we were at work on Christmas Eve, and we ran a very open laboratory at all times. Anybody who visited us was told exactly what we were doing and what we were planning on doing. We put our names on papers only if we had a meaningful level of participation, but never on papers for which we'd had the idea, but had done none of the work. We never thought that sharing authorship with junior people could possibly hurt us; we encouraged that. If these young doctors continued to do good research, it would be nice to know that we were associated with them at one time. If they quit doing research, then it was obvious that discovery would be identified with those who continued the work. Therefore, we were very liberal in incorporating anybody that had done any work with us into the credits. At the same time, we were careful not to take advantage of being a senior physician by putting our names where they didn't belong.
>
> I came on the scene when clinical research was just beginning to be appreciated. Patients themselves could serve as subjects for clinical investigation. There were very few doctors actually investigating patients and, therefore, nearly anything we did to obtain quantitative data provided information that had not been recorded previously. We experienced no real problems publishing data, and the now prestigious Journal of Clinical Investigation was not difficult to crack in my early years of work. However, I was really only an amateur laboratory investigator. I grew up in a time when there was no formal training for doing clinical research, no financial reward for doing investigation, and no anticipation that one would remain in the academic world long enough for research to be a major component of one's activity. So

while I thoroughly enjoyed the venture of trying to ferret out some of the things we didn't know, I was always limited by the drawback of having received relatively little precise laboratory training.

Stead was always willing and able to put his own work into perspective no matter how he was complimented by others or honored for his research discoveries.

He used the opportunity of being at Grady day and night to check in on staff and see how things were going. It was a practice that caught the junior staff off guard at first, and always made them feel a little uncomfortable. But the unpredictability of Stead's visits created an air of suspense and tension. An intern or resident could never guess when the Chief might stop by, and so they were challenged to be prepared always.

Dr. Heyman:

> With Dr. Stead's arrival it became apparent that we had to perform better. For the first time, somebody was looking over our shoulders and holding us accountable for our actions and our decisions. Paul Beeson and Dr. Stead were there all the time, making sure that patient care was up to their standards. Many times at night, sometimes in the wee hours of the morning, I would see Dr. Stead prowling the wards. I would be working up a patient and, while I was filling out some pages of the history at midnight or thereabouts, I'd look up from the desk to find Dr. Stead asking, "Have you got anything interesting?" After I recovered my composure I'd say, "Oh yes, great case," and then we'd talk about it a bit.

Residents were never too busy to work with the Chief. After all, these were exciting times—and they were getting paid five dollars a month to work night and day! The educational component at Grady before Stead arrived was primitive; the attending staff made rounds and a regular teaching staff taught students, but these were part-time people and education was not their strong suit. The situation was much the same at all large city hospitals. Heyman recalls that within six months of Stead's arrival, things had turned about completely. More importantly, the young doctors were exposed to a new way of looking at medicine. House Officers at Grady had always been fascinated by all of the disease they saw, but now they had someone to explain and to teach about those diseases and patients. The daily mixture of patient care, education and research was a nurturing one

Dr. Heyman:

> I was more or less engaged to my future wife, Dorothy Keyser, before I went to Atlanta, and very soon after getting there I said to her, "Come on, let's get married," which we did in February of 1942, soon after

Pearl Harbor. I had been living in the residents' rooms, which, of course, were not air-conditioned. Atlanta gets pretty hot during the summer, and I had the upper bunk of a double-decker bed in the hot and sultry summer when the heat rose to the top of the room. After complaining a bit the hospital gave me a room with beds on the floor, and after Dorothy and I married, we rented a small efficiency apartment on the outskirts of town. Dorothy got a job as a social worker at Grady Hospital and supported me on her salary. We hired a maid who lived in the apartment most of the day and cooked our meals for us; we paid her eight dollars a week, which we thought was a reasonable amount of money. There wasn't much to do in a small efficiency apartment. I didn't see Dorothy very often at home, but we were able to have lunch together because she was working at the hospital. We didn't own a car and we rode the streetcars together across town.

Most house officers were single in those days; in fact, most of the people I knew were single because none of us had any money with which to support a wife although we all depended on that five dollars a month to support ourselves to some degree. Even at the time it seemed like a terribly small sum of money, but internships in Boston and New York didn't pay anything at all. So really that five dollars was a fair amount of money to be receiving.

At Emory, the research fellows had teaching duties on occasion, but it was mostly Drs. Stead, Beeson or Hickam who discussed patient problems at Sunday School. It was the high point of the week, and the conference was extremely well attended. I don't think anybody ever said we *had to* go; everybody wanted to go. You would become absorbed in trying to make the diagnosis on a complicated patient or in stretching your mind in some new area of medicine that was unfolding around you. These were days for making discoveries, to be the first to know something, anything, of medical consequence.

The resident staff was subjected to a phenomenon known as pyramiding. Only a selected few interns were chosen to stay on as first-year residents, and of those, another few became second-year residents. There was just one Chief Resident, and that was a very desirable position because it meant you had been selected above the others. If you were chosen, you knew you had shown your ability to perform. The Chief Residents worked very hard, but they didn't resent the work. Despite the pyramid, there was so much camaraderie and so many opportunities for learning, and the faculty was so supportive, that one would do almost anything to maintain that. We dared not—would not—let our buddies down, and that is the spirit that carried us through.

Our work took on new meaning, too, under the informed guidance of our new mentors. Housestaff and young research fellows did not spend time in the lab. There weren't many labs then. Paul Beeson had a lab and Gene had his catheterization laboratory, but none of us did a whole lot of basic science or fundamental bacteriological work. We were doctors seeing patients and we wrote our papers on what we did best. We used the talent that we had. Of course, Eddie Miller made all the effort that he could to get the typhus organism cultured and the antibodies measured and all that, but there was no fundamental study of the biology of organisms like typhus. In studying syphilitic meningitis, I wasn't sure about the treatment or whether the spinal fluid tests were being done right, so everything we learned was a contribution in itself. Later on, when labs began to be developed, then the study of the physiology of heart failure and of blood stream infection and bacterial heart infection became more sophisticated. But in terms of what the average house officer or junior staff person did, we simply did what we did best.

Later, when the venereal disease epidemic was coming under control, Heyman switched to the study of brain circulation, at first in patients with neurosyphilis. He had help from the cardiology division who were not just interested in the heart, but also wanted to learn about the brain and its circulation. New techniques and people were now available at Grady, allowing Heyman to study people with neurosyphilis. Never before had anyone done any physiological studies in such patients, in part because there weren't that many cases, and in part because the people who knew about sophisticated circulation studies were cardiologists. Cardiologists and neurophysiologists never met except in Dr. Stead's Department at Grady Hospital.

The excitement of discovery was tremendous. A number of studies were taking place at one time, and as far as possible everyone worked together. One of Paul Beeson's major works concerned the bacteremia of subacute bacterial endocarditis, a deadly but difficult to diagnose heart infection. Beeson, the infectious disease expert, used heart catheters to get blood cultures from arteries and veins all over the body; Dr. Frank Engel, the endocrinologist, studied the effect of fever on hormonal blood levels. They all worked together, using each other's techniques; nobody was afraid that somebody would "steal" their ideas. Unlike most medical centers, Grady was like a big family where everybody shared. Nobody who had anything to offer was left out. As Albert Heyman noted, "You can't often go off to different departments and say,

'Could you help me with this,' or 'Would you be interested in that?' Very few people care what you're doing; they are interested in their own work. What we experienced at Grady was quite different."

From the time he entered academic medicine, Eugene Stead valued research, and attracted colleagues who wanted research to be part of their professional lives, wanted to honor scholarship and a spirit of enquiry. The young people Stead recruited were, as he was, well-grounded in clinical medicine but without formal training in research methods. Stead was ever on the lookout for young talent and that was how he came across one young man who was exceptionally skilled in an area that was new to him. During a conference on shock held at the Macy Foundation, Stead met C.N.H. Long, a professor of biochemistry at Yale, who had studied the pituitary-adrenal axis, and had prepared crude adrenal extracts. Long knew that stresses like shock produce a dramatic outpouring of hormones, including adrenocorticotropic hormone (ACTH), but the precise relationship of ACTH to shock was to become clear only in the future.

Dr. Frank Engel (twin brother of the George Engel who had corrected Stead's research when he was a visiting student at the Brigham) was working with Dr. Long at the time. He delivered an outstanding research paper on protein synthesis. Stead, who had been awaiting the chance to meet George Engel's brother, wrote to Long, expressing an interest in hiring his protégé. This led to Frank's taking a job at Emory after the war.

There were one or two hazards attached to Engel's appointment. When he first arrived in Atlanta, Engel and his wife, Mildred, rented an apartment that was being deregulated from rent control. In order for the landlord to meet the requirements of deregulation, the apartment had to be painted, and this proved to be a race against time because the Engels were eager to move in. The owner painted so fast that he didn't even wait for the roaches to get out of the way of the paintbrush. All along the baseboard, the Engel's had a bas-relief, so to speak, of roaches painted right into the woodwork!

Shortly after Frank and Mildred arrived, the Steads invited them for Christmas dinner. Sitting around the dinner table, enjoying the dinner and the festivity of the season, Gene noted that Frank looked yellow. He was in the process of coming down with hepatitis A, just as they were settling into the Yule Tide feast! Fortunately he made a complete recovery and eventually settled into a highly productive career.

Engel was well trained in biochemical aspects of endocrine disease, but his only clinical experience was in the care of people with adrenal insufficiency (Addison's disease). One day Frank announced that he was going to be an endocrinologist; Stead said "OK, since specialists are really made by practice rather than by formal training or anything else, we'll start shifting anyone who seems to have an endocrine disturbance in your direction, even the border-line cases, and before long you'll be an endocrinologist." This is how Stead's unconventional and unwavering support of goals and endeavors increased the productivity and success of his staff. Frank Engel became a leading endocri-nologist, despite the lack of formal training, by using his biochemical back-ground to learn as he went along treating the patients that came his way.

Dr. Stead:

> What Frank Engel and a number of other people did was to become knowledgeable in areas tangential to the specialty they were interested in. Instead of trying to be like other sub-specialists, they treated enough patients to become, at a slower rate than doing it full time, a competent clinical sub-specialist, but with a different (research) back-ground than they would have had if they had gone directly into the clinical sub-specialty.

In July of 1946, Dr. Jack Myers joined the team at Emory. He had been over-seas with the Brigham Unit early in the war, and was left in charge when the army decided to capitalize on the talent from Boston by spreading the young doctors around. No matter how many new people the army brought in under Myers, the unit retained its outstanding reputation. Stead realized that Myers must be the reason. Myers had the ability to instill good habits in his young doctors, so that they consistently performed in an efficient and successful manner. He realized that, under wartime emergency conditions, there wasn't time to intellectualize the practice of medicine. He wanted good habit pat-terns formed, so the doctors would make few mistakes. It didn't matter where they'd gone to medical school or where they had their internship or residency; if they got to Myers' unit, he'd make good doctors out of them, regardless. Stead recognized a winner in Dr. Myers.

His bristling crew-cut and pugnacious nature made him an unforgettable character, but it was his clinical intuition and great skill as a doctor that made him valuable to Grady. His diagnostic ability led other doctors to turn to him in particularly difficult situations. On one occasion he diagnosed hy-dronephrosis, kidney swelling because of blocked urine flow, just by manual examination of the patient. Feeling a big, fluctuant mass in the right flank, he confidently announced his diagnosis. It seemed unlikely that he could be right, seeing the patient for the first time on ward rounds, but indeed he was, and often was, over the years.

One of the exciting episodes at Grady Hospital concerned an allotment of new diapers bought for the nurseries. To prevent pilferage, they had been stenciled "Grady Hospital," but the aniline dye used to stamp them soaked through the skin of the babies. John Hickam and Jack Myers suddenly had a lot of infants with methemoglobinemia—the dye had converted the babies' hemoglobin to methemoglobin, preventing normal oxygen transport. As Myers said: "It was a God-awful mess! The children were pretty sick, but I don't think anybody died and we looked upon it as a clinical investigative opportunity because we'd never seen an outbreak of methemoglobinemia. The spectrophotometer had just come into clinical use, so we could get good spectra of hemoglobin; by checking the spectrum of absorbed light, we could determine that the hemoglobin had been converted to methemoglobin. That was exciting." These life-saving adventures represented great clinical research opportunities to doctors who were properly prepared. These Harvard-trained doctors had taken to heart the words of Louis Pasteur inscribed in the rotunda of the medical school dormitory there: "Dans les champs de l'observation, le hasard ne favorise que les esprits préparés."

In mid-1946, an Emory-affiliated Veterans Administration Hospital was organized in Chambliss, a suburb of Atlanta, by converting the existing army hospital there; Jack Myers was named Chief Consultant in Medicine. His four years as Chief of Medicine in the army gave him the necessary experience. Furthermore, his rigid performance standards resonated with those of Dr. Stead, so the philosophy prevailing at Grady was sure to emerge at the VA facility.

The whole reflects the sum of its parts. Gene Stead had chosen some of the right parts for Grady, and others had chosen him because they recognized in him the qualities that distinguish the great from the good. Grady Hospital had never before seen what so many well-trained, devoted professionals could accomplish on its wards. Even with the limited manpower and short supplies imposed by the war, these highly skilled, serious young doctors made a remarkable impact. Nevertheless, after about four years at Grady, the limitations of working in a city hospital system were clear. Even the careful training and supervision of staff could not solve problems that were, at bottom, socioeconomic in nature and immutable. Stead realized that it was time to look for new challenges. His influence did not evaporate, but remained at Emory in the men he left behind. Paul Beeson took over as Chief, continuing the Stead tradition.

Dr. Stead:

> By the time I left Emory, I had begun to appreciate the limitations of a city hospital. It was an ideal place for medical students and interns to see acute medicine, to follow patients from their admission to the autopsy room, and to discover the pathological basis of end-stage disease. But for students beyond the second year out of medical school,

the system became repetitive and the learning opportunities diminished. A city hospital is a place for doctors to learn about disease, not to learn about people. I think the best and most scholarly run city hospital I ever saw was at Southwestern Medical School in Dallas. Don Seldin was in charge of the medical program and, curiously, he simply gave up caring for patients. He made no effort to understand the impact of education and culture on the patients or the role the nervous system played in their complaints. He did not stress sensitivity as a special quality that doctors needed in caring for patients. He simply said, "Medicine is treating diseases; our patients have diseases; let's study and treat those diseases." And he ran their acute service in this way. If I had stayed at Grady, I think I would have been forced into the same position. There wasn't room for the careful study of people, for follow-up evaluations and the like. That simply didn't fit the circumstances or the short-term expectations of the patients. In private practice you can treat patients who drink too much alcohol for many years before they suffer liver failure and hepatic coma. And so, it is appropriate to treat the whole patient when you're able to have a long-standing relationship with him. However, at a place like Grady it becomes clear in a rather short period of time, when you only see alcoholic patients who already have cirrhosis of the liver, often in hepatic coma, that the patients are all going to die. The psychosocial aspects of health care are not very important when treating a person with a ruptured aorta or one in a hepatic coma. In that type of setting, a housestaff with a can-do attitude can take great pride in being able to fix what seems to be unfixable and then getting on to the next challenge. They sew up a man's belly in a five-hour operation at 3:00 a.m., and three months later sew him up again after another knife fight. Patients often returned to Grady with repeated traumas from knife wounds or car accidents.

Having worked in a number of city hospitals, I saw that it helped to provide the kind of care that could be administered at a relatively low cost. The goals and expectations had to be realistic, commensurate with circumstances. We provided a high volume of services to patients who were not going to be available for follow-up care and who were not likely to follow complicated instructions or buy expensive medication. The notion that a city hospital should have the most sophisticated x-ray with which to serve this population always seemed crazy. The laboratory should be simple and the services available to patients should be simple. This limits the opportunities for

teaching young doctors what care is like in the private practice setting where long-term relationships exist between patients and doctors. I've seen money thrown away by administrators who decided to
replace simple services with highly specialized services like elaborate
endocrine units or elaborate cardiovascular units, thinking they'd influence lives beyond the immediate. If one looked at the outcome
rather than the process, it was clear that even the very best technology would not produce the best outcomes.

I never claimed to be doing any great social good by running an efficient medical service on patients whose social structure had broken
down. It was a good, though limited, learning experience for the young
doctors, but I never said we made a big impact. There are a whole variety of people, admitted to the hospital for the fifteenth time, who
simply couldn't change or wouldn't change the ways in which they were
living. We required our housestaff to give the best simple care that
could be given, not for social reasons, because I don't think it served
any, but because if they effectively developed the ability to treat broken
down systems, they would be effective in systems that weren't broken
down. A sophisticated cancer service or a sophisticated neurology service didn't make any sense in that setting. The population we were dealing with was living such a hand-to-mouth existence that they really
couldn't follow any recommended schedule or program that required
continuous effort on their part. We'd intervene during a time of crisis
and finish when the acute episode was over. We would not see the patient again until the next crisis. And because of the restricted nature of
the patients and problems cared for there, I didn't think doctors at
Grady Hospital were going to be professionally satisfied over time.

During his four and a half years at Emory, Dr. Stead graduated a number of
people into community practice. He was impressed that they did very well in
terms of practice and money, but they didn't very much enjoy the great opportunity of being a doctor. In private practice, they saw middle class working people with none of the acute, catastrophic illnesses that had been the basis
of their medical training. Grady had been a court of last resort because there
really was no other place for indigent patients to turn, but now these doctors
had to deal with patients who would simply find another doctor if they were
unhappy with their care. The doctors often felt unchallenged because their patients weren't seriously ill or dying, and they missed the excitement of the city
hospital's rough and ready emergency practice. In a way, this turned out to be
an advantage to Stead's teaching service because doctors in private practice

would do anything for Grady Hospital (where they had experienced real fun in medicine). If Stead had stayed at Emory, he would have moved part of the teaching program to Emory Hospital so that students could see a broader spectrum of patients.

Emory Hospital, located on the Emory campus 5 or 6 miles away from Grady, was built in the depths of the Depression. It was supposed to have been the University Hospital, but Depression economics meant that the university could not support the hospital. As a result, it had no permanent university faculty on its staff and so had evolved into a community hospital. When Stead went to Atlanta, he realized that the doctors practicing at Emory Hospital helped it to survive financially but had no real interest in teaching.

Dr. Stead:

> Emory owed these practitioners something and, during the period when I was Chief, we had to decide how to pay off our debts to these doctors who contributed to Emory's survival. We had a difficult problem in that, over time, each of the practitioners had accumulated one or more assistants, and they wanted their assistants to inherit their practices and privileges when they retired or died. We finally agreed to take care of the older doctors, but prohibited their passing on their practices to appointed successors. Still, it was a long time before Emory became a true teaching hospital. The split campus posed a great logistical problem because Grady was far away from the medical school campus. The problems were inherent in the system, both at Grady and at Emory, so I decided to move on.

CHAPTER 9

CHAIRMAN AT DUKE— BUILDING DOCTORS AND PROGRAMS

Mistakes are at the very base of human thought...feeding the structure like root nodules. If we were not provided with the knack of being wrong, we could never get anything useful done.

Lewis Thomas

As his reputation grew and spread through the medical community, job opportunities began to cross Gene Stead's threshold. None of them seemed to offer more freedom or opportunity to deal with young people than Emory did, so Stead stayed put, waiting for something promising to come along. He did not have the wanderlust common to academicians; to the contrary, he kept busy being Chief of Medicine at Emory. Despite all limitations, the challenge in Atlanta was still absorbing. Then an inviting opportunity presented itself, sooner than he expected.

In March of 1946 Dr. Frederic M. Hanes, the Chair of Medicine at Duke University in Durham, North Carolina, died of a ruptured aneurysm. A search committee was leisurely looking for a replacement when Dr. Stead's name was introduced as a possible candidate by Elizabeth Peck Hanes, the late Chief's widow, who was active in the search process. Robert Lambert, the southern regional representative of the Rockefeller Foundation and a close friend of Mrs. Hanes, had visited the Emory campus. He told her of the exciting ferment in medical research and education there, and suggested Emory's young professor as a possible candidate, knowing that Duke would benefit greatly from the unique philosophy and approach Stead promulgated.

Dr. Hanes had been a good administrator, well liked by the staff, but he coddled Duke doctors rather than consulting them as colleagues. Hanes' paternalistic style had limited the influence of other staff members within the department. There were people at Duke who could have filled Hanes' shoes—

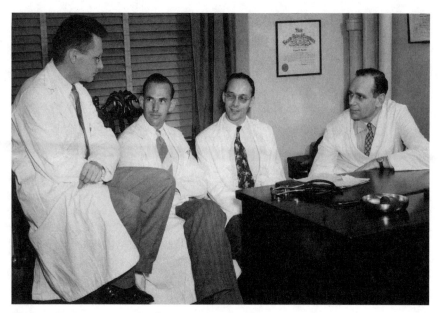

The young brain trust at Duke, 1947: Jack Myers, Walter Cargill, John Hickam, and Eugene Stead in the Chairman's office.

Dr. Davis Finn had handled administrative affairs for the Department during Hanes' absences from the campus, and Dr. David T. Smith served as Acting Chairman during the search for a permanent replacement—but it was Duke's intention to name someone from outside the system, someone with a fresh approach. Eugene A. Stead Jr. seemed to be that man. When he met with Wilbert Davison, the Dean of the Medical School, and the small group of doctors who comprised the Private Diagnostic Clinic (PDC) at Duke, Stead wasn't concerned about the impression he made on them. He was secure in his position at Emory, so he could afford to be a little cocky—and he was, perhaps more than a little. It was not in Stead's character to seek the approval of others or to curry favor among his peers. He spoke his mind freely, stating without apology his thoughts about what he saw and what goals he might have for Duke. And though he did not walk out of the meeting without stepping on a few toes, his qualifications and his vision greatly surpassed the question of social etiquette.

Dr. R. Wayne Rundles:

> At my first meeting with him, Dr. Stead mentioned that he was in-
> terested in some patients I had studied in the past (diabetics with or-

thostatic hypotension and orthostatic tachycardia). The fall in blood pressure and rise in heart rate that occurs when certain diabetic subjects changed from a lying to a standing position is a result of an altered autonomic nervous system. He said, however, that his experience with hematology had left him with little enthusiasm for the work I was doing at the present time. He underscored his point by telling me that a well-known hematologist at Emory had left and they weren't too sure that they would be looking for a replacement. It was not exactly what I would consider a propitious first meeting.

A number of things made Duke more attractive than Emory. The rural setting of the Duke campus and hospital, unlike Emory's, was very appealing. Atlanta was often shrouded in a veil of grey smog that hung ominously about the city, so the Durham landscape, its trees and grass seemed idyllic in comparison. For the raising of children, North Carolina had a wholesome appeal that Atlanta lacked. And professionally, Duke was attractive because it had room to expand its campus and research facilities. Emory had a split campus with two separate and distinct patient populations, which Stead thought would be a permanent drawback. Emory University Hospital housed private patients, but teaching activities were confined to indigent patients at the downtown Grady Hospital. Unlike Grady, where medical students had almost no opportunity to follow a patient's disease from onset through to its resolution, Duke Hospital treated paying as well as indigent patients. This meant that students would have access to a socio-economically diverse group of patients and broader exposure to various stages of disease.

The economic benefits were difficult to ignore. Emory paid its Chief $8,000 a year, and Duke offered a starting salary of $20,000. To a man with a wife and children, an additional $12,000 would make quite a difference. But the primary attraction at Duke was the flexibility it offered for research and teaching. Stead had hit upon an unusual formula for success. He recognized that academically affiliated doctors could, to an increasing degree, generate more income than was needed to pay their salaries. When this happened, the extra money was turned over to the medical dean or to the university itself. Stead thought that if a Chair could control at least a portion of the "free" money (that is, money not earmarked for salaries or fixed operating expenses), he would be able to recruit and develop bright young people and implement new ideas. Even then Stead realized that Duke's PDC would be a lucrative source of "free" money for important programs he wanted to promote. Laboratory work was a sidelight at Duke when Stead was asked to come, but that did not discourage him. The potential was great, and Dean Davison (unlike almost all his colleague deans) seemed receptive to Stead's ideas about money. Davison agreed that Stead could control half of any "free" money generated, and promised him the space and freedom that the new Chief of Medicine needed.

In October of 1946, Stead returned for a second visit, this time with his wife. It didn't take long to reach a decision, and at Christmas-time, they moved to Durham. Frank Engel, Jack Myers and John Hickam, the three key physician-scientists he recruited to the Duke staff, followed close behind, and eventually, a number of residents came from Emory. With this nucleus of Stead-trained people, he hit the ground running.

The Steads rented from the University a house that was only a seven-minute walk from the hospital. Being so close enabled Stead, for the first time in his career, to be home for dinner. This meant that the Stead family spent more time together, but that was the only change in his routine. It was otherwise business as usual.

Because housing was scarce, it was difficult to find a place for Hickam and Myers to live. As it turned out, the university building next to Stead's house— the President's House—was vacant, so Stead asked Dr. Davison if he could use it as temporary housing for his colleagues. However, the place was about to be remodeled and the President wouldn't let anybody live in it. After prolonged consideration, Stead realized that the housing shortage precluded any other solution. Back he went to the Dean, this time with another tactic. "My wife says there are a lot of rowdy and unpleasant activities taking place over at the President's house. Since I have a number of commitments on the national scene and will have to be out of town, I think it's perfectly appropriate for me to request that a caretaker be put in that house. And," he continued, "I've got two candidates—one named Hickam, the other, Myers." The Dean took the issue back to the President and the plan was finally approved. And since they were neighbors, Stead, Hickam and Myers walked to work together every morning.

Shortly after arriving at Duke, Stead noted the casual attitude and performance of the staff. He decided that the Department of Medicine had a "country club atmosphere." Not acceptable, socially or professionally, by his standards; he immediately set about to change things.

Stead was the first professional educator at Duke Medical School. He was interested in how people learn, retain, and use information. As a result, his approach to education and his attitude toward students differed vastly from his predecessor. Before his death, Dr. Hanes had become more and more distant from the students. He made ward rounds with the residents, but excluded students from those rounds and from the weekly medical conferences because he worried that they might discover that the staff didn't always agree on the plans for patient care. Stead, on the other hand, believed that exposure to the professional dynamic, including controversy and vigorous discussion, was essential to the students' education. He made it quite clear that he did not intend to participate in any educational exercise from which students were excluded. He would not require the students to come to meetings, but if they wanted to attend Departmental meetings or medical conferences, they would be welcomed.

One of Stead's more controversial changes concerned the on-call schedule. Under the new Chief, housestaff were expected to be on call five nights out of seven. At that time, most institutions scheduled their residents to work every other night, but Dr. Stead, whose training had consisted of living in the hospital without protected time, thought two nights off quite generous. Stead insisted on having more housestaff in the hospital than was necessary for ordinary clinical care. This freed up time so learning opportunities wouldn't be wasted. Most hospitals schedule just enough residents to provide adequate coverage, but that practice shortchanged opportunities for learning. Duke hospital could have gotten by with only one or two house officers in house, but Stead knew that much of the fun and excitement of medicine occurred during the evening hours. By being in the hospital at night, the house officers could attend their patients who got sick, and could share interesting clinical experiences with their colleagues. Often over a midnight supper, house officers would discuss the findings of patients admitted late at night; afterwards several would go to listen to an unusual heart murmur, palpate a vascular thrill, or feel an abdominal mass. Those learning opportunities would have been lost if only the minimal number of staff were on duty at a given time. Busy with routine tasks, they would never have a chance to explore new phenomena or exchange ideas.

It was clearly within Stead's domain to institute these changes, but they did generate resistance. Dean Davison thought that some of Stead's decisions were extreme or too demanding. He was concerned that such a hard-line philosophy would increase student tension and anxiety, and he said so. Stead was unmoved by the Dean's protests. He didn't believe in a low-key, non-demanding approach. Convinced that he knew well what students and young doctors needed to learn, and how to provide that education, Stead forged ahead. Unlike Davison, Stead believed that challenge would exhilarate the students who belonged at Duke; the others would identify themselves and leave.

Dr. Stead:

> I conceded that if there ever came a time when the students said they weren't learning more from our course in Medicine than from any other service, and Davison could demonstrate that to me, then I would change my methods. Until then, if the students didn't perform,

attention would be called to that fact. Our housestaff program was not for everybody and I knew that not everybody would meet our standards. In a large department store, there is a wide range of shoes to choose from. Some are good shoes, some mediocre and some fall apart in the first rain. We were only interested in one quality of shoe—excellent. If someone wanted to join up we were glad to have them, but if we didn't have the same standards, one way or another there'd be a parting of ways.

Stead declared that he would have "the most rigid service in the country," and that he would "maintain that rigidity as long as I can, because the natural tendency of anything is to weaken and become slack." Strong advocates like Hickam, Engel and Myers, made it easier to imbue the Department with a sense of how things were to be done and what was expected. But at first the older staff members resented the new, younger men Stead had brought from Atlanta. They threatened the way that the medical service had been run. Stead tried to be sensitive to the needs of the existing staff, but he was probably as sensitive as the proverbial lead brick. He was unequivocally committed to his ideas for developing the department, and the interests of old and new guard did not always run in the same direction. Stead took a hard line during his first year as he set about changing the status quo of the Department. He did not relax his standards for anyone. It was some time before the staff accepted the new Chief's goals and his methods for achieving them. In the meantime, the honeymoon was not without its difficulty.

Before Stead arrived, nearly everyone at Duke beyond the rank of Instructor in Medicine was expected to earn most of his income in the PDC. This meant that the faculty had no little or no free time for research; as a result, the Department of Medicine did very little laboratory work. Bill Nicholson, who was interested in endocrinology, had a small laboratory and a technician, but had published only one paper (on serum potassium in diabetic ketoacidosis) and that work had been done at Hopkins, before he came to Duke. By the time Stead took over, Nicholson's lab was not producing anything of significance. The only significant researcher in the Department was Walter Kempner, who had rented laboratory space from the Physiology Department. Kempner was to become one of the most famous of the Duke faculty, and one of the most controversial—more about him later.

The lack of research activity was in harmony with the Medical School's basic philosophy, which mirrored that of most medical schools of the day. The administration reasoned that, since students continually passed through the basic sciences into the clinical services, laboratories should be under the aegis of the basic science departments. Clinical problems that aroused research interest would be investigated in collaboration with basic science faculty, so clinical research laboratories were deemed unwarranted. Furthermore, there weren't enough hours in the day for clinicians to see large numbers of patients and maintain a close working relationship with basic scientists. Therefore, clinical medicine remained separate from the basic science activities.

Beyond the practical arguments, religious and political motivations limited Duke's ambitions and endeavors. Like Emory and Vanderbilt and many other schools in the South, Duke University had a religious foundation, and at one time received substantial support from the Methodist Church. From the very beginning, Duke struggled over whether it should be a secular institution (albeit with a Department of Religion), or a primarily Methodist school where religion guided administrative decision. The Medical Center might strive to be at the forefront of the medical field, but the rest of the campus was divided in its ambition because of Duke's ties to the Methodist church. As President of Duke, Hollis Edens decided that one way to solve the problem was to progressively loosen the school's financial dependence on funds from the Duke Endowment, a purely secular source of funds. He did not want the university to seek a national reputation, convinced that such a position was incompatible with Duke's church affiliation. Edens had grown up at Emory, which was then very tightly tied to the Methodist Church, and hoped to build an endowment large enough to protect Duke from becoming a merely secular institution.

Edens opposed expansion of the Medical School. He saw Duke as a sedate, regional university and didn't want another Johns Hopkins, where the medical school was so strong that it overshadowed the rest of the campus. He opposed the medical school's involvement in national organizations or taking federal support for buildings. Edens' ideas seemed provincial to the ambitious Stead, but his view was not unique. Indeed, at the time Stead arrived, many Duke faculty members opposed expansion of the Medical Center beyond its existing structure. Of course, outside opinion was unlikely to sway the new Chief, and he was not altogether alone in his vision.

Paul Gross, Chairman of Chemistry and later University Vice President, was a strong adversary of Eden's. He thought that stronger ties to the Methodist Church would inhibit Duke's becoming a great university. During his tenure as Vice President he fought to expand Duke's programs, reputation and influence. Dean Davison, on the other hand, was a complex person and far from single-minded about expansion of the medical school. When asked what he thought about research at Duke, he would say that it wasn't good for the school. One of his most impassioned speeches touted Duke as an important training-ground for family and general practitioners, but later that same day, he signed the papers approving the innovative Research Training Program, developed to foster training in research. It was impossible to tell whether what he said was for general consumption or whether it was what he truly believed. In the final analysis, however, Davison certainly tolerated all the special needs of the Medical Center, including research. Edens' ideas did not prevail. Douglas Knight, Eden's successor as president, made it clear in a variety of ways that the Methodist Church wasn't central to the life of Duke University. He instituted an Executive Committee, which bypassed the Board of Trustees and weakened the influence of those committed to a strong church presence. Knight felt that strong church ties limited the University's appeal to outside groups, but by the time he assumed office, the medical center was already well along the path of becoming a nationally recognized school—far ahead of the rest of the university.

Because research had not been a priority, the Department of Medicine had neither money nor space for this purpose. Stead had to create income that would foster research and provide laboratory space until grants were in hand and the research became self-supporting. After only a short time at Duke, Stead realized that the doctors working in the PDC created a great deal of income. The University contributed $2,500 a year, but each PDC member earned the remainder of his or her salary by seeing private patients. Stead recognized that the PDC had the potential to finance his plans for the department.

In the interval after Fred Hanes' death, Dr. D. T. Smith had overseen the department. In that capacity, he had instituted a tax system under which a portion of every dollar earned in the PDC was paid to the Department of Medicine. Stead maintained this system because it allowed him to hire full-time researchers and teachers and buy equipment until those staff members were able to support themselves with research grants. The PDC tax created a great deal of controversy among the older staff. The staid Southerners who made up the existing medical faculty didn't like change in the way the Department operated. They resented the Department being diluted with people recruited from the outside, people who were oriented toward teaching and research rather than practice. But the biggest bone of contention was that these new people, working in ways new to the regular staff, were being paid with money created in the PDC. This variation of taxation without representation rubbed them the wrong way. The old guard questioned using funds that they had generated to pay people who spent their time in the laboratory, and created only a small portion of their salaries in the clinic.

As time went on, the staff acclimated to Stead's ways, and controversy subsided. It was clear that the young Chief was strongly committed to Duke, and his educational and research programs had considerable merit. The Department of Medicine began to thrive, slowly evolving into a strong intellectual and academic enterprise, the likes of which Duke had not previously known. Its reputation began to spread. Even Ivy Leaguers, who knew nothing about Duke except that it was situated south of Philadelphia, were talking about Stead's innovative programs. There were minor confrontations with the Dean, but Stead gained the acceptance of his local colleagues—until 1949, two years after his arrival, when he unwittingly stepped into a brier patch of ill feelings about the budget. As it turned out it wasn't numbers that he miscalculated, but the emotions of his staff.

Calculating expenses for the Department, Stead surmised that eventually the University would look at the large income created by the PDC staff, and decide to cut off the $2,500 that it contributed to each doctors' salary. The administration would rationalize the cut by saying that the staff could earn the difference in the PDC, but the Department would lose $40,000 a year if and when the University cut back its contribution. Stead proposed taking pre-emptive action by not paying doctors who were working in the PDC from the University contribution, and using that money instead to pay the salaries of people who did not work mainly in the PDC. Of course, he didn't intend to cut salaries, only ask PDC practitioners to work a little harder. The plan made sense as a way to ward off a possibly considerable budget cut (Stead reasoned that if he were running the university, he would have cut out the payments to PDC doctors). What he didn't factor in was the symbolic importance of University money to the PDC members. They considered themselves full members of the University faculty, and felt they should therefore receive part of their salary from the University. Even a pittance would affirm their relationship with Duke. Misinterpreting Stead's intentions, the PDC Duke staff felt they had been discounted as members of the Duke community, and grew deeply resentful. It may sound trivial now, many years later, but a real confrontation was at hand.

Dr. Stead:

> Underestimating the feelings of the staff was the most serious error I could have made. If I hadn't done anything in the first place, the system just would have continued as it was. However, once the staff learned that I had initiated a change, the members of the Department took action against me, and I had a full-scale revolt on my hands. I decided, "the hell with it," and wrote a letter of resignation to the Dean.

Before Stead's resignation could be approved, it had to be read before the Executive Committee, which was scheduled to convene at an unspecified future date. In the meantime, the students heard what had happened and appealed to Dean Davison to do something to prevent Stead's leaving. "We just can't let him go," they pleaded, "he's given us so much." The students' opinion, voiced that way, was the first tangible evidence Davison had of Stead's impact on students. On a personal level, the Dean was not terribly fond of his Chief of Medicine, but he had to admit that the overall effect on the students was consistently positive. Still, Davison did not like Stead's teaching methods or Stead's ability to tirelessly argue his position on a matter. And the two men had different philosophies on how to run a department. Before Stead arrived, the Department of Medicine had been a sort of gentleman's club; Stead insisted that it be a working department. He preferred that his staff not be honored for their academic status or their personal connections, but for hard work at teaching and patient care, and for turning out good research. He wanted solid scientists, not amateurs or dilettantes. During his first few years at Duke, Stead tried to recruit the very best people he could, and the Dean did not always agree with Stead's choices. Dean Davison had Stead's resignation in hand and did not think that losing his Chief of Medicine would be a tragedy.

Walter Kempner, who had joined the Duke staff under Dr. Hanes, went to see Stead. He asked the Chief to retract his resignation, saying that the Department was just beginning to do well, and that a number of other staff members were upset with Stead's decision. Dr. Wiley Forbus, the rather crusty Chairman of Pathology, called on Stead as well. "You know, Gene," he began, "you've made a lot of difference here; just sit still and you'll do well." He continued on almost philosophically, "The time has come for you to eat some crow. You just go to Davison and withdraw that letter of resignation. I've been through this myself," he confessed. "I've eaten my crow; it didn't seem to hurt me any and it won't hurt you."

After thinking about it, Stead admitted that many things were going well, and it would be foolish to let misunderstanding change that. He wrote to Davison, saying he'd reconsidered and would like to withdraw his letter of resignation. Much to Stead's surprise, the Dean said he couldn't do that. The letter had already been turned over to the Executive Committee and would have to go through formal actions. In fact, Davison felt sure that Stead would be voted out of the chairmanship. Knowing how to make an oligarchy work, Davison had packed the Executive Committee with faculty members hand picked for their allegiance to him, and he thus felt assured about the outcome of all votes. It was some time before the Executive Committee was to meet, so things rocked along as they had in the past. When the meeting finally came, Davison arranged a long agenda with Stead's resignation as the last item. By the end of the meeting, when everybody was too worn out for a vigorous debate, Dean Davison introduced the question of Dr. Stead's resignation. All the members but one, who was momentarily undecided, cast their votes. Sur-

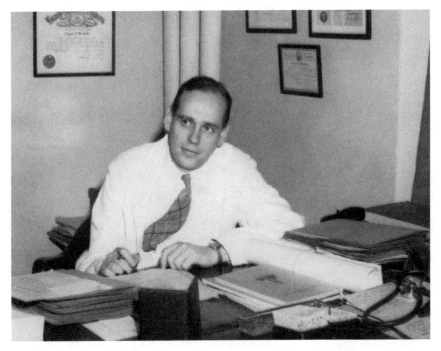

Dr. Stead in his office at Duke, shortly after assuming the Chair of Medicine in 1947.

prisingly, the vote was tied, with as many members in favor of Stead's leaving as opposed. Dr. Richard Lyman, the Professor of Psychiatry, held the deciding vote. Dr. Lyman, who was somewhat paranoid, worked largely at night because he felt safer then; hence he was around the hospital in the evening when Stead was also there, and knew the Chief of Medicine. Lyman must have thought that anybody who worked nights couldn't be all bad, because when he cast the deciding vote, it was in favor of Stead. Dr. Stead's resignation was the only critical vote by the Executive Committee on which Dean Davison was ever defeated.

Dr. Stead:

> It was truly a close shave. Thinking back over the years, I haven't been in any kind of serious disagreement with members of the staff that, in the end, wasn't my own fault. I always could have found other means to get what I wanted without doing what I did. And although it was a somewhat depressing realization for my ego, it was a valuable lesson to learn. I've always thought that the responsibility of a Chair-

man is similar to that of the doctor. The sign of a truly professional doctor is that he quickly senses and adapts to the needs of his patients. To ask the patient to be as professional as the physician means that the doctor is not professional. Whenever the medicine went wrong and a patient left me, I've always been willing to say it was because I made an error. This is because I'm the pro and really, there's no other possible interpretation. And it's the same thing with a Chairman. I can't ever remember not getting what I wanted when I'd set my mind to do so in an intelligent fashion. After the issue of PDC salaries was settled, I never raised any other major issues that were terribly important to the older members of the staff.

Or perhaps he never again raised controversial issues in ways that prompted the senior staff to take him on. Diplomacy was preferable to war. Later, a question arose over how doctors would be appointed to the PDC. Eventually it was decided that Stead could assign any part-time faculty member to the PDC, but that any candidate who would earn over half of his income from work in the PDC would have to be approved by a majority of the existing PDC members. It was perfectly clear to the Chief that anyone who was earning 50% of his income in the PDC would have to work closely with the PDC people and be integrated into the system. He never assigned anybody who wasn't immediately accepted, and, as it turned out, the PDC people often wanted new members brought in even more quickly than Stead did.

It was agreed that matters related solely to the PDC would be settled by those doctors who earned over half of their income there. On the other hand, decisions related to the curriculum, student assignments, residents' activities, and the like were decided by a majority vote of the entire medical faculty. For the first time, department policies were put in writing. This smoothed relations with the faculty, and Stead became more strategically adept about issues he considered important. When necessary, he lobbied for his point of view, and never lost a vote; in fact, few matters even came to a vote. The faculty all respected Stead, whether they liked him or not. They sought his advice on tough problems, a kind of court of last resort. Unquestionably, he was the brightest person in the Medical Center, and they were fortunate to have him.

Halfway through the 20th century, Duke University and Durham, North Carolina, were hardly advanced bastions of social change. Of course, the field of medicine has rarely been accused of excessive liberal tendencies. The South was segregated, so hospital wards and restrooms were racially separate. Black (and women) doctors were conspicuous by their absence, and there was little indication of the profound changes that were coming. How well medical (and other) institutions adapt to social change determines the kinds of people that want to work there. Gene Stead was a novice in these areas, but he was determined not to be left behind. His background was not progressive nor was he particularly sensitive to the rising tide of change about to flood the nation, but he understood that critical re-appraisal was required if his Southern institution was to survive and flourish. Stead started slowly but as we know, it's not how the race begins, but how it's finished that counts. And to Stead's advantage, he thought learning about human behavior was fun!

Dr. Stead:

> Before Henry McIntosh came on as an intern, we hadn't had any married people. The internship was such a busy time and required that people get fully immersed in it, so whether or not someone was married might have been a consideration in my selection. Obviously, when doctors in training started to marry younger, we had to allow for that on our medical service. Clearly, if everybody was married, we weren't going to have interns unless we changed our attitude. But we never had any problems in making the transition.

Dr. Henry McIntosh:

> I had a hiatus of five years between college and medical school, and I was married during that interim period. Upon applying for the Duke internship, Gene Stead looked at my application during the course of my interview and said, "I see you're married." "Yes," I replied. And he retorted, "I never had a married intern before and I'm not sure I want one." He said it that plainly.

Stead awarded McIntosh an internship despite his being married, but it set off a long, hard fight for full respectability. The conflict ultimately influenced both men and brought about great loyalty. Money was limited in the McIntosh family, so Henry decided on a residency at the Atlanta VA Hospital. "When I went off to Atlanta I was finished, as far as Gene was concerned. I told him that I would like to come back after a year, and even wrote him a letter saying that I wanted to apply for a position at Duke. He knew I went to Atlanta because of financial problems, but I did not get a job at Duke." The residency program was pyramidal, and Duke interns were given first priority for resident positions, but McIntosh says it was "not quite as brutal as it sounds. Although, from my vantage point, I had to fight my way back into the Stead group because that was where I wanted to be." McIntosh eventually became a major contributor to the Department of Medicine and Chief of Cardiology at Duke before being named Chairman of Medicine at Baylor.

Dr. McIntosh:

> I went back to Duke after the interviews at Baylor, and told Gene that I would be leaving in nine months. He asked me why I was waiting so long. I told him that I had to finish several things. Gene's reply was, "Well, if you're not interested in going before nine months time, I'm not sure you really want to go." He told me not to turn in my resignation for a while, and I didn't. He sensed that, if I'd had a really urgent desire to go, I would have moved more quickly. This is the kind of a man that he is. Although he had cut me off once, he later recognized that I had some promise.

Many years later McIntosh left academia to join the Watson Clinic in Florida and practice very high quality medicine there. In the meantime, many excellent married interns came to Duke and survived. However, the duty schedule was so demanding that many a spouse regretted the decision, for it surely put a strain on any marriage.

Dr. Grace Kerby was already a medical intern when Dr. Stead arrived at Duke, but she got low ratings by the staff and, therefore, was not offered an assistant residency in medicine. They did not think she was worth keeping. After Stead had been there a few months he decided that she was, in fact, the outstanding intern on the service. He persuaded the Chief of Dermatology to take her on into the Dermatology residency. She went through that program and then came back for a second residency, and eventually became Chief Resident in Medicine.

By the time Kerby became Chief Resident, Stead had become more relaxed about the military draft and did not appoint only draft-deferred residents. As a result, many residents were called to serve in the Korean War, but Duke found a very interesting group of substitutes, including some Canadians and Englishmen, who were not at risk of being drafted. Kerby had to indoctrinate these people from very diverse backgrounds. Since she lived in Duke Hospital even more than Dr. Stead, things went along surprisingly well.

Dr. Stead:

> I should have been brighter about appointing draft-eligible people in the first place, but in any event, I couldn't have had any other resident who pitched in as well as Grace did. I went to sleep about the possibility of war, and those residents were promptly called into serv-

ice. Korea came as quite a surprise to me. I don't know whether I could have anticipated the war if I'd not been in Duke Hospital as much as I was, but I do know I didn't anticipate it. We were very short-handed, but we filled in. However, I was always very careful not to let the resident complement fall below what we meant it to be, because that would have meant asking people to do more routine work than we had intended when we appointed them. Any residency that becomes short-handed but still tries to maintain a high level of service by doubling up, will go downhill.

As a woman supervising a predominantly male staff, Grace did well. She was a connoisseur of liquors and could, reputedly, drink any resident under the table. But she was always touchy about any genital contact when examining male patients. Perhaps this had to do with the difficulty of being a woman in medicine, and not treated as a peer by men, or perhaps there were other factors, unrecognized. Whatever the reason, she took care of herself, and she never had any trouble running the service. There were not lot of women doctors then, but Duke did have a number of female interns and they conducted themselves extremely well. There were no distinctions of female from male applicants for our internship.

Grace worked with Lee Cluff, one of the younger residents who went on to become a national leader in the field of infectious disease, and Sam Martin, who later became Chairman of Medicine at the University of Florida (Gainesville). Sam and Grace had worked closely together at Duke and they complemented each other's talents. Sam had an excellent support system at Duke, and he did some very nice investigative work. When he went to Florida, I calculated what salary to offer Grace, because what she was doing for me in the Department (running the housestaff selection program) was what Sam needed to have somebody do for him, and I didn't intend to give up my support system lightly. To my amazement, Sam never offered Grace a job. He would have been the greatest medical professor of his era if he had taken Grace Kerby with him so she could help him with the mechanics of running a medical service. Grace was not the most imaginative individual in the world, but she never turned in a bad performance. She not only ran our housestaff office and did very complex scheduling of resident rotations, she was running a lab as well. She had a number of very strong assets. She clearly knew how to set up a lab, she knew how to make instruments work and how to care for animals, and she could get cooperation from any of us. Grace was one of the few people who would always be allowed to borrow any piece of laboratory equipment because everybody knew it would certainly come back in at least as good of shape as it left.

Unlike Boston, New York, Philadelphia, or Baltimore, places with a great abundance of medical and scientific talent, there were only isolated pockets of medical excellence in the South. So Stead decided that the medical community in the South needed to be linked into a network of intellectual activity. But most of the leading people at Duke, including Dean Davison, didn't want competition from a second medical center in the Durham area. At the time, Chapel Hill had not yet been selected as the site for the University of North Carolina Medical School. Most Duke people wanted the school to go to Charlotte, far from Durham, but Stead took the opposite position. He wanted to concentrate scientific talent locally, and thought that Chapel Hill was an ideal spot for the school. He envisioned interchange between two medical centers that would provide jobs and educational opportunities for spouses of faculty at each school. Furthermore, he thought adding a second medical school would make the entire community more attractive to other scientific institutions. Of course, the remarkable scientific growth that occurred around Durham and Chapel Hill and Raleigh (the now famous Research Triangle) justified Stead's position. Besides, Stead thrived on competition—the nearer and keener, the better.

When it came to accepting black doctors, the Durham community was slow to change. Lincoln Hospital, an historically black hospital in Durham, was losing patients because the services there were not as good as those at Duke. Black community leaders were concerned about this. Dr. Charles Watts, a surgeon and Medical Director of North Carolina Mutual Insurance Company, worked at Lincoln Hospital and asked Stead to assign Duke housestaff to Lincoln Hospital. Stead wanted to help, but realized that any interns or residents he sent over would not return to practice at Lincoln when they completed their training. Stead suggested instead that Lincoln Hospital increase its patient services, and direct some money from this increased medical practice into an educational fund.

They developed a small prototype service, modeled on the Duke PDC, which used a part of the income generated there to pay a Duke intern or assistant resident to work at Lincoln. Because Stead was interested in training black leaders in medicine, he went to Howard and Meharry Medical Schools, and offered to provide internship appointments for students who wanted to participate in the Duke-Lincoln program. The program was highly successful; Duke senior residents and fellows were happy to be assigned at Lincoln for two to three months, and Stead went there often enough to show that the Chief was interested. Moreover, Lincoln Hospital provided great medical service to the community.

On occasion, Stead filled a vacant senior residency slot at Duke with one of the residents from Lincoln. Charles Curry, later Chief of Cardiology at Howard Medical School in Washington DC, came from Lincoln as the first black house officer at Duke. Around 1970, Louis Sullivan, a respected young black hematologist from Boston, was chosen to head up the Duke-Lincoln educational venture. He was to be paid partly from private practice income, partly from private contributions, and partly from Duke. Because Sullivan was an outstanding academic physician, Stead was happy to guarantee his tenure as a faculty member in the Duke Department of Medicine; if the Lincoln venture were not successful, Sullivan would be moved to Duke Hospital. Lincoln would largely underwrite his salary but Duke would back up the venture in case it didn't turn out happily for either party. Long negotiations ensued with Sullivan and his mentor (and Stead's former teacher), Dr. William Castle of Boston City Hospital and Harvard. Castle was very supportive, and things seemed to be moving along well until Durham Academy, a private school, denied Sullivan's son admission. The school had given the child a test and determined that he did not meet the admission requirements at Durham Academy. Stead, keenly aware of Southern biases, suspected that the boy had "failed" the test before he even picked up the pencil. Still sure the problem of the youngster's education could be solved, Stead proceeded with Dr. Sullivan's appointment as an Associate Professor at Duke. Since Duke University was responsible for only $2,500 of any professor's salary, the Chief didn't bother asking the Dean for approval. He just appointed Sullivan, as he did all new professors; no one had ever questioned such decisions because the Department of Medicine had the financial resources to provide for its staff. But when Taylor Cole, Provost of the University, learned of Sullivan's proposed appointment, he turned it down. He told Stead that Duke Medical Center could not guarantee tenure to a doctor who was working outside of the Medical Center.

The episode was extraordinarily embarrassing. Stead had to call Dr. Castle and concede that the South was not yet ready to move in his direction. In fact, it would be many years before the race barrier would be broken; only after Stead had retired as Chief of Medicine was the first black faculty member appointed in the Department of Medicine. Fortunately, these events did not interfere with Sullivan's career as a faculty member at Harvard, President of Morehouse School of Medicine, and eventually, Secretary of Health and Human Services. As Dr. Jack Myers said, "Dr. Stead had a real ability for recognizing good people. One of the most important attributes in medical education is being able to pick the right horses to start with; if you do, you're going to win a lot of races."

The Chief's innovations were wide-ranging. Rather than paying every faculty member a fixed salary based on rank, he set faculty income levels individually. Income was traded for free time for research, so professors who worked in the clinic made more money than those who worked in the laboratory. On the other hand, doctors working in the laboratory had great freedom to choose how they spent their time. That structure appealed to Stead, and he instituted this novel practice without a committee meeting or discussion. It was a general feeling that he paid you as little as possible, no matter who you were.

Doctor John Laszlo:

> He was always fair to me, and I had no knowledge of, or interest in, what my colleagues were earning. When he recruited me for the faculty I was still a resident. Walking down the hall he put his arm around my shoulder and asked me what I would need to join the staff the following year (1960). When I told him that the National Institutes of Health (NIH) would pay me $8500, he said that sounded right, and the deal was struck then and there for me to stay at that salary. The first year went very well, and the next year he spontaneously raised me by 30%, more comparable with others at my rank of Associate. I never had to ask for a salary increase. Probably he would have paid me $11,000 had I asked for that in the first place, but he took me by surprise, and there were no regrets.
>
> One young doctor, a full-time staff member who was earning $10,000 a year, learned that one of his contemporaries was making $13,000 working in the PDC. When the first fellow complained, Stead said, "If you want $13,000 a year, I'll pay you that. I've got job waiting in the Private Diagnostic Clinic, and you can start next week." This was the last thing this fellow wanted to hear, and so he dropped the issue. You could discuss anything with the Chief, but you couldn't bluff him in any way, shape or form. Staff members would approach him from time to time and say that they had received better offers from another institution. Dr. Stead would say in his southern drawl, "Wa'al, I guess you'll just have to take that offer."

Dr. Stead didn't want money and academic rank to be linked to one another, so he kept the two issues separate. He wanted young doctors to remain flexible enough to do what they wanted to do. He didn't hesitate to promote anyone whose performance was excellent; a reasonable academic rank within the Department was a reflection of their competence. On the other hand, basing salary on rank, would make it difficult for a faculty member to pursue better professional opportunities elsewhere. Taking another job with a cut in salary

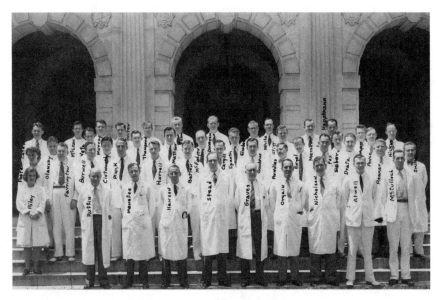

Stead with his senior faculty and house staff at Duke Hospital, 1947.

would be difficult for a man with a family. Doctors who were primarily interested in research and academics were welcome to stay as long as they were advancing, but the Chief also wanted them able to accept a better opportunity if one came along.

New faculty members were generally offered salaries that were lower than "the market." If someone was comparing a position at Duke with one at another institution, Stead suggested a careful weighing of the worth of uncommitted time, time free of other responsibilities to do what the candidate really wanted to do, versus what the other institution offered. Then Stead asked them to project how their careers might look after five years at Duke compared to five years elsewhere. Duke always looked good in this light. Harvard had reputation in its favor, but it was difficult for young doctors to grow rapidly there. Duke had a big advantage because the Department of Medicine could protect people, supplementing their income for a number of years until they got their feet planted firmly and their research reputations established. Other places might ask young doctors to be productive and fully independent more quickly than Stead thought appropriate. The ability to put a "floor" under young people during their formative years marked Stead's career as Chief.

Because doctors working in the clinic had relatively little time for teaching and research, while researchers like Jack Myers and John Hickam had much more, there was some strife among the older members of the staff. They couldn't reconcile the equivalence of a commitment to practice with a commitment to research and teaching. Not everyone shared Stead's vision of a symbiotic system in which various faculty members made different contributions to broad scope of activities, thereby strengthening the Department as a whole. John Hickam helped to smooth some of the difficulty between the old guard and the new. He was helpful, jovial, and people liked him. He was a new man on the team, but his presence didn't threaten anyone. He worked two days a week in the PDC and performed well. He was respectful of the other physicians, and even as a newcomer, aroused no resentment. Hickam always hung back a bit when he had a point to make, careful in his presentation and modest about his knowledge. "I've been thinking it over," he might say, "I'm not quite sure, but I think this is probably the way it is."

Dr. Stead:

> Of the people I've known, I guess I was personally more fond of John than anybody else. And I had an arrangement with him that didn't mature. When he left Duke I said, "John, during the next ten years, when you're in Indianapolis as the Chairman of Medicine, you've got to have somebody sign all those papers like recommendations for grants and awards saying you're a great man. And I'm the one you should send all those papers to. In return, when I get to be 75 years of age, I expect you to take care of me if I need any medical help or other assistance." And John agreed, but he reneged on that. Unfortunately, he died suddenly of a brain hemorrhage, similar to the one suffered by Soma Weiss.
>
> By contrast, Jack Myers was dogmatic and hard-driving in his assertions, which may have been tougher for the staff to accept. He was the antithesis of Hickam; he would pound on the table and say, "This is the way it is." But Jack Myers was an excellent doctor and a fine teacher. He gave many impressive performances in the CPCs; he was superb at teaching in that arena and quickly became a legend among the housestaff. When he first came to Duke, he gave a CPC on a patient who had contracted a rare infection, presumably by handling infected rabbits. Tularemia. No one had ever seen a case or had suspected the diagnosis. All the medical staff had been in on the case, trying to figure out what the infection was, but the patient died undiagnosed. Usually at a CPC, the medical staff is presented with a very complicated diagnostic problem but one person is assigned the role of discussant. He works his way through the case, suggesting possible diagnoses and explaining why some possibilities should be eliminated,

the whole time trying to make sense of the puzzle. Usually the discussant ends by rendering a differential diagnosis, a series of possibilities in order of their likelihood. Not knowing the answer ahead of time, they have to weigh the possibilities, often based on incomplete or even incorrect information. In his characteristic fashion, Jack analyzed the situation of the undiagnosed patient and said, "When everything is put together, there's no differential diagnosis to make, there's only a single diagnosis. Given the data you've presented, I would say that the patient died of tularemia." And he was right! And so if people were put off at first by his assertiveness, it was just a matter of time before they realized he spoke from a position of knowledge.

Myers and Hickam were popular with the students and housestaff. The style of one was distinctively different from the other and therefore they appealed to students for different reasons, but each made equally valuable contributions to the education of young doctors and both helped impress Stead's methods on staff and students alike.

The professional attitudes of Stead's inherited staff were only one level of response, however. The prejudices of the old South were clearly discernible in several of them, and had to be dealt as well as their provincial attitudes toward medical practice. For instance, Frank Engel, who was Jewish, worried about moving to North Carolina. The country club and other private facilities excluded Jews, and the Jewish community in Durham was very small. As it turned out, even some members of the Department of Medicine were reluctant to accept Dr. Engel. According to Stead, Engel might have had a more difficult time had cortisone not become available when it did. Engel's professional expertise made it obvious to all that he was an intellectual force with whom the Duke staff would have to deal. What did cortisone have to do with this social adjustment? Before it became available, people with adrenal failure (being unable to produce cortisone-like hormones) were very fragile. An infection innocuous to a normal person or the stress of surgery could prove fatal to these patients. With cortisone, they were able to surmount illness and stress, and thus lead normal lives. Extracted from beef adrenal glands, cortisone was very scarce and costly. The average doctor couldn't get it at all because it was still considered an experimental drug. Duke, fortunately had a limited supply, but it was rationed. Because of his work on the adrenal gland, and his association with treatment of adrenal insufficiency, Engel was chosen to oversee the distribution of cortisone. With doctors clamoring for this remarkable new drug, Engel found himself in a strategic and powerful position. Old time faculty members had no choice but to make their peace with Engel or risk not getting any cortisone. The prejudices of the older staff receded under the pressure of their professional needs, and the distance between them and Engel was bridged by their growing respect for their younger colleague. Indeed, Engel was a kind, gentle, soft-spoken intellectual who felt privileged to be a physician—a man without an ax to grind.

The significance of the many changes thrust upon the Duke staff was not lost on the new Chief. While implementing new programs, Stead had to be sensitive to the feelings of the older staff. He had achieved standing in the academic world at a young age, so he often dealt with people older than he, including most of his peer group. As a matter of courtesy, he decided to communicate with people in person rather than sending notes or memos. By so doing, he learned things he might otherwise not have known, especially how much was happening outside of his own office and lab. He knew that a talk with the Chief could make others uncomfortable, so it seemed to preferable to have the other person in his or her own surroundings. Most chairmen stay in their offices, removed from the world they are supposed to know and guide. As a result, they lead dull lives, but Stead got involved in the daily drama of the clinic, lab and ward—not only was it a lot more fun, but it helped him appreciate the dedication of his staff, something he took into account when dealing with them in other issues.

There were other favorable consequences of unannounced drop-in visits by Dr. Stead. He got a feeling for how various laboratories were organized and who staffed them, which boosted the morale of the ancillary people who otherwise might not meet the Chief. Moreover, the visits provided an element of quality control. His curiosity prompted him to look at data, to ask questions, to examine laboratory methods. He might not be an expert in the research at hand, but he brought his perspective—the big picture—to bear on each project. He had the knack of honing in on weak assumptions, noting inconsistencies with data from other fields, and suggesting important ramifications. If his faculty took a shallow approach to research problems, Stead's probing ferreted that out and called it to their attention. People paid attention to his counsel (not to do so would be professionally suicidal), and the next trip around he would pick up where he left off. His memory was phenomenal, and his attention span seemingly unlimited.

Scientific fraud was not a public issue at the time, but it's difficult to imagine falsification of results in that environment. A major transgression of research ethics, would not lead to lengthy hearings or appeals, just the next train out of town. There was no debate about this position; it was a given, and people were comfortable with such standards. Of course, the department was small enough that the Chief could see everything; and the Chair had fewer administrative demands then than today. These kinds of personal interactions are virtually unheard of today and may be impossible, even for Chairs who possess all the rare skills enjoyed by Stead. The price of complexity and bigness makes it quite unlikely that we will see another chairman with Stead's impact on a medical center.

When Stead first arrived at Duke Hospital in 1947 only the operating rooms were air conditioned. Unless they were actually in the operating rooms, Duke doctors had to endure the long, sultry Southern days and nights of summer— and so did their patients. At that time, Stead's research made use of the Van Slyke apparatus to measure blood oxygen levels. The instrument's stopcocks were sealed with grease, but when the room temperature exceeded 90 degrees, the grease liquified, the stopcocks popped out, and studies became impossible. It was essential that the lab be air conditioned, but Dean Davison objected, arguing that if he said yes to the Department of Medicine, he would be faced with one such request after another. But he finally conceded, and a very limited expansion of air conditioning began at the Medical Center.

The PDC was not air conditioned when Stead arrived, and it was soon clear to the Chief that the staff's efficient patient care sagged tremendously in the heat. He proposed to Deryl Hart, Chairman of Surgery, that they air condition the Medical and Surgical PDCs, but Hart vetoed the idea. His staff spent a lot of time in the already air conditioned operating rooms; he thought it wasn't worthwhile to air condition the Surgical PDC. Stead thought it might be a problem to air condition the Medical PDC but not the Surgical PDC on the floor directly above, but he went ahead. Soon thereafter, the surgeons complained about how hard it was to see clinic patients in the summer heat; Hart reluctantly agreed to air condition the Surgical PDC.

Dr. John Laszlo:

> Matters of personal comfort were not considered high priority items. When I came to Duke in 1959, the private wards had been air-conditioned, but the public wards had not. It was pathetic, using ice packs or alcohol sponges to cool down patients with raging fever from meningitis in ward rooms where the temperature could be 100–105ºF with the summer sun beating down on the roof. In the summer, the housestaff quarters were so hot that it was hard to sleep, although this was absolute necessary for the doctors. Later, air conditioning mercifully arrived, accompanied by great gnashing of teeth by tight-fisted hospital administrators.

In 1953, the Veterans Administration built a hospital across the street from Duke Hospital. It was not air-conditioned because of the $300,000 additional cost. In the early 1960s, when the folly of the original decision was clear, the hospital was air-conditioned over the course of 24 months and at a cost of about $3 million. Not only did it cost ten times as much, but the mess was incredible, requiring that Radiology or Surgery be closed for periods of time, Dialysis and Intensive Care Units moved, and so on. But living in the hospital greatly improved once the renovations were done.

CHAPTER 10

ENTERTAINMENT AND THE
SOCIAL SYSTEM

Humanity needs practical men, who get the most out of their work, and, without forgetting the general good, safeguard their own interests. But humanity also needs dreamers, for whom the disinterested development of an enterprise is so captivating that it becomes impossible for them to care about their own material profit.

Marie Curie

Dr. John Laszlo:

I first met Evelyn Stead at a 1959 picnic in the back yard of the Stead home in Durham. They lived in one of several houses at the edge of the campus, owned by the University and designated for use by the top Duke administrators and faculty. This house was provided to Stead as part of the chairman's job, with the stipulation that, when the job ended, the property would revert to the university. Every July 4 the Steads hosted a back-yard picnic for the Medical Housestaff; Gene and Evelyn were quite informal and very gracious hosts. They went out of their way to put the housestaff at ease and to make spouses feel welcome. A big keg of beer, an inexhaustible slab of cheddar cheese, crackers and pretzels, a friendly Dalmatian, and one or more Stead children helped break the ice, particularly for new housestaff who had arrived in Durham only a few days earlier. If Dr. Stead was still shy, he gave no evidence of that as he greeted one and all, and made appropriate small talk about the July heat in North Carolina, the local "institution" of foods like barbecue, black-eyed peas, and collard greens.

One subject never discussed by Dr. Stead was conspicuous by its absence. He had no interest in team sports and that alone, in a region known for its intense collegiate football and basketball rivalries, would have set him apart from most of the local citizenry. He was

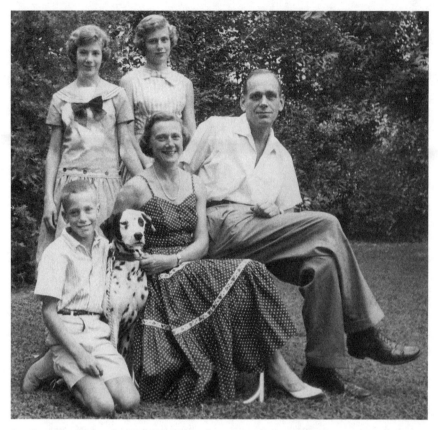

Family portrait taken in Durham, September 1958. Front: Bill, Evelyn, Gene Stead; rear: Lucy, Nancy Stead.

once asked if he would be attending the big Duke vs. Carolina game at the end of the season. The outcome would decide the league championship and seal a post-season bowl bid. No, he wasn't going. He said, "I've been to a football game."

It was a great treat to be invited to his house and see the personal side of the Chief. For one thing, it was difficult to be intimidated by a long-legged man in shorts. Spouses in particular found his informality and friendliness a sharp contrast to the larger-than-life stories they had heard. Interns and residents relaxed, secretly hoping he wouldn't take them aside to ask about a patient follow-up, or about incomplete charts of recently discharged patients, or other professional matters. But it was not that kind of occasion. House officers sometimes joked afterwards about the relatively spartan picnics—the beer was always Brand "X", costing a few dollars a keg less than name brands, but cold and refreshing.

On other occasions, the Steads entertained friends or visitors in their home with the warmth of Southern hospitality. Dr. Stead would make the first drinks for new arrivals; then you were on your own. The meal was prepared by Evelyn Stead and attractively served on beautiful place settings, often with the assistance of Duke employees who supplemented their income by serving at university parties and dinners. There was a feeling of stability in the household, a sense of clear purpose that conveyed to visitors that they were welcome in the Stead home, that their visit was not an imposition, no state visit. Not that the Steads entertained often; they did so only when they really wanted to spend time with their visitors.

Most of Duke's senior PDC staff belonged to the Hope Valley Country Club, located in an attractive area with the most elegant houses in Durham and a beautiful old clubhouse with golf course, tennis courts and pool. Many of Durham's affluent non-university people belonged. It was the social and power base of the Durham community, and the debutante ball, garden club functions and charitable events were held there. Of course, Jews and Blacks were excluded, although later a few token Jews were admitted to membership. Stead was not a member because he had no use for the facilities, but each year the medical PDC held a Christmas party there for the entire Department and to honor the housestaff and fellows This was the big event of the Medical Department's social calendar, held in the ballroom and side rooms of the country club. Some of the faculty dressed formally; it was a time to meet in a social setting people with whom one had worked or only heard stories about.

My first Christmas party was the least pleasant of the 27 that I subsequently attended. That December date towards the end of my residency year found me scheduled for duty in the Emergency Room. On such occasions, it was customary to divide the evening shift with a colleague and I had second duty. When the party began at 6:00 pm. Dr. Julian Ruffin, an aristocrat of old Southern tradition, welcomed each person with a glass of his own eggnog, which he poured with a flourish. He was splendidly attired, with a green and red waistcoat under his tuxedo jacket to mark the occasion. The waiters circulated martini and Manhattan cocktails; I had one of each. There was to be a big Christmas dinner but during the cocktails there were only tiny, thin, open-faced, cucumber or onion sandwiches on white bread (apparently a tradition, though why was never obvious to me). At 8:00 p.m. the dinner had still not been served and many of the housestaff were a bit tipsy, since we had little occasion to practice drinking during the year. My partner called from the hospital to remind me that I had promised to be back at 8:00 p.m. so that he could come to the dinner. Fortunately, the Emergency Room was quiet, so when I got back, I changed into my white suit and lay down on the metal cot in the hospital room where I lived. Then the nausea and vertigo began—alcohol was playing its tricks in my brain. There was no steadying the bed as it spun, but holding tightly to the frame kept me from spinning off across the room and into the wall or ceiling. Even though I knew I wouldn't take off, I was powerless to stop the sensation. At 10:00 p.m. the Emergency Room nurse called to report that an intoxicated patient had wandered in, but had no serious complaint. "Couldn't you send him home to sleep it off?" I asked. At 10:30 she called again, insisting that I come down to lend a hand. I wobbled to the bathroom to wash my face and compose myself. There was a moment of self-enquiry as to why I was brushing my teeth since this patient would surely not notice any alcohol on my breath. It was a very long walk across the length of the hospital; every step seemed problematic. The patient was drunk and unpleasant, and he seemed to be lonely, all of which the nurse had recognized. He was hard-pressed to conjure up a medical complaint; the best he could do was back pain of two year's duration. He chose to come in because he worked during the day and it was more convenient to come on a Friday night. He wanted a thorough check-up. For the only time in my life (I think), I was rude to a patient. He was summarily sent home to sleep it off (which was what I had hoped to do, too), and given an appointment for check-up in the Medical Out-patient Clinic the following week. But I was sorry for my actions then and am sorry now, recalling the event more than 45 years later. The long walk back to my room prepared me for sleep, and when the next call came at 2:30 a.m., the alcohol had been metabolized sufficiently that there was no further difficulty with functioning. I hoped my colleague had enjoyed the Christmas Party more than I had.

Toward the end of Dr. Stead's tenure as Chairman in the mid 1960s, I led a revolt against holding the Christmas party at the Hope Valley Country Club. We now had a black house officer and it just didn't fit the spirit of the times to hold official functions at a segregated facility (it never had felt comfortable, but now there was a critical mass of

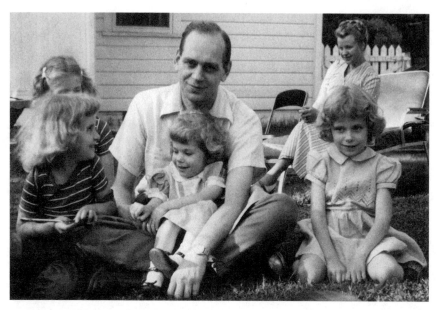

Backyard scene in 1949. Gene Stead is holding Lucy and Nancy is to his left. Unidentified children and woman in the background.

people, mostly young doctors, who were offended). Several members of the PDC old guard felt equally offended by young upstarts telling them where to hold their party. If the party were moved away from Hope Valley Country Club, they would refuse to pay for it. But I took the position that the whole faculty, not just PDC members, should impose a voluntary assessment on ourselves to pay for a party honoring our trainees. That position carried by an uncomfortable vote, and for a number of years thereafter, I chaired the Christmas party arrangement committee. We used a number of hotels, and the party was always successful, though the music was decibels too loud. There was a greater sense of faculty participation, though unfortunately we did lose a few of the old guard who felt unloved because they could no longer host the occasion. I was sad that the traditional eggnog was no longer served by Dr. Ruffin (at his choice to be sure), but no one ever complained of missing the onion sandwiches. I was most encouraged that a fairly conservative Medical Faculty had taken a positive step on a major social issue of the day. There was no turning back. The Medical Center and the University had still not moved very far in improving race relations, but the Department of Medicine led the way.

In order to set Duke on a research footing, Stead not only had to strengthen the department's few existing laboratories, but he had to expand its involvement in basic science. He needed a staff that would be productive, but he needed to be politically prudent with older doctors who were solid practitioners and deserved respect as such. Not satisfied with the lab work of Bill Nicholson, Stead decided to split the Endocrinology service into two parts. Bill Nicholson was named Head of Metabolism and Frank Engel, Head of Endocrinology. Engel was Nicholson's junior in years and clinical experience, but he was a superior scientist and knew how to design useful and productive studies that would appeal to grant review committees. By giving Engel a title, Stead not only recognized his contributions but made it easier for the younger man to get grant funds; by allowing Nicholson to retain control over part of the service, Stead preserved the senior man's ego. When the time was ripe, he eventually reunited both areas into a single Division of Endocrinology and Metabolism under Frank Engel. Stead later employed this same strategy when he gave Jim Wyngaarden, another outstanding young researcher and excellent laboratory scientist, responsibility for the Arthritis Unit while Bert Persons, one of Duke's original group, retained the title of Chief of Rheumatology. In this way, Stead could promote young people over entrenched senior people without too many hard feelings. The older people retained their titles and professional dignity, but the future belonged to the young. Stead was always clear about that.

His desire to avoid snubbing the older members of the Department never interfered with Stead's ability to effect change where it was needed. When he thought that someone wasn't an asset to the Department, he didn't hesitate to say so. He was always frank in his opinions, and he told people what he was going to do in a forthright manner.

Dr. R. Wayne Rundles:

> During Dr. Stead's first months at Duke, he proceeded to get acquainted with the staff and, as far as I was concerned, all seemed to be going along reasonably well. After about six months, however, he told me that he was bringing up several bright young associates from Emory, and that they would probably be too competitive for those who were already in residence. He thought that I shouldn't count on any long-term sojourn. The field of blood disease was moving rapidly, however, and it soon turned out that there was room for new work in the field, and that the competition he foresaw from the men he imported from Emory wasn't too severe. He was always supportive of innovative workers, particularly if their ideas panned out. We

developed a close relationship with a great deal of sharing and respect in both directions. For 20 years I had no concern about lack of administrative backing from Dr. Stead.

When it was clear that he had arrived at a hasty conclusion about someone (as in the case of Wayne Rundles), Stead did not hesitate to reformulate his opinion and support that person as he would any other promising staff member. He came to call Rundles one of the finest scholars he had known. More often than not, however, when the Chief made a decision, he did not waver. His decisions might be painful for some, but it was uncanny how often he turned out to be right.

Because he needed funds for the many projects he envisioned for the Department, Stead quickly clamped down on spending he didn't deem necessary. In this process, his eye lighted on the Neurology section. When Stead arrived, there were three neurologists at Duke, led by a Doctor Robert W. Graves. Graves contended that the sub-specialty area of Neurology could never be self-supporting and deserved to be subsidized by the Department. Stead felt otherwise when he found that much of the neurologists' time was spent doing preoperative evaluation of neurosurgical patients to save the neurosurgeons precious time. "You are just the handmaidens of the neurosurgeons— go out there and do some work," Stead chided. He told Graves to actively look for patients and not wait for surgical consultations to come to him. As incentive, Stead cut off any financial subsidy from the Department, which meant that Graves' neurologists had to earn their salaries and pay for their secretaries, just like all other doctors in the Department. Unhappy with those terms, Graves left Duke, taking the two junior neurologists with him. Stead was not unhappy with this result, but it left Duke without a neurologist for a long time. Eventually Stead brought in Charles Kunkel, as Chief of Neurology, and John Pfeiffer. And then he sent down to Atlanta for Albert Heyman, who had helped him when Emory needed a syphilis expert. Heyman had no experience in neurology, but Stead knew his capabilities. He offered his former resident six months of neurology training at the Massachusetts General Hospital before he came to Duke. That's the reverse of the standard procedure; people usually get training first, then look for jobs, but Stead invested in talented people, and arranged the training to fit. This unconventional method was usually successful, and Stead never argued with success.

Dr. Albert Heyman:

> When I went to see Gene, he outlined his proposal the same way he did with the VD program. Dr. Graves was leaving and he needed a

neurologist to see patients and do some research. Gene was aware that I did not know any neurology, yet he was willing to provide the necessary training if I would come to Duke. He was taking a big risk. After six months at the Mass General, I arrived at Duke. As it happened, John Pfeiffer was planning to leave, but fortunately decided to stay on. There was a tremendous need for patient care, and he provided most of that. Charlie Kunkel was there, and did much of the teaching. I learned from them what I hadn't learned at Mass General; without them I would have been lost. In time, of course, I got my bearings, but I always marveled at how Gene could couple people with areas that would provide them with satisfying careers, even paths that the individuals themselves might never have chosen. Certainly I would never have chosen neurology if Gene had not extended the offer he did.

Stead invested in quality people and he was willing to back their training if he could persuade them to go into the needed area. It worked out so well so often that he had no compunction about encouraging career changes as opportunities. As a corollary, he would leave even a key position unfilled rather than choose someone who wouldn't wear well over time. He wanted only the best people. This characteristic was occasionally frustrating when his Division chiefs wanted to fill a position but the Chief had reservations about the candidate.

Because he asked the best people to join his staff, Stead was bound to be turned down at times, and he had his share of rejected offers. But the rejections always came from bright and capable people, so they didn't bother the Chief terribly much. If he had asked less qualified people, he mightn't have been rejected, but he also wouldn't build a top-notch staff. And the very bright candidates who turned down Duke's offer would be friends of the institution thereafter—and that counted too.

CHAPTER 11

ROUNDS WITH THE CHIEF

The medical internship and residency program at Duke was designed
to give to the intern a knowledge of the factual material in the field
of medicine and a sound philosophical basis for a lifetime of learning in practice. What is done is important, but why it is done is even
more important. Duke was not just a collection of excellent doctors.
It was a group of doctors with a carefully thought out program of
training to allow maximum growth of people. The staff believed that
doctors exist to care for people, that patients can legitimately make
demands on doctors, and that, because the ill are not rational, these
demands do not have to be rational.

E. A. Stead Jr.

Stead's Teaching Rounds were planned with the care of a military operation. He made rounds on Osler Ward, where the house officer in charge was
a first-year (Junior Assistant) Resident or JAR. The JAR and two interns covered the 32 patients on the ward along with four third-year medical students
who were taking their first rotation in Medicine. Every patient admitted was
first evaluated by a student who took an exhaustive history and carried out a
thorough physical examination, including routine (blood and urine) laboratory tests. Then an intern performed a similarly thorough work-up, and the
JAR, a somewhat abbreviated work-up that focused on the "critical" issues.
Deciding what was a critical issue required experience and judgment, the latter to be validated only by subsequent events.

The medical student wrote the case history before others did, and then discussed the patient with the intern and JAR. A course of action would be decided based on the diagnostic possibilities, the so-called differential diagnosis
(a time-honored method of honing in on ultimate diagnoses according to the
order of their likelihood). A patient might have heart failure, headache, weight
loss, maybe ten or more different problems; each was evaluated and a differential diagnosis created. Decisions—sometimes difficult, sometimes easy—
had to be made about which possibilities were to be pursued and which were

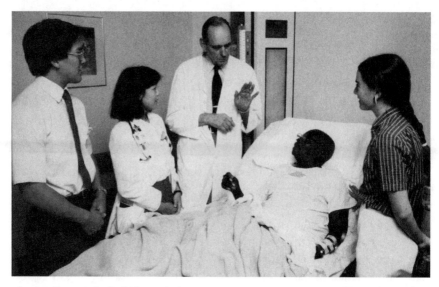

Always, always at the bedside, with the patient. Dr. Stead on teaching rounds with students Gregory Chow and Serena Chen and Junior Assistant Resident Kathy Merritt, circa 1985.

to be left alone. If the patient with severe heart failure had had headaches intermittently for 20 years and low back pain for 30 years, the plan would be pretty obvious: concentrate on the heart failure and simply note the other complaints without expending many resources.

Students and house officers learned to look at the patient, really look. They would feel the pulses in both wrists and ankles, listen with the stethoscope to the great vessels in the chest, neck, abdomen and groin—and in everyone, not just people suspected of having diseased arteries. Stead constantly stressed the wide range of abnormal findings in people who had no disease associated with those findings. Skin, hair, nails, eyes, ears were examined for color, texture, symmetry. The appearance of nails and underlying nailbeds might lead an experienced observer to diagnose illnesses as varied as chronic lung disease, bacterial endocarditis, lead poisoning, iron deficiency anemia, or protein deficiency. Careful examination of the eyes might reveal eye disease, but also detect diabetes, kidney failure, genetic disorders of connective tissue, malignant hypertension, melanoma, or leukemia. A doctor couldn't afford not to note the clues the patient brought along, whether from the history and physical exam, or from the laboratory and x-ray findings. Stead made it clear that the doctor's job was to obtain all available information, organize it into manageable form, and interpret it correctly. These steps were a prerequisite to recommending a sensible course of action for each patient. Such thorough and complete work-ups might seem, to the patient, highly repetitious, but comparison of the information obtained by multiple observers could turn up differences that proved valuable or at least provoked good questions.

The hallmark of Stead's rounds was that he always found something about a patient that no one else had thought of or asked about. Many times what he found didn't appear particularly germane until later in the course of the patient's hospitalization, or in discussions about the patient. But no matter how thoroughly the patient's case had been reviewed, he always found something new to ask that *was* important. He did not engage in a mere review of the literature or a discussion of the effectiveness of a particular therapy; Stead led a much broader discussion of the management of the patient or patients in general.

The ward team might be confident about the thoroughness of their preparation, but that confidence was never well placed. Stead always found questions that no one could answer. He would start his questioning at the bottom of the totem pole. If the medical student who had evaluated the patient couldn't answer the question, he'd then go to the intern; if the intern couldn't answer, he'd then go to the junior resident; if there was a visiting professor, he was next. Right up the ladder until it was clear that there were aspects of the case that no one understood or had thought about (and many were the JARs who heaved silent sighs of relief when the intern or the medical student gave a satisfactory answer just ahead of the resident's turn).

When Dr. Stead began his relentless questioning he always had something in mind. These were not exercises in trivia, but even knowing that, it was often hard to guess where the questions were leading. And it didn't help to know that Stead was in hot pursuit of something that should not have been overlooked. These bedside lessons often made lasting impressions on the entire ward team, but particularly on those who had prime responsibility for the patient.

Dr. John Laszlo:

> I remember one patient from my resident days. This 40-year-old man had felt well until shortly before admission, when he began to tire easily and feel short of breath. He had bruises of his skin from the most minor trauma, with no knowledge of having bumped himself. He had an enlarged liver and spleen, and unique abnormalities of his blood cells that meant this otherwise robust-looking man was suffering from acute leukemia. I had no doubt in my mind; we had made the correct diagnosis. On the night of admission, the student rehearsed the presentation he would make to Dr. Stead in the morning; the tell-tale blood slides were set up in the doctor's office on the ward;

all was in readiness. During the case presentation, Dr. Stead wanted to know more about the patient's single prior hospitalization at Duke. We had not yet received the old medical records, but had not worried because the patient told us that 15 years earlier he had been hospitalized for about 48 hours for dysentery. That didn't seem important in light of the stark current findings, but Dr. Stead persisted. Why hadn't we searched out the old chart in the middle of the night? Things seemed to be getting pretty ridiculous. Were we to spend precious rounding time chasing an irrelevancy for the sake of having a "complete" record? Weren't we supposed to treat the patient and not his chart? Sensing our impatience, he dictated one of his famous cryptic notes for transcription into the chart: "Just say for me that the patient's present illness is related to his past hospitalization." The Chief had finally flipped!

Later in the day, a resident from Pathology ran down to Osler Ward, all excited. Had this patient ever received Thorotrast? Thorotrast was a very long-lasting radioactive material once used as a radiographic contrast agent. It has a characteristic microscopic appearance that the resident had found right in the midst of the leukemic cells in the bone marrow sample taken from our patient. Theoretically, Thorotrast might cause leukemia, but what a strange suggestion. Then, when the old chart was recovered, it turned out that, during the hospitalization so many years earlier, a diagnosis of amebic dysentery had been suspected, and Thorotrast was given to determine whether there were any amebic abscesses in the liver. Use of Thorotrast was eventually abandoned when it was realized that it stayed in the body indefinitely, and increased the risk of cancer and leukemia. True enough, the man had leukemia, but the radioactive Thorotrast was probably responsible, and we had been unaware of his exposure. Well, Stead was right again, and we were humbled. It didn't make any difference to the patient's outcome, but the students and interns and I became much more thorough in perusing *all* data pertaining to our patients. A thorough history and careful study of all related material is crucial—and you have to do that time after time.

Stead was able to teach different levels of "students" at the same time, so the medical ward was like a one-room schoolhouse. He had medical students who were new to clinical medicine, interns, seasoned veterans like junior residents, and sometimes visiting professors, all around the patient's bed. Everyone had a chance to participate. Obviously, he expected more of junior residents than of junior students, and, although all might at times tremble in his presence, he was really pretty gentle with them. True, he became less gentle as he went up the line to his faculty and even full professors.

Another of Stead's teaching sessions was his "Morning Report." At eight o'clock on Monday through Friday mornings, JARs crowded into Stead's tiny office for Morning Report. Each resident quickly reviewed all patients who had been admitted the previous day so that everyone would know what was going on. Stead might ask questions about a patient but the whole summary took only 15–20 minutes. For the next half hour, the residents could talk about any subject with the Chief. The conversation might touch on the philosophy or ethics of medical practice, ideas about teaching, the role of sub-specialties in medicine, or other broad topics of general interest. This was Stead's time to offer something extra to the residents: his thoughtful perspective on issues of importance to the profession, where it might be headed, and what individual physicians might do to improve their world. The breadth and range of these impromptu sessions were fascinating.

Dr. John Laszlo:

There were two rules for morning report:

Rule 1) Be punctual! 8:00 A.M. did not mean 8:01 or later. Dr. Stead considered it an intelligence test for his young doctors to figure out how to be on time every day. There were no excuses. If someone came late, he simply stopped talking and the group might sit in silence for the balance of the session. And what long and painful silences they were!

On the very first day I was scheduled to attend this meeting, I was detained on the ward, helping my intern draw blood from a very obese patient. No one had told me how important it was to start at 8:00, and I arrived ten minutes late. There was a shocked silence, but on this occasion Dr. Stead picked up the conversation quickly. I sat unaware of the importance of unflagging punctuality until we left the office and the other JARs took me aside. I was told in no uncertain terms never to be late again and now, being aware of the rules, there would be no excuses.

Rule 2): It was up to the residents to start the discussion. If nothing interested them, Dr. Stead would sit in silence, twirling a pencil. He wasn't angry; he was content to wait. In order to avoid these long, uncomfortable silences, each resident kept mental notes of one or more topics that could be introduced if there was a pause. They took it as a challenge to keep a discussion going. From Stead's point of view, this was his absolutely undisturbed time with this resident group, and they could use him or not, as they chose. He happened to believe that these "thinking sessions" gave his residents a flavor of their profession that other programs did not offer—and he was certainly right!

Stead taught as much by example as by pronouncement. He always looked at the primary data himself; he didn't rely on the radiologist to interpret the x-rays or on the authors of a research study to draw conclusions. He might not keep track of every single thing going on in his department, but he certainly knew what was happening in the Cardiology Laboratory. Not only was he interested but this was his area of expertise. At the same time he could be both very supportive and very critical, in the best sense of the word.

Dr. Robert Whalen:

> Before we could submit a paper for publication, we had to defend it like it was a doctoral thesis. Compared to a review by Dr. Stead, peer review by a medical journal was nothing; we figured if we could get it past Stead, we could get it past any editorial board. He took a very active interest in our work that way, but he absolutely never put his name on a paper we published. He wouldn't even let us acknowledge his critical review at the end of the paper. This is the way I learned that the Chief of Medicine is not supposed to be out pasting his name up all over the world. He is supposed to be motivating his young people and be certain that they produce good—and defensible—data.

The Duke Hospital world was divided into "private" and "public" wards. In the 1950s and 1960s, the private wards consisted mainly of double and single rooms, and these wards were air-conditioned. Public wards (where indigent and low-pay patients were treated) had a large, central 16-bed ward, a 6-bed unit on a closed-in porch, and some 1-, 2-, or 4-bed rooms, none of which were air-conditioned. The small rooms were used mostly for patients with infectious processes like active tuberculosis, typhoid fever, etc, but sometimes the single rooms were used for patients with delirium tremens who screamed day and night from alcohol withdrawal, or paralyzed or comatose patients who required intensive nursing care. In these days before intensive care units, all patients were hospitalized on the general medical wards. Stead served year-round as attending physician on one of the public wards, Osler Ward.

There was little or no privacy on a public ward, although curtains would be drawn around the bed if the patient was being examined or was sitting on a bedpan. Naturally, examining a patient in the middle of the night was noisy, required lights, and generally disrupted the sleep of other patients. Those who were mentally disturbed or delirious might talk to themselves or to imaginary visitors day and night. Public wards were places of active treatment around the clock, but the setting was not conducive to healing and to rest. In many ways, the public wards at Duke were similar to those at Grady or other public hospitals. What differed was the attitude at Duke, where private and ward patients were cared for by the same staff.

Certain trademarks of excellence are universally recognized: companies strive to be another Rolls Royce or IBM. Institutions strive to be another Harvard University, Metropolitan Opera or Getty Museum. Programs of quality take many years and a total dedication of human resources to build. Great medical programs are no less demanding, and the miracle is that this was accomplished at Duke over a mere 20 years.

Not all Stead-trained doctors are excellent, but a remarkably high percentage is. And not only Duke students but those at Ohio State, Galveston, Pittsburgh, Yale, Indiana, Florida, Baylor and other medical schools who were taught under similar philosophies by his star pupils. When he retired as Chairman of Medicine in 1967, he had trained 33 other department Chairmen, an incredible statistic that has since grown even larger. The generational dimension thus created multiplied Stead's effect on American Medicine. His tenets included an unvarying demand that the doctor meet the needs of the patient, whatever these might be. He emphasized that open and honest communication establishes the basis of trust, and no smokescreen of elaborate laboratory procedures or complex medical terminology will substitute—now or ever. The human aspects of medicine must keep pace with the dizzying rate of technological advance; the crucial decisions of when and whether to use the available technologies should be born out of the doctor's skill, wisdom and compassion. In Stead's eyes, it was always important to meet patients on their terms or to turn them over to someone who could. It never meant ordering a galaxy of tests, or summoning a consultant for each of a patient's separate complaints. A well-trained internist was expected to diagnose and treat patients in intelligent, efficient, cost-effective and personalized ways. A well-trained internist should know how to locate and engage outside resources for the benefit of the patient, how to follow through after treatment is begun, when to change treatment strategy, and how to evaluate the effectiveness of treatments. A well-trained doctor must understand that some time has to be set aside each week for reading, attending conferences and learning. It is easy to become obsolete and of no value to your patients. Critical thinking is the most important single yardstick by which the internist should be judged. Deciding when to work all night with a very sick patient and when to simply console the patient and loved ones were the philosophical and medical values that Stead imparted to those willing to work hard under his tutelage.

Dr. Stead was Duke Medical School's first professional educator. He was interested in the processes by which people learn, retain and use information. As a result, his philosophy of education differed vastly from that of his predecessor.

Dr. Stead:

> I spoke with all of the students who came through our program. In over 20 years, there were quite a few, and 95% of them appreciated the fact that they had to put forth effort, but that we put forth considerable effort too. We would help students during the course in Medicine but did not pass them until we thought they had gained the competence they were going to need, and we didn't care if some people repeated Medicine as many as four times. If they came to Duke, then it was our responsibility to see that they got to the accepted level of competence.
>
> My successor, Jim Wyngaarden, worried that bright Harvard medical students wouldn't want to come to Duke to intern because they would have to work too hard. I was never concerned by that, however. I knew that if they didn't want to work hard, it was irrelevant how bright they were. We would be any better off not having them at Duke if all they were going to do was sit around and talk. I still don't believe it hurt the Department to have a reputation as a hardworking unit. If someone really wasn't seriously interested in medicine, I wanted them to know in advance that they'd better not come to Duke. In the end, that reputation did us a lot more good than harm. We saved ourselves time and trouble by attracting only those who wanted to be here.
>
> Dean Davison thought I was too self-serving in my approach to the Department of Medicine, but my attitude was that if I succeeded in establishing a strong department, in due time I would have greater influence in the school. If I did not run a first rate show, however, I never would have influence in the school. I believe that subsequent events bore out the wisdom of my decision for the school as well as the department.

Early on, Dr. Stead determined that students and interns on his service would receive a broad menu of experiences in medicine. And as Chief, he would determine the items on the menu. He was not concerned that students might prefer to sample only one portion of the program. He believed strongly that medical students ought to be exposed to many things. He valued depth of knowledge and mastery of a topic, but felt that students who restricted their menu too early might pass by areas that could provide a great deal of satisfaction. And so, to get off the ground, students were expected to go through a general medical service, and to take good care of patients with many different medical problems. This would allow students to see and discuss and think about a broad range of issues and help young doctors determine where their true interests lay. When the time came for these young doctors to enter practice, they would be in a position to determine the things they enjoyed doing and arrange their practices accordingly.

Dr. Stead:

> When I made ward rounds, I always spent most of my time on the patients that the housestaff were least enthusiastic about, urging them by example to get involved. If a doctor was obviously on top of a case, enthusiastic about the challenge the patient presented and going to the library to read up on the disease, there was no reason for me to spend time with that patient. I'd go see those patients in whom they exhibited little interest. That kept the staff alert and ready for anything. On one occasion, a resident said to me, "I really don't want to work up this stroke patient. I've seen three patients with strokes already this week." We saw many, many stroke patients in the days before anti-hypertensive medications, but I believed then, and still do, that there are things to be learned from each patient, regardless of the diagnosis. The ward was busy that day, though, and I knew the resident could make himself useful on any number of other interesting cases. "Fine," I replied, "I'll look at the patient." I'm not quite sure if I was lucky that day, or the resident was just unlucky. When I sat down to take the history of the "stroke" patient, I asked what the last thing he remembered was, and he said, "I fell out of the automobile." The patient hadn't suffered a stroke at all; he had a subdural hematoma! The house officer missed the diagnosis because he hadn't bothered to work the patient up. The patient might have died without surgery to remove the blood clot adjacent to his brain. Making a diagnosis is one of the most important steps in the process of rendering care. You can never assume anything, because if you're wrong, it's the patient who suffers. I'm thankful that resident wasn't me!
>
> The medical history ought never be a mere mechanical recording of data. Each statement must be scrutinized for its possible bearing on the present status of the patient and particularly for any light it may shed on the symptoms of which the patient complains. The mind of the doctor must be constantly alert to the possibility that any

event related by the patient, any symptom, however trivial or remote, may yet hold the key to the medical problem.

Stead was compulsive in his pursuit of information and knowledge, a quality he believed every doctor needed in order to provide optimal care for his patients. One method by which he encouraged young doctors to aggressively search out and understand medical questions was the famous nickel bet. In the midst of a vigorous discussion on the ward, Dr. Stead would challenge students or house officers to solve a clinical problem by waging a nickel against them. In his mind, the nickel bet was one device to stimulate the student to perform as well as he could.

Dr. Stead:

> One has to lead by example, and I don't know any better way than to "ace" the housestaff now and again. A doctor should be able to do that if he's been around a long time. In addition to my experience, however, I had one other advantage over the younger doctors: I knew almost intuitively what a house officer hadn't done. For example, I knew he'd probably never find out if a patient sweats—it's not something house officers think to ask about. Under certain circumstances, however, sweating could be the key to a severe imbalance of the autonomic nervous system, and that might strike me as a possibility. Conversely, there were many things I knew the house officer did ask, which I didn't have to bother asking. So you can appear better than you are, once you know the routine in which you're working.
>
> Every once in a while the tables were turned, and a member of the housestaff pulled a coup over even the more seasoned professionals. One such occasion involved a very bright house officer named Hal Silberman. He later went on to become Chief Resident and then a long-time member of the faculty at Duke. Early each summer we had a housestaff picnic; the housestaff were released from their duties and the senior staff ran the medical service, from Emergency Room to Intensive Care. I was acting as resident on Osler Ward that year, and I worked up a patient who had a remarkable series of abdominal, psychological and other complaints, and a complex socio-economic background. She'd had a gall bladder operation some months earlier, but after thinking about her complaints for a long time, I was not sure how to diagnose her rather involved medical story. Hal came back that night after the picnic, spent ten minutes with the lady and said, "She's got a stone in the common bile duct; we'll make arrangements

to get it out." And he turned out to be quite correct. Our house officers were pretty smart people, who could ace us at times—and I liked
it when they did!

It's true that everybody is going to be wrong at times. That's a
given. So I wouldn't criticize a bright doctor who missed a diagnosis.
We can all find times when we were that bright guy. You can't practice clinical medicine, or interact with a very smart staff at all levels,
and be right all the time—it's a neurotic goal and it's absolutely impossible. Very early in my life, I decided I would like to be right rather
than wrong, but even more I'd like to learn rather than protect my
ego. The best way to learn is to admit that you're wrong and then try
to determine why. To be wrong and not learn from it is crazy, but to
pretend you're right when you're wrong is sinful. The right to fail belongs to everyone, and when I fail, I prefer to come out being smarter
in the end. That way I won't fail the same way again.

Not only is it impossible to be right all the time, but to pretend to
be denies the intelligence of others. Any intelligent developer of people discovers very quickly that even if you could be right all of the time
you wouldn't want to be. Ego strength is developed in the younger
people when they see they can best you. They've got to win a nickel
bet from you now and then to develop confidence in their own skills
and knowledge. And it's important, as their superior, to set an example by tolerating your own defeat and enjoying their triumph.

Winning a nickel from the Chief was no small victory, and it was greatly cov-
eted. And while the money at stake was of little financial consequence (although it would free a Coke from the vending machine in the basement), it
represented an opportunity for intellectual enrichment, regardless of who
ended up with an extra five cents in his pocket. More than one such nickel
hangs framed on the wall like the trophy from an intellectual big-game hunt.

George J. Ellis, III, MD (Dr. Stead's last Chief Resident):

One thing on which all house officers could agree that they learned
from Dr. Stead was the meaning of a nickel bet. Nickel bets were Dr.
Stead's stock-in-trade since his intern days in Boston. They became
the cornerstone of medical education at Duke. These nickel bets were
made during discussions of clinical problems that usually took place
after leaving the bedside of the patient. The bet was not a frivolous
gamble on the patient's fate. Instead, the nickel bet served three functions: first, it stimulated a meeting of the minds by defining differ-

ences of opinion; secondly, it stimulated data gathering in support of the arguments; lastly, it provided a time limit for settling the question.

Believe me, Dr. Stead's nickel stuck to the blackboard was a great stimulus towards answering clearly defined questions. It was not surprising that the loser of the nickel gained more than the winner. After all, he invested more energy in trying to save his nickel, and in the process he learned something he didn't know before. (Ann Intern Med. 1968;89:990–1)

Dr. Stead made many significant changes in post-graduate training. By the 1950s stipends for fellowship training were readily available, which made it possible to have both general internal medicine residents and sub-specialty fellows on the clinical services. The senior staff were eager to have the residents working with them, as long as the staff could limit the residents' responsibility. This did not jibe with the Stead notion of connecting responsibility to learning. In order to insure the residents' direct involvement with patient care, Stead established a rule that senior staff could not have a resident working with them if the resident didn't take care of the patients. Residents were not simply to observe what the sub-specialty fellows or senior staff did; they were not a second-class trainee in a specialty program, but were to have defined roles with real patient responsibility. In exchange, Stead assured the faculty that the resident rotations would be sufficiently long for them to learn enough to be helpful; this would justify the responsibility they were to have. Three-week rotations, for example, were so brief as to be chaotic, whereas three-month rotations were comfortable for everyone. If the rotations were any longer, the residents' experience would have been limited to too few specialties, and they wanted to experience as much as possible. One-year rotations were reserved for people who were already settled into a sub-specialty fellowship after having completed a residency.

It was not possible for every resident to rotate through every subspecialty. Therefore, they were allowed to request the rotations they wanted and were guaranteed a certain number. As a result, one resident's service rotations over the year were often quite different from those of another resident.

The opposition to resident responsibility quickly died down. In the end, there was only one holdout, a faculty member who didn't want residents in charge of his private patients. As a result, Stead removed senior residents from his service, which piqued him greatly because he lost the work power of a third year resident, but Stead would not compromise.

Of course, when Stead came to Duke, a number of faculty were so accustomed to their ways that they were unlikely to change, no matter what the Chief said—physicians like Julian Ruffin or Walter Kempner, both of whom were intolerant of doctors who knew less than they did. The two men were worlds apart in their backgrounds: Ruffin was a son of the old southern aristocracy and Kempner was German-born and Berlin-trained. Both were good didactic teachers, firmly set in their ways, and unlikely to teach students the way Dr. Stead wanted. If the student had a patient with a peptic ulcer, they gave a lecture on peptic ulcers rather than teaching at the bedside about *that* patient. They never let themselves stray from the mode in which they had always performed. Stead, on the other hand wanted the student to learn about the particular patient at hand, not some vague "average" patient or a medical statistic. Stead was always more interested in the particular rather than the general; he preferred that the student see how *this* patient differed from (or was similar to) others with peptic ulcer so that the student could tailor his approach to the patient. With Stead, one needed information but, more importantly, had to use it appropriately. Manipulating information and putting it to proper use was Stead's rare stock-in-trade.

For Stead, clinical responsibility was the keystone to learning. This meant that students should learn the most during their last year of medical school, when they could assume the greatest responsibility. With this in mind, Stead arranged teaching rotations on the private wards so that students and residents could participate in the care of private patients. This gave both groups more responsibility and closer contact with faculty. However, getting the senior staff to agree was tricky. Before Stead's arrival, senior medical students worked in the Out Patient Clinic, which gave them limited responsibility, but eased the workload of the senior physicians. Not surprisingly then, the senior staff objected to Stead's changes. They wanted to write all orders and determine all plans, thereby limiting the students' and residents' responsibility (and, according to Stead, their learning). In order to assure his plan was carried out, Stead personally ran the clinical service and thereby assured the quality of the teaching experience. He met daily with the residents, reviewed admissions, and discussed with them his vision of the medical world.

Once full housestaff coverage was in place, all medical orders had to be written by the intern assigned to the patient. This was the rule on all private and public wards without exception. Even full professors like Ruffin or Kempner (or Stead for that matter) could not write orders for their own patients. If the professor wanted something done, he had to find the intern on his service, explain what he wanted done and why. The 30 or so interns didn't always agree with their attending doctors, but that was part of the learning experience. This system meant that all ideas about a given patient were funneled through a single doctor, which minimized conflicting orders. For the first time since he had come to Duke, Kempner's patients weren't fully under his control, and that worried him. He didn't like having to justify what he wanted to do before the orders could be implemented. He attempted to skirt the rule by claiming that his patients were too sick to be examined by the housestaff. Stead didn't believe that was so, but told Kempner to make a note in the chart each time a patient was "too sick" to be examined by the housestaff. Kempner said he would.

Dr. Stead:

> Dr. Kempner had a huge patient population in the hospital at any given time, and I knew he couldn't handle so many people without making some errors. So I just sat back and waited for him to make the first serious mistake. When I discovered that he had given dicoumarol (an anticoagulant) to a patient with a bleeding peptic ulcer, I lowered the boom on him. I said from then on I'd have to be the one to certify that the patients were too sick to be examined. Dr. Kempner was so busy he didn't have time to argue with me about it and eventually his patients, like all other patients, were taken care of by housestaff.

Of the educational changes instituted by Stead, teaching assignments in the Out Patient Clinic caused the greatest conflict with the old staff. Because senior students were to be assigned to the medical wards, Out Patient Clinic assignments were given to junior medical students. Stead knew that this less-experienced group would not perform brilliantly, but he expected that they would still ease the burden on the senior doctors in the clinic. The students would learn how to talk to patients, carry out an initial examination, and begin to taste some of the bread and butter of clinical medicine. The staff objected that the junior students would provide less help than the seniors had—that is, the faculty would have to work harder in the ambulatory clinic. After a prolonged debate, Stead was unable to convince the staff, and so he contrived a compromise: no student would be assigned to the Out Patient Clinic without at least one ward rotation on Surgery, Medicine or Pediatrics. Student schedules were rearranged to give third-year students a taste of ward experience before they went to their medical rotation in the clinic. As a result, the junior students were seasoned enough to be a real help in the clinic, and most of the time on the medical ward was still reserved for fourth-year students. The deadlock was resolved.

Dr. Jack Myers:

> Gene's service was different from that at Duke before he arrived. His teaching was structured to engage the students as part of the team

and to get them involved in solving the problems of patient diagnosis and management. Shortly after we moved to Duke, Gene announced that there would no longer be separate rounds. Up to that time, there had been one set of teaching rounds for housestaff, another for third-year students, and yet another for fourth-year students. Gene decided that we were going to teach them all together. As far as John Hickam and I could tell, the idea was revolutionary! We had never heard of such a practice and so we wondered, how could this possibly work?

"There's not much difference in education between a third-year student and a fourth year student or even between students and residents," Gene observed. "I've seen many instances in which a third-year student knew a great deal more about a case than the second year resident. I'm not worried," he assured us, "there's no significant difference. Of course," he added, "we'll have to target our teaching up and down the scale, but we can teach them all together. It's going to save a lot of time, because we'll only have to schedule one set of rounds." He was firm in his decision and, although we had our misgivings, we didn't try to dissuade him. We had learned from experience that you have to pay attention to what that fellow thought and said because he was so often right. Even though you might be certain he was wrong, be careful! And so Gene set the policy in force, and it's done in many places now.

When third- and fourth-year students finished their clerkships, they were given an oral examination by several members of the Department of Medicine: Gene, John Hickam, and a few others, including myself. It was a little intimidating, but as teachers we learned an awful lot about the student. Of course, we took their anxiety into account and would make a few introductory remarks, starting out with some fairly simple, straightforward questions to build up the students' confidence.

As far back as his time at Emory, Gene had the habit of appearing on the ward at all hours. There was no way of knowing when he might stop by to see what was going on; it might be midnight when he showed up. He did it to keep people on the ball. It was not done to drive people to work nonstop, but to instill the house staff with a sense of responsibility and dedication to their patients. Abandoning a sick patient on the ward at 11:00 was simply not tolerated. As a result, a real spirit of work was quickly inculcated in the resident staff, and they didn't abandon their patients. Many people considered the schedule inhumane, but Gene believed that it was more educational for a doctor to stay with his patients, see them through the course of illness, and learn medicine by being the central participant. Shortly after Gene left Emory, his successor announced that he was going to inaugurate a new, less rigorous schedule. Within a week or two, the residents asked to go back to the old schedule. They said they weren't learning as much as they had before.

By the mid 1950s, Stead's influence on Duke was taking noticeable shape. Word spread through the medical community that Duke's previously weak Department of Medicine had become a competitive and challenging environment in which to learn medicine. Although aware that medical education was becoming quite expensive, Dr. Stead took a hard line against paying students and residents for off-duty ("moonlighting") work in emergency rooms. In those days, most of the money that funded fellowship training in medical sub-specialties came from tax-supported governmental grants from the National Institutes of Health. Those grants were hard-won, and Stead was determined that their recipients should make the best possible educational use thereof. Students were inclined to take moonlighting jobs because they needed the money, but working outside meant decreased resident/faculty contact. Stead wanted the students to get as much out of Duke's unique educational system as possible. Stead and his colleagues formed a very sophisticated faculty; most students would never again be exposed to that kind of intellectual stimulation and excellence. As Stead saw it, the medical students and residents were building up a store of intellectual capital. The concepts and notions being learned were not just for the present, but for their medical practices 10, 15 or 30 years in the future. Years after leaving their intense contact with the faculty, they could draw on that capital. The more capital a doctor had when he left the medical center, the more likely he was to be an excellent practitioner 40 years downstream.

However, Stead's opposition to moonlighting did not mean that he was insensitive to the housestaff's need for money. It was not uncommon for senior physicians to look on the plight of young doctors and think (or say): "If we could do it, so can they." Stead, however, had quite a different take. Duke ran a busy ambulatory clinic where patients were evaluated by interns and residents. To satisfy their educational needs, he believed that interns and residents needed to see a certain number of patients in a day. Beyond that number, however, he thought that the doctors were providing service to the Medical Center and should be paid a fee for any patients they saw beyond the educational quota. Since it was much more efficient for a patient to be treated in the hospital by the doctor who had seen him in the out-patient clinic, Stead proposed also to pay the doctor for the work performed beyond that required in the ambulatory service.

The plan worked for about a month, but once other departments heard about it, there were vociferous protests. One distinguished and very popular Professor of Radiology was among Stead's more ardent opponents on the issue. Once he caught Stead by surprise in the hall and marched up, sputtering his objections to the program. "I regret that the Department of Medicine recruits such poorly motivated housestaff that they have to get paid for their services to patients." He continued, "I think it's a disgrace for such a system to be introduced into the Medical Center," and furthermore "that any doctor who had to be paid for work done during his training years was unfit to be at Duke." The Radiology faculty argued that the medical housestaff was deteriorating, and Stead was trying to prop it up with money. Stead responded: "The irony of this claim was that the medical housestaff was always in the hospital and available at any time of the day or night, 365 days a year. The odds of unearthing someone in the Radiology Department at 2:00 on a Saturday morning were much less of a sure thing, as the staff routinely quit at 5:00 P.M. on weekdays." Eventually, though, Dean Davison decided that paying interns and residents was not permissible policy. Since the Dean refused to discuss the issue any further, the matter was closed and never raised again. But Stead continued to lobby for increased pay for residents and eventually succeeded.

Dr. Henry McIntosh:

> Gene Stead was one of the leaders of American medicine who worked to improve the salary structure for interns. When I was an intern at Duke, the housestaff were required to live in the hospital 5 nights a week and for this we got $12.50 a month. In exchange for our rooms, however, we paid our $12.50 back to the hospital as rent. We never even saw our checks. Within a matter of two or three years, though, Dr. Stead changed that. By 1954 or '55 it was clear that he was a leader in raising salaries for housestaff. Certainly he championed the cause at Duke.

Stead had no Chief Resident lined up when he first arrived at Duke, although this key role would set the tenor of the training program. As it turned out, in January of 1947, shortly after he arrived at Duke, the hospital's chief anesthetist, Dr. Ruth Martin, asked him about a position for her husband. Sam Martin had graduated from Washington University with an outstanding record as both a medical student and a resident. He had been in the army and done very well, and would return from the service in a few months. His wife hoped that he might become the Chief Resident at Duke. Stead agreed to meet with him, and liked what he saw: Sam was quite bright; he was aggressive; and wanted to do well in medicine. Since his wife already at Duke, his reasons for wanting to come there were obvious. Stead, of course, had good reason for wanting Sam: being new at Duke, he needed a strong, intelligent first Chief Resident.

Sam Martin joined the Duke staff in July of 1947, and was an excellent Chief Resident. He lived in the hospital, and set a high standard of performance for interns and residents, which was critical during Stead's first year. He was good at patient care and interested in teaching, but had a broad range of interests and pursued learning wherever the opportunity presented itself. If he found himself working with expert consultants in particular fields, he learned what they had to offer, and went about caring for his patients without being intimidated.

Among his many responsibilities, Sam ran the morning outpatient clinic. In the course of work there, he saw many patients, some of whom had vague complaints without any obvious medical basis. It became clear to Sam that the complaints were related to the patients' jobs, their bosses, or other factors not susceptible to cure by technical medicine. In caring for these patients, Sam came in contact with the psychiatric residents, and asked them who on the psychiatric service provided the most help during their residency. They all said "Bingham Dai," who was a sociologist and practicing psychoanalyst. Sam introduced himself to Dr. Dai and, over time, developed a relationship that resulted in a unique program for the Department of Medicine's Chief Residents. As part of their training they would undergo psychoanalysis!

Stead was supportive of the idea. He spent a great deal of time in the hospital and had watched how the residents reacted to various situations. Many of the young doctors, Stead observed, exhibited behaviors that reflected hostility. For example, they might not like patients who arrived after 5:30 P.M., and then had to be taken care of throughout the night. Such reactions, Stead knew, were not determined by intellectual, but by emotional or "feeling" states. The residents may have become angry about subordination to authority, or the hospital rules, or whatever, but their hostility clearly had no intellectual basis. Stead believed that the residents would be more productive if they could use their energy to do what needed to be done instead of being angry about things they could not change—like the hour at which patients came into the hospital. Stead reasoned that if the residents could learn how they picked up certain attitudes and behaviors, they could begin choosing how they wanted to spend their energy. He viewed education as a way of producing slow and positive change in people, and considered the Chief Residents' experience with Bingham Dai a rung on the ladder of education. Each person, he knew, would profit from a psychoanalytical experience to different degrees, and in different ways, but he was sure that all would benefit.

Dai made only two stipulations: He insisted that his interactions with the residents be totally confidential, so that they never could influence the recommendations Stead might write for them. And he, Dr. Dai, would be the one to determine when it was appropriate to terminate the resident's analysis. Stead assured him that he would pay for the sessions for as long as Dai felt they would be profitable. In return, Dai charged the Department of Medicine the same fees paid by his poorer patients.

Dr. Stead:

> No one has ever found a way to quantify the total wear and tear on the body from nonproductive activity, particularly when that activity involves hostility. All you can say is that the people who put in long days that also involve a considerable amount of hostility and anger have one complaint in common—they're always tired. There's obviously a tremendous amount of energy expended in anger. But the Chief Residents never believed this when they started with Dr. Dai. As they began to work through how they grew up however, and went back and wrestled with some of their earlier developmental problems, they discovered that they were also tired. There wasn't any doubt in their minds (when they got through the experience) that emotionally-determined activity could be as exhausting and debilitating as any disease. That's a very valuable piece of information for a doctor to have.

Psychoanalysis with Dr. Dai (affectionately known by the Chief Residents as "Dai-alysis") formed a unique aspect of Duke's medical residency. And it had a palpable effect on the medical service. Not only were the Chief Residents better able to cope with their own problems but, over time, the housestaff in general learned more about the health impact of non-disease-related factors than doctors on most medical services. Without Sam Martin's influence, that program would not have come to be.

Dr. Stead:

> I did think Chief Residents learned a lot, but I did not think any of them changed fundamentally. When my daughter Nancy was in high school, she was a very critical young lady, and furthermore, she had the annoying habit of being right. However, she didn't have a very good time while operating in this mind-set, nor did it make for anyone else having a very good time. So I used to pay her a reward every time she said something nice about somebody. Nancy has always been

very conscious of money, so money was an appropriate reward system. If you can persuade people that it would be nice if their colleagues enjoyed them more, and then you help them figure out how to make somebody enjoy them more, people discover that they're happier being liked by their colleagues. This occurs at the intellectual level. They finally decide that it's more profitable to have the telephone switchboard operator like them or the head nurse like them, than to have these people not like them. And the amount of energy used in converting the system isn't very great.

When I watched people perform after their experience with Dr. Dai, I thought that they were going to have fewer problems. They were more willing to say, "Hostility is expensive; I don't think I'm going to indulge in any," and more willing to say, "If I'm depressed today, rather than depress everyone around me, I'll go home." These are some of the simpler decisions you can make with the IQ portion of your brain.

Throughout his tenure as Chairman at Duke, Stead made teaching rounds three mornings a week on Osler Ward, and he did this eleven months a year. This schedule seems virtually impossible to modern academicians because department chairs now find the burden of serving as attending physician so onerous that they cannot accommodate even one month on service. But, in addition, he had another truly unique activity. He single-handedly conducted, without the interposition of faculty assistants or residents, two weekly clinics. In one of these clinics he saw paying patients who, despite—or because of—their wealth and many medical consultations, continued to have symptoms. With these patients, Stead usually stopped all of the many medications that had been prescribed by the multitude of preceding consultants. Then, he began to teach the patients how to live with (and despite) their symptoms. To the other clinic, he invited mainly indigent patients who, for one reason or another—usually because they either did not fit into a simple diagnostic category or had symptoms that arose from disordered life circumstances rather than organ pathophysiology—were not popular with the resident staff. Once again, his aim was to help these patients find a way to fit their lives around their symptoms.

Dr. Stead:

At Duke, I always ran a small private practice in which I acted as a private physician. I didn't have any opportunity to do that at Emory, where my experience was purely city-hospital. There are no niceties in a city hospital, I can guarantee you. You know, there's no courtesy in a city hospital; if you try there to show that you can take care of the patient as an individual as well as a sick person, you'll fail. The city hospital is a place of last resort; if you're excluded from the city hospital, there's no place to go. Of course, if you practice medicine at a city hospital, you are an absolute god. Gods aren't always nice. This is what broke the heart of Gene Ferris. He had worked with Soma Weiss for two years, and he did have a feeling for people. He thought, and I thought of course, that if you took care of the disease and at the same time took care of the patient, you got a much better result than if you just took care of the disease. So, when he was appointed chief of medicine at Cincinnati General Hospital, he made every effort to show that care of the patient as well the disease would produce a much better outcome. But nobody in the city hospital was really interested in anything they could avoid, so they certainly weren't interested in taking care of the patient. If they took care of the disease, they thought they'd done their part. Gene made every effort to show that he could teach people to practice better medicine than was the norm. But you can't practice good medicine when the social system is broken down. A doctor in a broken-down system can't do anything. He can't prescribe medicine, can't give physiotherapy; all he can do is, when you die, say "I wish things had been different." The city hospital is absolutely brutal.

So right from the beginning at Duke I ran a private practice on my own, and I did it for two reasons. In my own heart I knew that I was an effective and useful doctor, but that meant that I needed to have at least a few patients. In the Duke system, everybody could say when he wanted his vacation, and nearly all of the PDC people wanted August or September vacations. I told the admitting office people that I was always available for patients during those months, so I picked up enough patients during the summertime to provide an active practice for at least the next 24 months. And I carried on simply as a private doctor, without any support from residents or fellows.

This plan served two purposes. One, with most of the people wanting their vacations at the same times, it was nice to have somebody like me who never took a vacation then. And, two, it provided me some self-protection. You see, the Duke Board of Trustees never really knew what the medical school was about. I'd watched other medical schools and knew that every now and then their trustees would set up programs so different from what I wanted that, if I were there, I would simply have to leave. I wanted to be able to leave the medical school if I suddenly felt that I was wasting my time. I wanted to be independent, to be able to leave the medical school without any fear as to whether I had remained a physician.

Now, my patients were private patients, and the money from the fees I charged went through the PDC to the medical school. As Chairman, I determined the income of everybody in the Department of Medicine, and I had decided when I came to Duke that I would simply have a fixed salary. I didn't want to compete for patients with the rest of the staff, many of whom depended on patient income for existence. To put me above the fray, I fixed my income at about a third of the average PDC doctor, but not with any resentment because in my way of running things I only worked for Duke half-time. The rest of the time I was just working for Gene Stead, doing things that most professors of medicine would have done if they had the freedom. I just made sure I had the time. And the arrangement allowed me to know that I was a good doctor, and that I could leave Duke at a moment's notice without gaining or losing anything except my university housing.

And I ran my practice without residents because, if I had left Duke for practice, all such support would have gone away. It seemed to me the sensible thing to do was to look at myself as an individual private practitioner, perfectly capable of earning a living and independent of the Duke Board of Trustees. Fortunately for me, during my years they never raised their heads to do anything, but that began to change a little bit when Jim Wyngaarden came and a lot when Joe Greenfield came.

You see, I used to think I was a pretty good doctor. Whether I was or not, you could argue, and I could show you some terrible mistakes I've made. But at least I was a conscientious doctor, and I knew that the two components of medicine had to be put together. If a man needed vitamin B12 because he was anemic and had the whole pernicious anemia syndrome, to not give him what he needed was bad medicine. On the other hand, if most of his problems arose from his position in society and everybody wanted to keep him down, like many of our black patients, I tried do something to mitigate some of the discrimination. Not all of it. I believed that taking care of the disease would be the simplest piece. When the social system is completely broken down to the point that you can't even get any medicines, doctors became irrelevant, can't do anything. In the end, I was always aware that when you knew what drug to give but you couldn't get it for the patient, then you had to use other options.

I really did carry on an interesting private practice. See, on account of my position in the medical school and the community, if a patient had wealth and had been to 35 doctors and spent half a million dollars and wasn't any better, I would be asked to see the patient. I always took those patients. They were a fascinating group of people because poverty didn't enter into the equation. They might have been disturbed by the fact that their spouses didn't like them, or their children didn't appreciate them, or whatnot. But it's always easier if there's money around, and I simply charged these people whatever PDC was charging. I didn't make enough money in a year to be an important source of funds for the school, but I had a good time, and I really worked out finally a satisfactory way to take care of these people.

I learned this partly because I'd been a lonely intern at the Brigham. I was away from home. I didn't drink, I didn't smoke, I didn't have any money, I lived in the hospital because they clothed me and fed me, but they didn't pay me any money. My colleagues and fellow interns didn't have the time that I had, you know. None of them had wives, but they had girlfriends, and they had money, and they went out on the town. I couldn't do any of that, because I didn't have any money. But I didn't have any inclination, so I never felt gypped. I didn't have a single date during that period, but that meant that I was available in a way that the average intern wasn't available. And by chance, some of the patients tried to engage me socially. I did occasionally go to their houses and have dinner and whatnot, and I began to see that how I'd been taking care of these patients, usually without much profit, came down to two things: the disease and the patient.

Much of what Stead took with him to his own clinics at Duke he had learned under Soma Weiss's tutelage at the Boston City and Peter Bent Brigham Hospitals.

Dr. Stead:

Soma was a humanist of a high order. He was the first person I knew who was interested in why the patients had the symptoms they had. He grew up, as I did, at a time when pathology dominated medical thinking. But if you had fainting spells the pathologist didn't add anything. There are whole lots of things that happen which remain mysterious if you are a pure pathological doctor. Soma was always interested in why patients experienced what they experienced. And therefore one of the first things that we studied was how to make normal people faint because we wanted to see what happened to the circulation, what happened to a variety of things. We also wanted to know what the patient's experience was. And we did a lot of the very simple things that I liked to do because I always did simple things. I never was profound enough to do complex things. But I was interested in how much blood you could take from a patient before he fainted. The person knew he wasn't going to die when I took the blood, and a month later when the blood volume was back to normal I re-bled him. The second time I could take twice as much blood before he fainted. So the fainting was a function of the nervous system, not of the circulatory system. Very simple illustration, but to me it was kind of interesting.

I also worked with John Romano in the purely patient-care-related things, which were not psychiatric. I did the work and shared the credit with John who taught me how to write the message. See, all of us who went to the Brigham with Soma Weiss were paid a low salary. After we'd been there five or six months, Soma said, "I want to give you people a secretary and I want each of you to do some private practice. You'll learn a lot, and you'll help me because you'll put a little money into the system. You're not going to be big earners, but when you're poor like the Brigham is, any kind of money helps." So we all began to do private practice, and I immediately discovered that the people who only knew about diseases were of no use to me, because I knew about diseases too, and mostly I knew better than anybody else. But I was at a loss when people clearly had some piece of disease, which made a diagnosis possible, but the disease was a relatively small part of why they were not happy. I didn't know what to do with those people, so I sent them to John to find out what to do. And of course, 90% of the time what he did was just listen more acutely to them, so that he heard things that I hadn't heard. So I joined up. We'd sit down and talk about it; we were right in the same office and had the same secretary. John was always a psychiatrist. He grew up in Milwaukee, went to medical school there and was interested in the mental state of the patient, what could be done about it. John was helpful, and every time we saw a patient together I really learned something.

In his afternoon clinic, Stead gathered patients who were not attractive to the house officers. When asked why he did this, he replied that his position as Chair meant that he was designated as "the best doctor in Duke Hospital." He assumed that being the best meant that he should take on the most difficult cases. Quite typical of Stead, though, he did not define "difficult" as meaning those patients who defied diagnosis or in whom standard therapy offered no benefit to the march of pathophysiological processes. He took on in his "hypertension clinic" those patients whom others found it difficult to care about or for.

Dr. Stead:

> Well, I used to go down to the medical clinic close at closing time, and one thing that impressed me was that I always saw the same people on the benches. They were the last people seen in the clinic, time after time. I didn't have to be a genius to figure it out. The resident staff just didn't like these people. These were essentially nice doctors, but they saw those patients begrudgingly, if at all, and they sure didn't see them promptly. You know, those people clearly had illnesses, but what they needed most was somebody who wanted to care for them. And for a variety of reasons the house staff just didn't want to. This was what was happening at the bottom, at the last part of this clinic.
>
> Now, another fascinating thing about the clinic is that every now and then we had a time in which the house staff was off duty and the senior staff took care of the people. Sometimes Dr. Ruffin would be the only doctor to see all those people in the afternoon clinic. Everybody felt very sorry for him, because he was going to have to do something for every patient. Actually, Dr. Ruffin would have seen everybody in the clinic by 4:00 rather than 5:00. He was a man who was extraordinarily good at deciding whether the problem was how the patient lived or whether the problem was the disease. Mort Bogdonoff had a little of this ability to quickly sort out all of the other factors and to appreciate that, although you might have a hard time doing anything about the illness, you would have an even harder time doing anything about the patient because the system wasn't set up to be kind to patients. It was set up to be kind to doctors. All medicine operates that way. So I knew that, because the same people were always the last to be seen, it meant that somebody didn't like them.
>
> And so I began my little clinic. I ran it, too, all by myself, on Wednesday afternoons. I think I called it a hypertension clinic because

hypertension was very common in that population, but most of the patients were just being rejected. And I didn't take house officers or fellows because they weren't interested. I was interested. Now, you've got to remember that the house staff was not sitting around doing nothing, but I thought I'd reached the stage where I understood how to take care of the patient as well as the disease. This population had very few resources, but I got a few of these people jobs, which nobody else would have ever done. And I managed to have a group of disadvantaged patients who felt less disadvantaged when they came to my clinic than if they went anyplace else. I kind of liked to see what I could do. I was not, obviously, universally successful, but I remember one lady whose husband refused to let her drive, which was a considerable handicap to her. I was the only doctor who really found out one of the sources of her discontent and aggravation with whatever illness she had. I finally broke her husband down to where she was allowed drive the car. That made a lot of difference. I got some of these people jobs in the hospital, because being a clerk in the hospital didn't require being very advanced in knowledge. Some of my patients could fit into the hospital if I took a little time and whatnot.

CHAPTER 12

RESEARCH AS THE
ENGINE OF PROGRESS

When the war finally came to an end, I was at a loss as to what to do.... I took stock of my qualifications. A not-very-good degree, redeemed somewhat by my achievements at the Admiralty. A knowledge of certain restricted parts of magnetism and hydrodynamics, neither of them subjects for which I felt the least bit of enthusiasm. No published papers at all.... Only gradually did I realize that this lack of qualification could be an advantage. By the time most scientists have reached age thirty they are trapped by their own expertise. They have invested so much effort in one particular field that it is often extremely difficult, at that time in their careers, to make a radical change. I, on the other hand, knew nothing, except for a basic training in somewhat old-fashioned physics and mathematics and an ability to turn my hand to new things.... Since I essentially knew nothing, I had an almost completely free choice.

Sir Francis Crick

In the 1960's, NIH support provided rich opportunities for scientific research, and the government made money available to schools that were prepared to expand. However, new funds from the NIH had to be applied to new ventures, not merely be substituted for funds that were already supporting projects. One way around this stipulation was to hire all faculty on a yearly basis, rather than committing to pay anyone in the future from NIH or other funds, and this is what Stead did. That way, the Department was not supporting promised salaries with NIH funds. Prior to the advent of NIH funding, Stead had paid each year's salaries from income created in the PDC during the previous year, but NIH funds freed PDC income that could be used for other ventures and initiatives, like new buildings or developing important scientific areas. This was precisely the "free-money" that Stead needed.

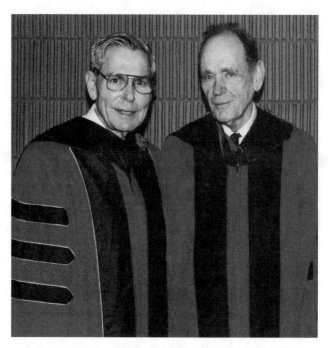

Henry McIntosh and Eugene Stead at the American College of Cardiology meeting in 1995.

The ready availability of research grants led to an explosion of important clinical studies at Duke and elsewhere. The time was ripe. Henry McIntosh, trying to develop a cardiac catheterization lab, was already performing trans-bronchial catheterization; gastroenterologists were biopsying livers to learn about different types of liver disease; the nephrologists and hematologists were using kidney and bone marrow biopsies to redefine old diseases and discover new ones. The cardiologists, however, were particularly short on space. They had only a crowded little laboratory in the Radiology Department; in order to slide a rigid, hollow, metal bronchoscopy tube into a patient's airway, the doctors had to maneuver themselves and the patient in an awkward manner. McIntosh went to see Stead about getting more space, and learned that the Chief had already given a great deal of thought to the situation. Stead had decided that the Department of Medicine needed to carry out organ biopsies and kidney dialyses, and needed a team that could train doctors to do these things. Stead would convert a student laboratory for the purpose if McIntosh would assume responsibility for developing the program.

Henry McIntosh went to Boston in the late 1950s to learn how to run the kidney dialysis machine, a Rube Goldberg contraption in those days, and then he was given the space. Within three years, Dr. Bill Gleason became one of the few young doctors trained to do both heart catheterization and kidney dialysis. Dr. Bob Whalen became the first person to make arteriographic images of the four major blood vessels going to the head and neck. McIntosh's lab used renal arteriograms to visualize the kidneys, and learned how to place catheters in the heart to measure pressure in the heart's chambers, permitting precise diagnosis of heart disease.

These catheterization techniques were born of the desire to visualize the blood vessels and patterns of blood flow in the brain, or kidneys, or heart. As a result, the doctors discovered new diseases and new ways to treat diseases. Knowledge in cardiology and nephrology had been limited until then, but within three years both areas were blown open in the United States. The team at Duke contributed significantly to the new insights

Dr. Henry McIntosh:

> Before the war, I attended Davidson College, an excellent pre-med institution. My advisors there recommended that I go to one of the eastern medical schools, and suggested the University of Pennsylvania, Hopkins or Jefferson. I was interested in Duke, but was told it was a second-class institution. So I applied to the others and was accepted at all three. By then, however, World War II was underway and, while I could have gone to medical school and stayed out of the service, I volunteered to go overseas instead.
>
> Four years, later when I came back to the States, I went back to Davidson and talked to the same people I had previously talked with about getting into medical school. I was still interested in Duke, particularly because they had a three year course which would have better suited my needs as I was older than most beginning medical students. Once again, I was told that it was a second-rate institution, so I went to the University of Pennsylvania.
>
> After completing medical school in 1949, I inquired about Duke for an internship. At that point I was told that it was an outstanding institution, especially in internal medicine, and it was recommended very highly. The difference between Duke's reputation in 1945 and 1949 was that Gene Stead had taken over as Chief of Medicine.
>
> Later, Dr. Stead offered me the opportunity to run the cath lab, and it was the most exciting experience I ever had in my life. Within three years we had gained important new insights into catheterization and into kidney dialysis. We were learning things that other people didn't know. Nothing can reproduce the exhilaration of plowing

new ground in understanding the function of sick and well organs. We studied patients with hypertrophic subaortic stenosis, a rare heart condition in which enlargement of the heart muscle impedes the flow of blood out of the heart. The disease could not be detected by usual means because the blockage in the heart was dynamic; it came and went as the heart contracted and dilated so it did not show up in standard x-rays and couldn't even be found in postmortem examinations! It had to be demonstrated by using a catheter to inject dye into the heart and observing the outflow of blood by means of rapidly taken x-ray pictures. Bob Whalen was the first person in the world to demonstrate the dynamic nature of the syndrome, and he did this while he was still a fellow in training. They were exciting times.

In looking for an animal model that would simulate human hypertrophic subaortic stenosis, we sent down to Florida for some greyhounds that had failed at the track. We thought that their hearts might function like our patients' but that didn't work out, so we looked at turkeys, and finally decided on alligators. Alligators sound like a peculiar choice of animal for a research study, but I had read in an article describing three cases of hypertrophic subaortic stenosis that the condition might have something to do with the embryonic development of a portion of the heart called the infundibulum. I didn't know anything about the infundibulum, I hardly knew what it was. So I looked a little deeper and learned that the infundibulum was particularly well developed in the alligator. So we had several six-foot alligators shipped from Silver Springs, Florida. Sure enough, when we catheterized them, they really did have functional hypertrophic subaortic stenosis, which resembled the abnormality seen in our patients.

Of course alligators are poikilothermic, which means that their temperatures rise and fall in response to the surrounding environment. In order to handle them, we put them in the walk-in refrigerator to lower their body temperatures, and while they were hibernating, we tied them down. The first time we did this, we didn't appreciate the physiology of hibernation. The heart rate fell to about one beat every two minutes, and I thought I had killed the alligator. So we opened up his chest to study his heart, but as he warmed up his heart went blip and then another blip. Pretty soon his heart rate was up to 30 and he wasn't tied down. He opened up his gigantic mouth, and I had a vision of the next day's newspaper with my obituary on the front page! Fortunately we were able to restrain him and tie his mouth shut. Subsequently the reptiles were cooled and then fully anesthetized with phenobarbital, but it was hazardous work until we got the hang of it. So much for alligators.

Clinical research began to open up on a number of fronts. Special, pressurized rooms such as those used by the Navy for diving experiments had potential in medical research as well. Duke had one of the first at a medical school, housed in a "temporary" Quonset hut behind one of the medical buildings, and later in a very large and fancy facility. The Department of Medicine conducted most of the pressure chamber studies, although surgery, physiology and others participated. New pressure records were set in simulated "dives" conducted by professional divers; there were experiments to help stroke patients get more oxygen to the brain, and studies with new surgical or radiation techniques. It was research and application day and night.

Dr. John Laszlo:

> I tried to reverse the episodic crises that occur in patients with sickle cell anemia by taking some of these very sick patients to three atmospheres of pressure with high oxygen concentration. At high pressure, oxygen dissolves in the bloodstream, and we hoped that it would preserve tissues that were marginally viable. To our disappointment, it didn't help sickle cell disease. But the surgeons found that they could use the technique to salvage a trauma victim's partly severed limb, even when it was hanging by just a tiny bit of tissue and fed by an inadequate blood supply. In the hyperbaric chamber, the severed tissue got enough oxygen from the highly oxygenated blood to prevent gangrene while the limb was being repaired.

In the Duke facilities, whether the hyperbaric chamber or the angiogram suite, there was a merging of research and clinical applications. A monkey might come out of the laboratory ahead of a stroke patient going in, or a patient would come out and a pig or dog would be brought in. That was standard operating procedure for Stead's faculty.

The hyperbaric oxygen program opened up so many new possibilities for clinical research that, under the leadership of Dr. Herbert Saltzman of the Department of Medicine, Duke obtained funds for a huge new building. This facility was better equipped for high pressure research, containing a pressurized operating room, and chambers to simulate high altitude or modify the humidity. Because of the facilities, new talent came to Duke, and that was always an important part of such programs, not just a casual by-product. Still, Stead was always mindful of the marketability of the people he recruited, of whether they possessed the skills to change directions if interest in the current field waned. This was a conscious strategy on his part, and it helped to keep the faculty viable.

In addition to paying the salaries of researchers, government grants underwrote the construction of new facilities, including new research buildings. The institution had to put up matching money, usually about one-third of the total cost, and Stead carefully saved his "free money" for such opportunities. Nevertheless, there was continuing resistance from the older staff who, among other things, liked the way things were and did not want to change floor plans in any way. The only expansion that the old guard could envision was a major addition to the main medical school building (Davison Building), which housed the classrooms and laboratories for medical students. The emergence of technology-intense research, however, demanded new facilities that could not be accommodated in the hospital or Davison Building. There were limits to what could be done inside Gothic-style structures with three-foot-thick stone walls and archaic wiring. Such buildings might be fine for classrooms and offices, but they were most impractical for high technology laboratories. Because the older staff was reluctant to expand beyond the confines of the original structures, there was little chance of getting government funds. Without new facilities, they could not carry out the kind of work that would earn grant support. Their views were highly restrictive, but cooperation still came, hard and slow.

Interestingly, the person who gave Stead some of his ideas about how to expand the research program was not a member of the Department of Medicine. Dr. Joseph Beard, of the Department of Surgery, had initiated the research thrust at Duke Medical School, and he was quite a character. To meet him was to meet a farmer from the deep South, irreverent, charming, and self-confident. Trained as a medical doctor, he practiced medicine for only a very short period. He was really a research scientist at heart, but during World War II, when so many doctors were in the service, Deryl Hart, Chairman of Surgery, enticed Beard out of his research lab to work in the Surgical Clinic. On the very first day there, he was asked to remove a cyst from the neck of a patient. Beard carefully cleansed the skin with antiseptic solution and properly draped the area with sterile towels, but when he picked up the scalpel and confidently made the incision, the patient jumped right off the table! Beard had forgotten to anesthetize the skin before making his cut! Shortage of doctors or not, Beard went back to the laboratory that day. Fortunately, he was a remarkably productive researcher who made a number of truly important discoveries including a pioneering study of cancer-causing viruses in animals, and a vaccine to protect horses against the deadly equine encephalitis virus.

As the most professional researcher in any of Duke's clinical departments, Beard had organized his cancer study program into a biological unit, a chemical unit, and a physical unit, all staffed by good researchers. In addition, Beard was quite enterprising about finding ways to expand his laboratory and fund his research. Royalties from the sale of his vaccine went into the Joseph and Dorothy Beard Fund, which he controlled, and this gave him great flexibility in his activities. He once said that he would have been in really great shape if only tractors hadn't superseded horses, sharply curtailing his source of private income. However, he got grant funds to construct the first research building at the medical center, the Bell Building. Situated about 150 yards northwest of Duke Hospital, it represented a break from the connected cluster of hospital buildings, and provided new laboratory facilities that others could emulate.

Philip Handler, PhD, Chairman of the Department of Biochemistry at Duke and later President of the National Academy of Sciences, was the first of Duke's basic science Chairmen willing to break loose and join Beard. He moved his whole department out of the medical school complex into the Bell Building. Other basic science department heads thought he was foolish, but they were grateful because his move freed up space for them. Handler's biochemistry group also had room in which to expand, and so they were able to compete successfully for the funds that were being poured into research. In turn, getting research funds made it possible to build new facilities, recruit more scientists and develop a growing research program. Success breeds success, but Duke was slow to use such opportunities in the early days.

Biochemistry took over part of the Bell Building, but in and amongst the biochemists there was still space available for Medicine. Previously, Medicine had been land-locked by the hospital's design and unable to expand. Since biochemical discoveries opened many of the new frontiers in medicine, it made sense to look for medical scientists who could profit from working next to the biochemists and thereby complement the Bell Building's research community. Frank Engel, the endocrinologist, was the first of a subsequent stream of Medicine faculty to move into the Bell Building. These researchers learned a great deal from the biochemists in the adjoining laboratories. Each helped the other and collaborated well, bringing the two departments closer together and proving that geographic proximity is a too often ignored component of intellectual productivity. To cement the bond, the Department of Medicine paid for some activities controlled by basic science departments (such as electron microscopy and genetics). Over time that investment paid off handsomely in research collaboration and training. As conservative as Stead was in using "free money", he was farsighted in his support of basic science departments with less financial flexibility. Protecting the well-being of basic science disciplines was in Stead's interest, and having his researchers located close to the biochemists was a great opportunity for everyone concerned. The physician-scientists became better teachers of medical students, and their research success gave Duke the luster of a good place for working and investing in research.

Once Biochemistry made the break from the old building complex, building additions grew like Topsy. Research became an accepted role as the staff competed for and won funds from the NIH (especially the Heart and Cancer Institutes), private foundations, and local sources. Decisions as to who would occupy new space were based on who raised the funds for additional laboratory facilities. Free enterprise was at work. As it turned out, the Bell Building became the model for future buildings. Scientists from several departments housed together under one roof created a symbiotic system; this made the planners look smart, even though it really did come about by serendipity. The system seems obvious now though still not widely practiced, and it was certainly unique for its time.

Dr. Robert Whalen:

> Stead was always modest about his own accomplishments and those of his Department, but he didn't want modesty to be misinterpreted. On one occasion he had to organize an on-site visit by the NIH to review a cardiovascular training grant that he held, and he was having some problems defending a request to continue the grant. The first problem was that he had already used up all of the money for non-cardiovascular projects. It wasn't stealing from Peter to pay Paul, it was stealing from Uncle Sam to pay for Peter and for Paul, both of whom were worthy. Parenthetically, he used to make us cardiologists all get our own grants and fellowship awards, and he would take the money awarded by the NIH, and go out and hire a new gastroenterologist or dermatologist. His defense was that if you want to have a good Division of Cardiology, you have to have a very good Department of Medicine. But on the occasion I recall, he was under the gun because the NIH had scheduled the site visit to see where the hell all the money was going since Gene couldn't name a single cardiologist who had gotten money from the grant. That would be a devastating problem for the average doctor. But not Stead. He rounded up the 32 young members of the Division of Cardiology, and we all sat around a long table in one of the conference rooms, together with the outside reviewers. Stead sat at the head of the table and said, "Now I want all these young people who work in cardiology to tell you what

they're doing and we'll just take one minute apiece!" We had all been told that we had 60 seconds to speak—like presenting a medical history at Grand Rounds—so we got it out fast and then got out of the way. And as he went down the table, there unfolded an unbelievable description of work being done in our labs and in collaboration with others. Stead summed up, "Between North Carolina's Research Triangle institutions and Duke, we will, in the future, have a magnificent intellectual campus for biological sciences." One of the site visitors said, "This is terrific! Why the hell don't you just tell the NIH to move down here?" And Stead said, "Well, you know, I did recommend that, but for some reason, they weren't interested." Naturally, this bold gambit got us our money.

The outcome was felicitous for Duke, but the methods were unorthodox, even then. Now they would be out of the question.

Dr. Stead:

I'm one of the few people honest enough to say to a site-reviewer, "You're going to site-visit me on a three-million dollar, three year project grant next month, and I'm going to visit you on a $100,000 project in your institution, and you can be damn well sure you will get a favorable report!" I think there is a series of human interactions, some call them conflicts of interest, that are absolutely impossible to control. Sometimes a reviewer is biased in favor of the applicant because he is doing similar work that he believes is important. Sometimes he is biased against the applicant because they are competitors. These are situations for which we have no good solutions because we have to rely on people with expert knowledge of what a person is proposing to do. This is what peer-review is about. It was rumored that I wrote my grants by stating in the application only that next year I was going to do more of what I did last year. But there was no truth in that. We did stay a cycle ahead, however, because we were working on fairly simple things and we did our work quickly. We got up early in the morning every day. And 90% of the time, what I proposed to do in my new grant requests were things we had already done but not yet reported. We simply described things that were already done and were going to be published six months after the grant request was funded. By using this system we stayed ahead of the game. We were awarded money based on what we said we would do and, in fact, had already successfully done; then we had the freedom to do what we wanted. It seemed to me to be a very sound way to operate, because one of my rules was to never take money for something I didn't want to do. That can just be a disaster. I've always believed that if you really want to do something, you'll do it whether you have the money for it or not. To stay out of the bureaucratic trap wasn't always easy, however. If, for example, you wanted to do something you thought was going to be highly productive, and six months downstream you said, "My God! How ridiculous!" it wasn't always easy to make the changes you wanted to make. But if the work proposed in the grant had already been done, then you were doing whatever you wanted to do. Thereby you gained the reputation for completing the things you set out to do. So it's a very sound way to write research grants.

A famous physicist also employed Stead's strategy. He wrote a grant application describing work he'd already done, but the other physicists who reviewed it turned it down. The reviewers were sure that his proposal wouldn't work! Fortunately that never happened to Gene Stead.

CHAPTER 13

GROWTH AND DEVELOPMENT

Students, interns and residents came to us for training. Each was different and each gained satisfaction in a different way. Our role was not to stamp out residents from a common mold. Our goal was to identify the best use of the man and to find the limits imposed by his structure. We honored the man who did excellent general practice as much as the specialist, research scientist, and doctor with administrative talents.

E. A. Stead Jr.

The Research Training Program (RTP) evolved from the collaboration of Stead and Handler and was a joint effort of the Departments of Medicine and Biochemistry. Before the program began, young researchers tended to learn scientific techniques that were needed to solve the problems they were studying. Once the original study ended, the researchers looked for other problems that could be analyzed with the skills they already had rather than finding new problems that would require learning new techniques. Handler and Stead questioned the value of this pattern, and asked why bright researchers did not learn new methods to attack new problems. They wondered whether learning a narrow repertoire of skilled techniques early in a career might inhibit the later learning of new methods or the tackling of new problems. Such stunting would be a serious limitation that would forever restrict scientific growth.

Stead and Handler determined that young researchers needed a program that would provide sophisticated techniques in four or five different scientific areas, such as growth and development, bacterial genetics, enzymology, and electron microscopy. To break out of the restricting mode, such a program would require the latest and best equipment, like electron microscopes, ultracentifuges, and radiation counters. To prevent students from being limited to a single discipline, they structured the program so that each student would examine a specific research problem from several vantage points.

The RTP was embedded in the normal medical school course, but available only to the most gifted students, who were allowed to take the one-year program free of charge. It provided an opportunity for those students to explore scientific research in a broad and unrestricted way. Providing stipends for tuition and living expenses proved to be a good incentive, but in addition, senior requirements were waived in the field in which the student would intern. For example, students who planned to intern in Medicine were exempted from senior medicine requirements. Roughly one-half of the trainees who enrolled in the program were medical students, and most of the rest were postdoctoral fellows of one kind or another. However, people at all levels were accepted, including the Chairman of Medicine from the nearby University of North Carolina, who enrolled during a sabbatical year. Undergraduate and postgraduate students benefited from exposure to one another, and when the undergraduates finished, most knew clearly the discipline they would go into. (Overall, four out of five went into medical specialties, the rest into surgical).

A clinical researcher was given supervisory responsibility for the program, and additional basic science faculty were hired whose teaching responsibilities were entirely satisfied by their work in the RTP. To head the program, Stead and Handler recruited Daniel Tosteson, who later became Chairman of Physiology before moving to Chicago and then Boston to become Dean of the Harvard Medical School. James Wyngaarden joined the RTP and later became its Director. The program was staffed with excellent research scientists who were eager to teach, and formed as high-powered a group of young faculty as could be found anywhere. Stead and Handler funded the program through grants from the NIH and private foundations, and raised enough money to hire the necessary staff and to expand the Bell Building to house the program.

Dr. Stead:

> Dr. Handler was always looking out for the larger interests of the medical school, and he did it extremely well. He put Duke on the national scene in biochemistry by having high quality faculty in his department, by helping to establish the Research Training Program, and by alerting the rest of us to the kind of people who would be very helpful to the basic science area of the school and who also fit into our clinical departments. Hiring Dan Tosteson was a joint venture between Phil and myself, but if Phil hadn't been here, I don't think Dan would have come. I don't think I could have hired him alone. Handler had the prestige in basic research that I certainly did not, and he spoke that language effectively with young, ambitious recruits like Dan Tosteson.
>
> We were aware that we had a number of students with the potential to pursue distinguished careers in research, if only they had some knowledge of research and the opportunities available in that field.

They otherwise might never know of their talent. Therefore, we wanted to provide them with an introduction to research. The Research Training Program was designed to give them much more exposure than the usual apprenticeship in a single laboratory where they'd be trying to get on their feet and simultaneously trying to discover whether they had an aptitude in that specific area. We didn't think that they would be ready for a research career after one year in the RTP, but we thought they would know whether they wanted to continue their research activity and become sufficiently expert.

Dr. John Laszlo:

I was privileged to participate in the Research Training Program. I came as a young faculty member (Associate in Medicine) who had completed formal clinical training and had done extensive lab work for two years at the National Cancer Institute. However, the research techniques that I had learned were narrow in scope and specialized, just the kind of limitation that Stead had recognized. As a faculty member trying to run a laboratory program as well as see patients and teach, it was difficult to find the time to learn new research methods. Dr. Stead saw that my potential in academic medicine would be enhanced by the RTP experience, and I was very glad to have the chance to take this intensive, nine-month program. The arrangement took planning because we had to recruit another person to handle my other duties. The RTP experience served me well in my subsequent research career and kept me ever-willing to learn new methods while maintaining proper respect for the nuances and limitations of technology. I also recognized the desirability of teaming up with basic scientists whose work would not be interrupted by the need to care for patients and their families. That arrangement, which I was to use extensively in my research career, grew out of lessons learned in the RTP.

The research program at the NIH in Bethesda, Maryland, expanded considerably from the mid-nineteen fifties through the sixties. The NIH took bright young medical doctors into the Heart, Cancer, and other Institutes where, protected from the draft by an appointment in the U.S. Public Health Service, they learned about and contributed to medical research. The best medical schools in the country wanted to take advantage of this resource; Duke and Dr. Stead were particularly well known for the high caliber of doctors they sent to the NIH. The "shuttle" ran in both directions, of course, and many NIH-trained people came to Duke to pursue their aca-

demic careers. I was one of the first of these, and many others followed. Everyone who had been trained in research at NIH brought
something new to Duke, and that was always a welcome commodity.

CHAPTER 14

A New Departure—
The Physician Assistant

The discovery by the doctor that his assistant can do, on any one day, the majority of things that he himself does raises some interesting questions about medical education. Why does it take so long to educate the doctor and so little time to educate the assistant?

E. A. Stead Jr.

The physician assistant program that Stead began at Duke represented a new concept for health professionals. As he wrote: "Persons with high-school education, a reasonable rate of learning, and a tolerance of the unavoidably irrational demands often made by sick people can learn to do well those things which a doctor does each day. Under the wing of the doctor, such a physician's assistant can collect clinical data, including the history and physical examination, organize the material in a way that allows its use in diagnosis, and carry out any required therapeutic procedure that the doctor commonly uses. He can, of course, master any technical procedure that the doctor uses frequently. In fact, as part of the doctor's team, he performs so well that the patient cannot tell who is the assistant." (*E. A. Stead, Jr.: What This Patient Needs Is A Doctor*, pp 90–1)

It is very rare that a single individual can be identified as the architect of a whole new career field, one that allows people with lesser training to carry out, and carry out well, many of the duties hitherto reserved to highly trained doctors. In conceiving the idea of the Physician Assistant (PA) Program, Eugene Stead was precisely that. He not only conceived the idea, but he developed the educational program to be undertaken, fought the battles that led to acceptance of this new category of allied health professionals, and nurtured the fledgling profession as it developed standards for licensing and credentialing. And he carried out this tour de force while continuing all his other duties and responsibilities. Although PAs are now widely accepted throughout America, few people know the role played by the Stead in creating the field. It is interesting to examine how this program arose out of necessity.

Dr. Henry McIntosh:

On a number of occasions Gene would take someone from one area
and put him into another area, often with dramatic effects. This was
particularly true with the Physicians' Assistant Program, which he
began. It came about because we were trying to develop a Coronary
Care Unit at a time when nurses were in very short supply. We were
also trying to develop skilled technical assistants to work in the Catheter
Lab. The Nursing Service directed a great deal of hostility toward us
because we recruited some of the best nurses to work in the Catheter
Lab. It seems that nurses are always in short supply, but in 1963–1964
we were trying to get special nurses. The very first Coronary Care Units
were developed in three places around the country in 1962, and we
were developing ours sometime around 1964. And not only was there
a terrific shortage of personnel, but we needed one nurse for every two
patients. We thought that there must be people who could be quickly
trained to watch patients. We hit on the idea of using firemen, and
went down to the Durham Fire Department to recruit them.

It seemed to us that firemen had experience with risk, with life-
and-death sorts of things. They were medically uneducated, but they
were used to moonlighting and they were reliable people who were
getting good fringe benefits from the city, so they could be hired reasonably cheaply. So we trained firemen to monitor blood pressure
and heart rate in the Catheter Lab, and to talk with the patient while
we were catheterizing. We recruited eight people, as I recall, and six
of them did quite well; these were the people we selected to work with
us. Their loyalty was to us because we paid them and we had trained
them and certified them, but somewhere along the line it was politically feasible for us to let the Nursing Service take a couple of these
people to work in the Recovery Room. So for a period of about four
of five years there was a small cadre of firemen being used either in
the Coronary Care Unit or in the Recovery Room.

About 1960, we had made arrangements to provide consultation
at the Catheter Lab at Portsmouth Naval Hospital about once a
month. It was there that we realized what outstanding people medical corpsmen were. And so, since we were still experiencing such a
real personnel shortage, we decided not to use nurses in the Catheter
Lab, but to use former medical corpsmen instead. Gene got his idea
from seeing how corpsmen worked, and he must have all the credit
for the development of this program.

Look Magazine heard about what we were doing and came down to interview us about the PA program. They wrote an article (nobody thought of looking at the title) and they called it "Less Than a Doctor, Better Than a Nurse." That headline was devastating! The nurses were furious! Eventually we were able to satisfy the local nursing groups that we had nothing to do with the title, but it did compromise the relationship between medicine and nursing.

The reason that we used corpsmen, and then PAs, was that Gene felt doctors had to have somebody who could be an extension of themselves, someone not restricted to eight hour shifts and who could be on call 24 hours a day. At that time, it seemed logical that these people should be men because women nurses were often raising families and, though they might get away for eight hours, couldn't be on call 24 hours a day.

Dr. Stead:

Thelma Ingles, R.N., was in charge of the Nursing Service on Medicine, and was never a great supporter of the PA program at Duke, for the simple reason that she felt the nurses should have been the ones involved in it. She appreciated that, at the time we started the PA program, no nurse was going to do it. So she wasn't angry with me about starting it, but she always felt that it was regrettable that there had to be a PA program at all. Almost all the other nurses were frightened of the PA program and its potential to supplant nurses. Kay Andreoli was the only nurse at Duke willing to say that a nurse could conduct certain aspects of PA training better than a doctor, but she was an unusually talented person who did not feel threatened.

Perhaps my biggest contribution to the Physician Assistant Program was showing the nurses that there's a lot of turf out there, and if they didn't want to claim it, somebody else would. In the end, what the PAs do with the training they receive is probably going to have more impact on the whole health care business than what the nurses decided to choose for themselves.

Henry McIntosh was the first man to recruit the personnel that allowed us to implement the PA Program. Henry looked through the telephone book to see what kinds of people wouldn't sleep on the job, and he found firemen. That was his approach.

In the 1960s Dr. Stead wrote about the Physician Assistant Program he had begun. Like George Orwell's *1984*, much time has passed, but the points are still profound and worth repeating here:

A doctor's education consists of four parts: 1) preparation to function as a citizen; 2) language preparation to allow the doctor to obtain content as needed from books written in part in symbolic languages; 3) development of problem-solving abilities; and 4) application of known knowledge to medical practice.

Society wishes its doctors to have a reasonable knowledge of people, history, social sciences, literature, and art because the doctor must relate the mysteries of the human body to the rest of society. Doctors care for the leaders of our society in times of trouble and, because of the nature of the doctor-patient relationship, doctors can influence the course of the society out of proportion of their actual numbers.

The natural and, hopefully, the social sciences are taught to our doctors because a knowledge of the symbolic languages developed by these disciplines makes a wide variety of content available over the doctor's lifetime. The specific content taught is not important; the ability to read books written in the language of the particular science is important.

The preclinical portion of the doctor's experience serves a third purpose—namely, to increase problem-solving abilities. Again, the content used to modify the nervous system by having it engage in problem-solving is not important. Practice in problem-solving will modify the nervous system in a favorable way so that problems, regardless of their nature, can be approached more effectively.

The application of known knowledge to the care of people is taught by the apprentice method. This method is very effective for teaching the medicine of today. If one paces the learning correctly and teaches what is not known, one can intersperse apprentice learning with problem solving, use of symbolic language, and acquisition of new content related to the medicine of tomorrow.

The overall purpose of the long educational program for the doctor is to prepare him for a lifetime of good citizenship and a lifetime of learning. The intent is to create a thinking doctor who is completely protected against obsolescence regardless of the changes in the social and technological scene.

One can make a first approximation of the success of the educational program by watching the doctor at his daily work. If he has time in the day to be thoughtful, if he can gain new content by the use of his training in symbolic language, if he is continually preparing for the medicine of tomorrow, the educational system is justified. If he is harried, tired, handling patients in a routine, non-thinking way, the educational system has failed.

I am confident that the PA can put time back into the day of the practicing physician, provided the doctor is able to organize his own day and is capable of being a good supervisor. We do not select medical students for this talent, and our clinical support system may founder on this hidden reef.

The time has come for medical schools to broaden the intake of students to include those who have done well in the areas of economics, business administration, sociology, information sciences, and bioengineering, and those who wish to continue their development in these areas while they are becoming doctors. The present high and inflexible bioscience hurdles keep out of medical schools many students with special aptitudes in other areas who are unwilling to spend two years memorizing a large number of facts in bioscience in order to pass the required medical school examinations. Those who are willing to undertake the memory work usually turn out not to have been particularly interested in the areas of their undergraduate work, and do not continue to develop and use those areas. For example, the engineering graduate who comes into medicine has usually rejected engineering before he enrolls in medical school. Medicine needs an input from engineering students who maintain an interest in engineering while they are becoming doctors.

In the near future, some medical school is going to convert its medical center into a true university laboratory. Doctors, medical students, interns, and residents will live with the information scientist, the economist, the professor of business administration, the sociologist, and the bioengineer. They will learn the culture of sick and well persons, the ways of doctors, and the culture of medicine. The doctors in turn will know these new colleagues and will be willing to use their talents in the education of doctors. We will continue to produce our current bioscience-based product, but also we will produce equally good practicing doctors with a wide diversity of interests and skills. The paths for learning the disciplines underlying the health field and the delivery of health care will be varied. At the research level, the student's experiences will reflect his interest, and the doctor with a bioscience base will engage in quite different areas of research than the doctor with the information-science base. The non-bio-science-based doctor will be as effective in patient care as his bio-science-based colleague (*E. A. Stead, Jr.: What This Patient Needs Is A Doctor.* pp 91–3)

CHAPTER 15

LEADERS AND LEADERSHIP

An army of a thousand is easy to find, but, ah, how difficult to find a general.

Chinese Proverb

The issue of staff mobility concerned Stead from the beginning. He was aware that the Department was in for trouble if all its members grew old in unison. And so, as Chief, he wanted to provide incentives for his staff to move on. And mobility would not be helped if people were making so much money at Duke that they couldn't afford to take a job they really wanted in another institution. At least that was his rationale for paying low salaries to his staff; it is also true that he was a tight man with a dollar, as Dean Davison and others learned.

Dr. Stead:

> I was interested in the wellbeing of Duke's social system, and I thought that staff should be free to go on to new opportunities. I don't remember ever feeding somebody a major increase in salary in order to keep them when they otherwise would leave. I've given major increases to people who deserved it, based on their productivity, but, if someone told me he had been offered more money from another institution, I was not likely to make a counter-offer. Anybody who left Duke was clearly going to have an increased income. And I knew, from the salaries at other schools, that someone would tempt them away. I thought in the long run, that it was to our advantage to let them go when they decided the time was right. More than once, I urged a person to take the other offer. On the other hand, I also believed that I should know which school was likely to court our faculty members, so I could make the first move if I didn't want them to get away.

Even after years of friendship and productive collaboration, Stead made no effort to keep his faculty. If he already had the best ten years of somebody's

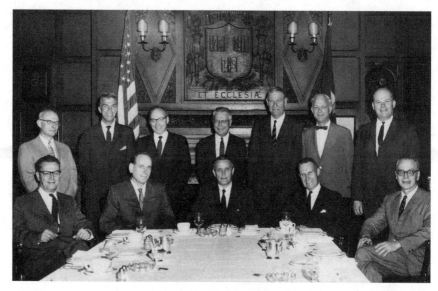

Dinner at the Harvard Club in honor of Stead and Beeson, who was about to assume the Nuffield Professorhip at Oxford. New York City, 1965. Front: John Romano, Eugene Stead, Paul Beeson, Charles Janeway, Walter Sheldon. Rear: Philp Bondy, Louis Hempleman, John Hickham, Jack Myers, Gustave Dammin, Max Michael, James Warren.

post-graduate experience, it would make Duke stronger yet if they moved on, leaving behind two or three bright young people whom they had trained. This kept the Department of Medicine refreshed with young staff whose most productive research years lay ahead of them. Everybody at Duke was going to be nationally recognized as a clinician, a research scientist or an educator.

Dr. Jack Myers:

> By the time I left Duke, I was a member of the "Old Turks" (the Association of American Physicians); everything I could do to build academic recognition, I'd already done. The same was true of the several colleagues who had joined Gene when he started out at Duke. It was time for some new blood, and time for us to move onto the next rung in our careers. Gene believed that when the people he had brought to Duke had matured, it was their responsibility to become chairs of medicine and guide educational programs elsewhere. It was what he expected. Stead knew it would be more productive for Duke, and more fun for him, to bring in a new team and build it up. I moved to Pittsburgh in 1955, and over the next several years, John Hickam went to Indiana and Jim Warren to Ohio State. Many other

people went on to become chairs, too; we scattered about and did our damnedest to emulate him, because everybody respected him very highly. That was the way he extended his influence throughout American medicine—via the people he farmed out.

As time went on, even his closest friends found opportunities elsewhere that allowed them to expand the roles they had begun at Duke. Whenever members of his faculty were ready to leave for new positions, Stead did his best to counsel them. He not only wanted his protégés to be successful in their careers, but satisfied as well. Still, not everyone who decided to move elsewhere was ready to become chair or ready to perform effectively. Sometimes the issues were subtle and the decision was hard, but Stead had his own way of thinking about solutions to problems.

Jack Myers:

> When it came to deciding if somebody would remain at Duke, either on the housestaff or on the faculty, Gene was direct and sometimes brutally honest. He'd tell them he thought Duke might be too difficult for them. Gene used to make hard decisions, as in the case of Gerry Rodnan, a rheumatologist. Gerry went through the Chief Residency at Duke and wanted to stay on when he finished. But Gerry was obese, and Gene bluntly told him, "I think your health situation is such that I'm not willing to invest in it. You're not going to provide your real capabilities for enough years that I want to invest in you." Rodnan was only about 27 at the time. Well, that was when I was planning to move to Pittsburgh, and Gerry asked me to take him on in a junior capacity. I did and Gene's prediction was, at least in part, correct. Gerry did die of obesity-related hypertension and diabetes, but 30 years later, after he had become one of the most productive and respected rheumatologists in the country.

Dr. Stead:

> When someone came to me seeking advice on whether or not to take a chairmanship position elsewhere, I first asked them whether or not they really wanted to be a chair. I knew there was no sense in taking a job you didn't want. They had to realize that instead of working in the lab creating information and knowledge as they had been doing, they would be working with people and creating medical professionals. They probably would not be elected to the National Academy of Science because they would be involved in another kind of work. There are just so many hours in the day and you can only spend them once.

I also counseled them about my concepts of "free-money," about getting the necessary commitments to create new programs, hire new people, expand laboratories or buy equipment. And finally, I urged them not to leave Duke unless one way or another, a cadre of people would go with them. When you have a job that you're really excited about doing, and you know some good people are going to join up with you, you're bound to be successful. One person really has an almost impossible job at a new institution unless they have other people with them who think like the do. And taking colleagues along with you is a way of testing the availability of "free-money." If you say, "I'd like to come, but I'd like to bring these people along as well," you quickly discover what free-money is available. If the institution can't offer you the funds for your associates' salaries, you can take it as a pretty good indication of the kind of support you're likely to get with future requests.

A new chairman needs somebody he can let his hair down with and talk to, somebody who knows what can be accomplished under a different system. He needs the support of a group of loyal people who are committed to the same work ethic and goals. If you can't get the new folks in, you might as well not be chairman. It would be crazy to think the established people whom you will inherit could really adapt to a new system and provide the support you need to make it work—it's just asking more than humans can do. I tried to impress that on them as well.

During the entire time Stead was at Duke, his departmental budget was smaller than at any of the departments his people left Duke to run. However, he had the most "free-money." And from the chairman's point of view that is what really counted. To Stead it didn't matter how big the budget was; if the money were already committed to ongoing salary and building expenses, then there would be none left for new initiatives. When Dr. Michael De Bakey offered Henry McIntosh the Chair of Medicine at Baylor, Stead gave him his characteristic counsel.

Dr. Stead:

Henry made 15 or so trips down to Houston to look at the Baylor position before taking the job, but nevertheless, I thought he went too soon. I'd been down there for two months helping De Bakey, and had arranged for Salih Wakil, to go down from Duke as Chairman of Biochemistry, which was one of the positions they really needed filled. Baylor also needed a Chair for their Department of Medicine. But everybody knew that matters had to be worked out in advance, because the place had never really been properly institutionalized, and there weren't any rules as to what the Dean or Chairman of Medicine did. They just did what Mike De Bakey said—that was they way the institution was run. But I couldn't keep Henry from accepting too soon. He did make a lot of visits to Baylor, but Henry never solidified his arrangements with De Bakey. If he'd waited longer and gotten his requirements and the promises made put in writing, he would have been much better off. Mike had a very rigid sense of honor. If he had put something in writing, he'd execute it. And he could, because he had the resources.

Henry could have set up a PDC-type of system at the Methodist Hospital, which was part of the Baylor system, because Mike was desperate, but I couldn't get Henry to stand firm on this demand before he accepted the offer. Such an arrangement would have provided Henry with the wherewithal to generate the "free-money" to develop new programs. Instead, he accepted without this concession and went down there based on a series of word-of-mouth promises, which eventually evaporated.

I was always concerned with the huge salary that he was offered. I said, "Henry, you shouldn't take that much money," because you can't be both academic and wealthy. At least I don't think you can. If money means that much, you've got to go out and make money in private practice. If instead you say, "I want a life with different kinds of satisfactions, I want to live at a different pace, on a different time schedule, and do what I want to do," then, unless you were born with a silver spoon in your mouth, you're not going to have as much money. I warned that if he went down there, he was going to have to sustain that salary and he would be responsible for raising the money. And Henry explained, "Well, I've been poor a long time." And I said, "Yes, but you've been happy a long time." I thought the administrative set-up at Baylor was not congruous with academic goals. It was too money-oriented rather than productivity-oriented.

Dr. Stead had an uncanny ability to recognize unusual talent. Conventional wisdom might run strongly against an individual or an idea, but Stead was able to cut through the bias and see beneath the surface. Having always thought of himself as a little unusual, he was never put off by the unconventional. He welcomed people whose behavior or ideas breached the normal limits of acceptability, as long as they had something worthwhile to offer. As a result, Stead embraced people who would otherwise have been limited by a system intolerant of anything foreign or overly daring. He served as a catalyst, fostering medical advances that otherwise might take years to achieve. Dr. Kempner was one of the people whose stories Stead helped write.

Walter Kempner came from a distinguished scientific background in Germany. His scientific mentor in Berlin was Otto Warburg, Nobel Laureate in 1931, whose laboratory produced a number of famous biochemists. As a young man, Kempner studied fundamental issues of cell metabolism, using special instruments developed by Warburg to measure the uptake of oxygen and generation of carbon dioxide. Stead's predecessor at Duke, Frederic M. Hanes, helped Kempner get out of Nazi Germany, and rumor has it that Mrs. Hanes smuggled out his money. At Duke, he was given a small laboratory that included a Warburg apparatus with which he continued his metabolic studies. Beside his research work, Kempner taught medicine, and he became one of the more popular clinical teachers. Yet he was very Prussian in his mannerisms, with a thick German accent and medical associates who spoke with him in German. In short, he was very different from the largely Southern doctors at Duke. Stead claims that Kempner did not make ward rounds in a satisfactory manner, though he did quite well on a one-to-one basis in the clinic.

At first, Kempner did not have a private practice, but laboratory studies led him to surmise that kidney cells would change their metabolic activity if exposed to an increased concentration of carbohydrate and a lowered concentration of sodium. He thought that patients with kidney disease might respond to a diet that increased the carbohydrate content and lowered the sodium intake far beyond the usual. He propounded his thesis until some of his students said, "If you say that you know how to take care of such people, why don't you take care of them?" And so he did. Kempner became a specialist the treatment of hypertension and kidney disease in that way. He had an idea he wanted to try out, patients came to him, and before long, he was extraordinarily knowledgeable about vascular and metabolic disease.

In the late 1930s there was no known treatment for advanced kidney disease, and most kidney patients eventually died of uremia, the build-up of metabolic wastes that could not be excreted. Neither was there any treatment for high blood pressure, the most lethal consequences of which were kidney and heart failure; these patients all died as well. Kempner began his work on the public wards at Duke, which housed patients who couldn't afford private medical care. He carefully measured how much protein leaked out in the urine, and the blood levels of nitrogen waste products that accumulated in patients whose kidneys could not excrete such material. Then he treated these patients with a low protein-diet of his design, using rice and fruit as the main constituents. Rice consists largely of complex carbohydrate so, unlike meat, it produces very small amounts of nitrogen waste. The ultra-low salt rice diet led to improvement; patients with kidney disease and hypertension experienced a dramatic drop in blood pressure, and in those who had heart failure, the edema went away. Kempner recorded all of these responses and over time he was able to demonstrate the successful treatment of kidney and heart failure, hypertension and even diabetes. He had the data to prove it, but the whole idea was so heretical that most other doctors mocked him.

As Stead was running his clinic for individual patients, he and Kempner practiced medicine side by side in the medical out-patient clinic. Within a very short period of time, it became quite clear to Dr. Stead that Kempner's patients always did better than his. In fact, it was difficult to ignore that fact because the interns and students commented on the difference. Being curious about it himself, Stead decided to look at Kempner's practices.

Many of the senior staff were angry because Kempner used so many hospital beds for the patients he was treating with his new rice diet. The leaders of the old-guard—Julian Ruffin, William Nicholson and Edward Orgain—were very antipathetic to Kempner: they thought he used too many of the institution's resources, they thought his work was scientifically unsound, and they particularly didn't like his record keeping system (an unusual complaint about a doctor, but Kempner's method of recording medical information was foreign to them). There were numbers and measurements in Kempner's charts, but no detailed verbal descriptions of the patients. He often made photographs of the optic fundi of patients with high blood pressure who were going blind from hemorrhages and exudates in their eyes. He had pictures before, during, and after treatment, but no verbal descriptions of what he saw when he looked at the eyes with an ophthalmoscope. For him the pictures were worth a thousand words. He had x-ray measurements of heart size, but none from the physical examination. He had ECG's on his patients, but didn't comment on how they reflected (or didn't reflect) heart disease—he simply put the test results in the right place on the chart. Stead pointed out that most medical records merely recycle information that is already there, but Kempner didn't do that. The letters he wrote to referring doctors were very complete and contained all the necessary information, yet there was little or nothing in the chart of a verbal nature.

The staff thought that Kempner's "poor" record-keeping reflected a lack of knowledge and judgment. So Stead was asked to review Kempner's record system in hopes that Kempner would be removed from the staff as incompetent. When Stead looked at the records, he realized their format was novel, but by the time he finished his investigation, he had decided that Kempner's records, in fact, surpassed those of the rest of the staff. Instead of firing the unorthodox Dr. Kempner, Stead promoted him to full professor. This rankled many of the medical staff, but in Stead's mind, his action was justified.

Dr. Stead:

> Dr. Kempner and I always got along well. But many people saw only his eccentricities, like driving to work in the winter, dressed in a blue blazer, with the top down on his convertible. Their general mistrust of him was increased by the fact that he was markedly private about his personal life, even where he lived, and he was conspicuously absent from the social functions his colleagues attended. They did not recognize the intellectual depth of the man. I knew who he had trained with, and I knew that the results of his lab were highly reproducible— there wasn't any argument about the figures that were coming out— so he had to know something about running a laboratory.
>
> Many doctors were actually antagonized by the fact that their patients did infinitely better under Kempner's regimen than under their own care. And instead of being appreciative of the fact that their patients were much better off, they resented the fact that Kempner was practicing a style of medicine that was unfamiliar to them and which they didn't like: his low-salt rice diet. In those days, however, he took care of more cases of destructive cardiovascular disease than anybody else in the world. Knowing that cardiovascular disease eventually would cause strokes, heart and kidney failure, and death, he believed that treating at an early stage would prevent organ destruction before it was irreversible. Therefore, he treated patients with mild hypertension as aggressively as he did those with severe or malignant hypertension. His patients would be asked to eat at one of his "rice houses" and stay in town for months to take his treatment, even if they were feeling well at the time. They and their doctors didn't appreciate the potential seriousness of the hypertensive state.

The interns and residents who worked with Dr. Kempner had a mixed reaction to him. Many people were interested in what Kempner did, and learned a great deal from him, but not everyone could work with him. He was brusque and rigid about the care plans that he prescribed for his patients. His patients often had illnesses that would prove fatal unless treated aggressively, so Kempner expected them to adhere to his rigid program. The rice diet was bland and monotonous, and many people found it hard to follow faithfully, but they did so because it meant the difference between life and death, and because they were afraid of being scolded by Kempner if they "cheated." He checked patients' urine daily, and finding a high sodium excretion meant the patient had deviated from the prescribed path. There was no guessing involved. One day, Kempner confronted one of his cardiac patients, a nun for whom he had prescribed the strict low-salt diet. Her urine tests showed that she had not done as directed. But when Kempner queried the good sister, she denied any deviation. They went back and forth for several minutes, Kempner all the while holding her test results—the proof of her transgression—in his hand. Finally, angered by her attempt to veil the truth as well as her failure to comply with his instructions, Kempner lost his temper and yelled, "Sister Agnes—you lie!" The frightened nun clutched her rosary in disbelief and the housestaff, distracted from their immediate work, stood agape. Dr. Kempner, however, saw to it that she properly atoned!

In spite of his harsh manner, Kempner was widely sought after and became perhaps the best known doctor at Duke because of his enormous following of rich and famous patients. Stead and Kempner developed a deep and mutual respect, although from time to time they had minor conflicts because Kempner's entire practice, laboratory included, was supported largely out of funds generated by his patient fees. Stead believed that Kempner should find grant support for his work, and urged him to apply to the NIH. As it turned out, however, the US Public Health Department peer review process didn't work well in Kempner's case; grant reviewers who judged his work were unhappy that he didn't see the world or behave the way they did. In Stead's opinion, though, Kempner never would have succeeded with all those patients if he were a mere carbon-copy of the doctors who reviewed him. Hardly a diplomat, Kempner was arrogant, self-assured, and argumentative—qualities that don't fare well during grant reviews. He didn't care what others thought of his work, and he was not about to compromise or negotiate. He promised to do things that had not been done before, which made him seem boastful and pigheaded. And like the Duke colleagues who mistook his unique style of record keeping for incompetence, review committees found it difficult to objectively assess the work he was doing. His grant applications were turned down.

In spite of the initial failures, Stead continued to prod Kempner to apply for grant funds. Stead figured that, if Kempner got grant support for his work, more of Kempner's PDC earnings would become "free-money" that would allow Stead to put a financial floor under other young people. Kempner's enormous practice did generate a lot of money for the Department—he made as much as the rest of the staff put together—but running his laboratory used a lot of what he took in. And because his research was plowing new ground, in theory, at least, Kempner was an excellent candidate for grant suppport.

Dr. Stead:

> Interestingly enough, we managed to get Kempner funded by the
> NIH outside of the peer review system. It was the only time in NIH

history that such a thing ever happened, and it was not without its consequences. Oscar Ewing, Administrator of the Federal Security Agency that directed the United States Public Health Service, had lived in Chapel Hill, just down the road from Durham. His wife had been a patient of Kempner's, and so Ewing was aware of Kempner's pioneering work. He knew also that each time the review cycle came around, the NIH rejected Kempner's proposals. Being a man of influence, he decided to use persuasion to see that justice was done. In his mind the work deserved to be funded, but simply was not receiving a fair evaluation because of Kempner's unorthodox attitude and manner. "The NIH is going to yell like hell," he said, "but we're going to support Dr. Kempner."

He had the power to overrule the peer review process, which had denied Kempner funding, and order the NIH to award him a grant—and he did. When Thomas Parran, the Surgeon General, learned what Ewing had done, he became incensed. To ignore the decision of the review committee was heretical and a blatant display of contempt for the system. His sense of honor made it impossible for him to continue to align himself with an administration that tolerated such a transgression. In an act of protest he resigned his post and joined the private sector.

Time passed, and I forgot all about the episode. I had had nothing to do with Ewing's action in the first place other than persuading Kempner to apply for a grant. One day—years later—I went to Pittsburgh to visit the Mellon Foundation in an appeal for funds. When I arrived, I was ushered into the office of the Director, and offered a seat. Unbeknownst to me, there on the other side of the desk from where I was sitting was Thomas Parran, whose career the Kempner issue had so strongly affected. Although 15 years had passed by the time I met him, time had stood still for him as far as that event was concerned. He leaned across his desk with a satisfied grin and said, "You seem to have forgotten about me, Dr. Stead, but I haven't forgotten you. You see, I was Surgeon General at the time Dr. Kempner was awarded NIH money without the consent and approval of the review committee. I resigned my post over that issue." I knew when luck was working against me, and so I stood up, extended my hand and said, "I appreciate your reminding me of this event and I don't think I need to take up any more of your time." "You're quite right," he replied. And so I quickly left, got back on the airplane and returned home.

Kempner was a member of the PDC, and like everyone else, his income was taxed by the Department of Medicine. The more he made, the more "free-money" he created for the Department. Over time the Rice Diet Program became internationally famous, and his practice became an enormous success, financially as well as medically. Many of Kempner's patients were rich and they were consumers, so they were a boon to the economy of Durham, as well as to Duke. The money Kempner generated helped the Department of Medicine construct new buildings and recruit faculty, both of which greatly contributed to the further growth of the department. But Dr. Kempner's work impacted the entire University. It was Stead's opinion that, in time, the source of this impact would be recognized. Duke was a state and regional school until Walter Kempner came; he made Duke visible on the national and international scenes.

Stead nominated Kempner for the CIBA Pharmaceutical Award, citing his identification of the role of diet and cholesterol in heart disease. Kempner had demonstrated that you could drastically reduce the intake of nitrogen in the diet if you had adequate carbohydrate intake. He showed that the electrocardiographic pattern indicating heart strain could be reversed and heart size reduced in adequately treated patients. He showed that a high carbohydrate diet improved diabetes and reduced insulin requirements, and that it was possible to normalize high blood pressure even when it reached its dreadful malignant phase. These were very important clinical advances, and Kempner was the person who had achieved all these firsts, argued Dr. Stead.

The Committee agreed that Kempner had made a tremendous contribution to the field. It was decided that the award would be given to two people that year: a geneticist who had identified a strain of hypertensive rats, and Dr. Kempner. However, Kempner refused to go to the banquet to receive the award. He wrote to the committee, thanking them and saying that he'd like to be there, but that he would be in Europe on the date of the ceremony. The committee mailed the award money ($7,500) to Dr. Stead to give to Kempner. But Stead was angry. He had gone to considerable trouble to put forward the nomination of his colleague, and Kempner hadn't even shown the simple courtesy of attending the banquet. "I want you to sign this check over the Department of Medicine," Stead told him, "and I want you to do it this morning." Dr. Kempner calmly replied, "Don't yell at me so loudly, Gene. I'll process the check in my account and write you a check for $15,000." "OK," Dr. Stead agreed, "and I won't remain annoyed."

Dr. John Laszlo:

> I knew Dr. Kempner as well or better than most other members of our Department. That is, not very well. However, I had extensive experience using the Warburg techniques to measure tissue oxygen con-

sumption, had used it in my own research, and had read all of Kempner's papers, even the German ones. This pleased him because no one
else was familiar with the work he did before coming to this country.

In 1959, while a medical resident at Duke, I developed a research
interest in young people who were morbidly obese—those weighing
upwards of 300 or 350 pounds. After carefully reading about various
approaches to treating obesity, it was clear that nobody knew how to
help these people; weight lost by "dieting" would eventually return
because most patients were unable to maintain restricted calorie intake. I wondered whether, if we hospitalized such people and gave
them no calories for a prolonged period, they would "shrink their
stomachs" and make them content to eat much less.

It was a serious question because total starvation is risky—but the
prognosis for a 350-pound 18-year old is also dreadful. Dr. Kempner
was skeptical, pointing out the dangers of total calorie restriction, such
as ketosis and acidosis. This was uncharted territory, but I did arrange
to treat one patient at a time, monitoring their blood tests closely over
a 3–6 week period. During the fast, my patients exercised, drank
plenty of fluids, had some nutritional but non-caloric supplements,
were taught about their dietary problems, and received some psy-
chotherapy. It worked like a charm; at the end of the fast, patients were
barely able to eat even 800 calories a day because that much food was
"just so filling." Of course, that situation was transitory and, unless they
had gained some basic behavioral skills, the weight gradually returned.
But I learned a great deal about obesity and metabolism in the process.

Kempner said little more to me about my approach, but some time
later, as he began to treat increasing numbers of obese people, he too
began by fasting them. Always the dogmatist, he still was willing to
change the dogma as he saw fit. Stead saw that I was trying a new approach to treating obesity and, although Kempner was the local diet
authority, there was no directive that all nutritional research had to
be approved by him. In Stead's book, the world belonged to those
willing to work and no artificial pecking order should get in the way
of progress. What was good for the goose, was good for the gander.

Kempner made many enemies in his career and he rarely thanked his friends,
except perhaps Eugene Stead. Still, Kempner saved many patients in his career, patients whose doctors had given up on them. Stead recognized that, if
Kempner had been like other doctors, his program would never have existed.
"He was honest and uncompromising, and never spent a single hour of his

life in any society or even in a committee meeting." Those differences enabled him to accomplish what he did, but without the support of a chairman like Stead, Kempner's accomplishments might have been limited. Again and again, Stead took risks on people others might never have noticed. He saw differences as assets, and used them to his department's advantage. He never insisted that a person conform to popular beliefs, if there was a good reason to take the road less traveled. The wisdom of this philosophy was proven by what men like Walter Kempner achieved under Stead's aegis.

CHAPTER 16

GROWING UP IN THE SYSTEM

[The master word] is directly responsible for all advances in medicine during the past twenty-five centuries.... And the master word is *Work*.

Sir William Osler

All doctors who spent time under Stead's tutelage have their share of "Stead Stories" to tell. Dr. Robert Whalen rose from intern to Chief Medical Resident to Professor of Medicine and prominent cardiologist at Duke under Stead. His perspective on Eugene Stead, and what it was like to grow up under his eye is both singular and universal:

Robert Whalen, MD:

> I ended up at Duke in 1956 by default. I had gone to Cornell Medical School planning to become a pediatrician or a surgeon, but I wanted the preparation of a good medical internship. I listed Duke as my fourth choice for internship, though I didn't really know anything about its medical service. Fully expecting to get one of my first three choices, I didn't bother to research Duke. As luck would have it, however, I was turned down by the other three schools. I never thought that would turn out to be a lucky thing—indeed the best thing that could have happened—but it did.
>
> I had just gotten married, and my wife and I went to North Carolina on our honeymoon. While there, I arranged a last minute interview at Duke, not because I was so terribly interested in the program, but that day the greens were frozen at the Pinehurst Golf Course, so we couldn't play golf. I called the Department of Medicine and was invited to talk with John Hickam in the same laboratory that I would later direct for 10 years.
>
> I was struck by the fact that the senior staff I met were all doing much of the same sorts of things that I had done. I had spent most of my senior year at Cornell in a research laboratory at Memorial Hospital, involved in studies on hepatic coma and other things. Duke

was the only place I interviewed where research just seemed to be part of everybody's day. At the more traditional programs, like Columbia and Rochester, I was interviewed by clinicians who had no real contact with research. I hadn't really noticed that fact, though, until I saw how things were run at Duke.

Duke's was a relatively easy residency to get into when I applied. I started in 1956 and the medical service wasn't a particularly "hot ticket" at that time. As a matter fact, only four my twenty-two co-interns had been medical students at Duke; most Duke students went elsewhere. Over the Stead years, however, Duke became an increasingly attractive place, and the competition increased significantly. Its reputation spread as junior faculty left Duke for jobs at other medical centers and Stead-trained interns and residents filtered out into the medical community. During my first few years at Duke, Sam Martin, John Hickam, and Jim Warren all left to chair departments of medicine at Florida, Indiana, and Ohio State, respectively. They took with them Stead's philosophy and high standards. In turn, they imbued a host of young people with Stead's principles and his standards for running a medical service. Within a very short period of time there were a lot of Duke-trained people across the country, and they talked a lot about Duke and the Stead system. They liked the way they had been trained, hard as it was, and they liked Durham. Suddenly there was a whole host of salesmen promoting Duke, which had never happened before. Since Stead turned out so many good doctors, the word spread that his service provided a unique caliber of training.

I arrived on a Sunday night and although my internship didn't officially start until Monday morning, I went to see where I was going to be stationed. It was a typical Sunday night on the Private Medical Service. There were 20 or so admissions, half of whom had flown in from Florida, and everybody was running around frantically. I met Marty Liebling, who was just finishing his internship, and out of interest and curiosity I asked him, "Tell me, how do you like this service?" He used a few vulgar words to describe the whole experience and said "I'd never ever come back to this jungle." But about two years later, after a tour at the National Cancer Institute in Bethesda, Marty returned to Duke for a junior residency. As I was about to learn, there was something about the place that couldn't be duplicated elsewhere.

At 11:45 on the first day of internship, a junior resident who had been shepherding us through the system suddenly said, "OK every-

body, noon conference." "My god," I thought, "what's this noon conference stuff? I've got 15 patients I've never seen before and 3 new
admissions." But the residents all insisted that everyone, interns or
not, go to noon conference. So we did and did so routinely throughout the year. I think that was when I first really understood what an
educational experience Duke was going to be.

We had an excellent teaching system on the private service, although I only really appreciated it many, many years later. We spent
2 hours with a senior faculty physician, presenting patients to him,
and he would give us a little different view of the patients' problems
than we got during our work rounds with the attending doctor who
was in charge of the care of the patients. In retrospect I think it was
a much more valuable experience than I ever realized at the time. Trying to explain a patient's problem to somebody who wasn't directly
responsible for the patient seemed a little like playing house to us. But
Jim Warren, who ran rounds early on, was really excellent in providing an overview of what was happening to the patient.

Dr. Stead believed in vocation and medical commitment, not "education," as a way of teaching anybody to be a doctor; this meant performing habitual or repetitive tasks, the way a biochemist is trained,
for example. When I first arrived at Duke, I didn't know how compulsive I was. I had gone to a Jesuit college where memorizing and
knowing all the facts that there were to know was part of the game.
The Duke internship was sort of like returning to the Jesuits. As pre-
med students we worked every minute of every day except Saturday
night, which we took off. But we still went to bed early Saturday night
because we had to be bright and alert on Sunday to do all our homework. The five nights on call out of seven that the Duke housestaff
worked was much the same. We worked hard throughout the week
and then took one weekend night off to enjoy ourselves and our families. It was a lot like college in the sense that we lived in a dormitory
with our fellow sufferers, and we commiserated together. Spending
that much time together, we interns became a closely-knit group. A
friendly competition existed among us, but there were also deep
bonds and a sense of *esprit de corps* because we were all in it together.
The most beloved of my group was a bright young doctor who came
to Duke with both MD and PhD degrees. He had trained in one of
the country's leading biochemistry labs and actually spent three years
setting up a surgical research laboratory at Yale before coming to
Duke. He had a bibliography of something like 38 papers and the

most impressive credentials of any intern there. Ironically, as it turned out, he was incompetent clinically. He was all thumbs. He had the bibliography and he had plenty of facts, but he just didn't have what it takes to put everything together to solve a patient's problem. On top of that, he lacked the one ingredient that you had to have as a house officer at Duke: he was not compulsive. We weren't asked by Dr. Stead to be intellectual giants, we just had to do things the same way over and over again, and to be sure we didn't miss anything. The system was almost anti-intellectual, and this man fought it because it was not a totally intellectual system. In spite of the poor fit, however, he did manage to get through. His colleagues understood that he wasn't going to be a superstar clinician, but that he had other strong assets. And because we all loved him, we picked up behind him and did a lot of his work for him. In the end, he went on to be successful in a more appropriately suited career. There was room at Duke for people with many different career goals.

Perhaps the most amusing story I recall about Dr. Stead occurred early in my internship. A house officer named Alex Kisch was working with me at the time, and it was a difficult time for Alex who was preoccupied with the war between the Israelis and the Arabs, the Israeli-Sinai campaign, and the sweep to the Red Sea. Alex had relatives in the Israeli army, and he worried about them. One day, Alex presented a patient to Dr. Stead who asked him what the cholesterol level had been on an admission in 1949. Alex said "high," and Dr. Stead asked, "What was the blood urea nitrogen in 1951," and Alex said, "It was normal," and then he asked for some other data; Alex's answers invariably were qualitative terms like "high," "low," and "normal." When the rounds were just about over, Stead paused in the doorway and said, "Dr. Kisch, I really think you ought to become more familiar with an Arabic custom." Alex said he felt heartsick. "I never thought that Dr. Stead was anti-Semitic," he said, "but here my relatives are being shot by Arabs and he's asking me to get involved with an Arabic custom, and just as my worst thoughts were percolating to the surface, Stead finished off the remark by saying, "You know they invented a famous system called numbers." He wanted quantitative information and not generalities.

During my time, interns were paid $25 a month at Duke, and during the half of the year that we worked at the VA, we were paid the equivalent of about $120 a month. On that salary, of course, it was necessary for my wife to work. She had been a school teacher, but she went to work as a technician in the catheter laboratory, and learned how to do blood analyses and that type of thing. We had our first child in March of my second year at Duke; then we had another child after that. In order to survive economically we had to borrow on savings that my wife and I had. We also borrowed money from the Department of Medicine's so-called Hanes fund, which was set up for this type of need. I think all my fellow house officers took loans because nobody had much money. I went to Dr. Stead and told him that I needed money to pay the rent, and was loaned money from the Hanes fund at 6% interest, the repayment of which began a year after I finished at Duke. By the time I finished my medical training, I had borrowed six or seven thousand dollars. We didn't live very high off the hog and we didn't have big expenses. We didn't buy a television set until I was Chief Resident and then it was a black and white set bought with money I got from filling out medical insurance forms at $5 a head. But we all lived reasonably well in the sense that we were comfortable in our homes or apartments. Originally my wife and I lived in a furnished apartment because we thought I was only going to be in Durham for one year. When I moved to North Carolina we brought down some kitchen utensils and that was it.

In other programs where house officers weren't paid much, they moonlighted in emergency rooms, but there wasn't any moonlighting in the Department of Medicine. First of all there was no time for it. Being on duty five nights out of seven, we were pretty well bushed on our nights off, but we never really thought of moonlighting. It was not a custom and there were few part-time jobs in emergency rooms. It might even have been against the rules, but I don't think that we would have paid that much attention to rules unless we were threatened with death. I just think nobody moonlighted because we literally worked too long and hard.

We did not have many defectors from the Duke training program. We had a relatively happy internship, which I think is attributable partly to the boot camp atmosphere. Because the system was demanding and competitive, we had a sense of pride and loyalty that kept us fighting to succeed. Few from my group left because they didn't like Duke, although some left for other career reasons.

Each week the residents assigned to the ward services met at "History Meeting" to review the chart of every patient discharged during the preceding week. We were looking for shortcomings or inadequacies in care. When he first came to Duke, Dr. Stead personally ran the

History Meeting, but by the time I arrived it more or less ran itself. The junior residents had been indoctrinated into the procedure when they were interns, and they took responsibility for making sure the charts were in good shape. And they *were* in good shape. It's amazing how this compulsive approach to making sure that "t"s were crossed and "i"s dotted and everything was in the right place worked. If an intern were asked at History Meeting about a patient's test results—for example, whether the stool had been tested for occult blood—he or she would never give an indignant or arrogant response. Anyone who said "I did a good job working up this patient. If there is no stool test, it's because I didn't think it was important, and I'm not going to do anything else about it" earned an invitation to talk things over with Dr. Stead. And he would explain in fairly explicit terms that certain things were required. He never rushed to find you a job elsewhere, but you knew that his recommendations really were dependent upon playing the game in accordance with the rules.

Housestaff were on call five nights out of seven; everybody thinks of that as overwhelming and brutal. Quite frankly, though, I still think it's the best way to train house officers. We spent a lot of time together and discussed our cases over late night supper. We really learned medicine by seeing patients and practicing medicine. We were there when our patients got sick and when they improved. It turned out to be an excellent way to learn. There was a good bit of complaining, but it wasn't that hard on families. Our marriages survived reasonably well. Two nights out of the week the families would come to the hospital for supper, and the dining room would be filled with kiddy-carts and the paraphernalia of young families, and we'd fill our trays with enough food for the whole family. There was a lot of togetherness among the housestaff; wives socialized and formed bridge clubs and knitting clubs; everybody survived reasonably well. When I went back to visit some of my medical school friends who were housestaff at Cornell a year or so later, I realized that they really had almost the same thing as our five nights a week. Technically, they were "on" every other night, but they stayed until everything was finished. So they would get home tired at 11:00 at night, which was no better.

Since we were going to be in the hospital all night, we didn't have to rush to work up a patient who came in at 1 or 2 in the afternoon. We had time to roam the Medical Center to see what was being done with our patients. For instance, I felt free to go to the Catheter Laboratory with a couple of my patients to watch them being catheterized because I knew I was going to be there that night; if I had two or three admissions, I could work them up after supper. I think that our interns got more sleep than most other interns in the country at the time. If there were two of us on call, then both of us were admitting. We weren't taking care of the other interns' sick patients and also admitting. Therefore, we were able to get plenty of sleep.

The transition from medical student to intern was easy intellectually. In the Duke system there was always somebody around to help us with difficult problems or medical challenges. Our faculty was very young and they were often in the laboratory at night so we could call on an expert when the need arose. Like the interns, junior residents were in the hospital five nights out of seven, and a senior resident, who was really the Officer-of-the-Day in charge of the Medical Service, was around checking each ward to be sure everyone was "tucked in." Usually the Chief Resident dropped in later in the night to find out who had been admitted and who was very sick. So those doctors, plus the young faculty provided a tremendous support system for the intern—you had only to ask.

The scary part about being an intern was taking charge of the care of patients, as real doctors have to do—the feeling that a patient's life and well-being were in our hands. One patient in particular contributed significantly to my initiation as a doctor. Late in the fall of my intern year, an optometrist's wife was referred to Duke, suffering (supposedly) from an hysterical illness (the patient said that she couldn't swallow and couldn't breathe normally). Once Mrs. X was rolled onto a stretcher, it didn't take us long to realize that we had a case of bulbar polio on our hands. I had never before seen polio, let alone bulbar polio, but I knew that if the paralysis caused by this viral infection progressed from the feet up to the muscles that control respiration or even higher, the patient might die. As fate would have it, I was assigned to her case. We put Mrs. X in an old-fashioned iron lung respirator, which was the primary method for keeping patients like her alive, and the treatment proved to be a very stressful experience for her and for me as well. In order to keep her breathing, the surgeons made a tracheostomy (a direct opening into her airway), and we had to struggle perpetually to keep the cuff of the iron lung away from the opening of the tracheostomy itself so that air could move in and out. Nobody on the regular staff knew anything about the mechanics of the iron lung, so I had to become an instant expert. The patient was admitted just before Thanksgiving and we had private duty nurses taking care of her, but a new practical nurse was assigned each shift. I didn't dare go to sleep because I knew that at midnight I was going to have to teach a new nurse how to use the manual air bellows provided for emergency use in the event the power went off. Every eight hours I taught a new nurse not to be afraid of the iron lung. It was actually very simple to operate, but it was emotionally draining. It was the first time I realized that a patient might die if I made a mistake or if I didn't make sure that everybody involved in her care knew what to do.

When I look back on Mrs. X, I know that she's the patient who made me a doctor. I think every intern has that kind of transforming experience, some patient who makes him realize that he is a critical cog. Of course there are times when patients die regardless of what we do. For the interns who want to see themselves in shining armor, those occasions represent undeniable defeat. But we learn to go on, hoping the next time to save the burning castle. The amazing thing is that we sometimes succeed.

The middle of the 20th century was a unique time in American medicine and in American politics. Doctors were subject to the military draft unless they had a Berry Plan deferment, which exempted them until they had completed specialty training. I did not get a deferment, so I was liable to be drafted at anytime. I told Dr. Stead that I planned to go back to Cornell after my internship for a medical residency, but I really didn't want to leave. I was very happy at Duke; I liked the program, it met my needs and I was learning a tremendous amount of medicine. On the other hand, I felt drawn back to my alma mater and, since my family lived in New York, it seemed like a good move. I pointed out that I didn't have a Berry Plan deferment, and Stead was quick to say that he didn't much worry about that. He told me if I wanted to, I could stay on as a junior resident. Having a job no matter what relieved me greatly. Then I talked to the people at Cornell and told them that I didn't have a deferment; they said they wouldn't to take me without one because if I were drafted, it would leave the program short-handed. Stead's willingness to take a chance on me is really indicative of the way in which he operated. He took chances on all sorts of people and all sorts of situations. Looking back, I can see he was a wise administrator. If you lose a junior resident, you can always appoint somebody else or tighten the service up a little bit. Dr. Stead knew that he could run the service without the housestaff if he absolutely had to because he had done that at Emory.

And it was a tremendous vote of confidence to know that he believed enough in my skills at that time to take a gamble on me.

During the 1950s and '60s, postdoctoral training in medicine consisted of twelve months of internship followed by 12 months of Junior Assistant Residency. After that it was possible for candidates to sit for the examination given by the American Board of Internal Medicine. Young doctors who elected to continue their medical training went from Junior Residency into subspecialty programs as fellows, or they elected to continue for another year as Senior Assistant Residents (SARs) before entering practice or fellowship. In addition to JARs and SARs, each year Dr. Stead chose two Chief Residents—one based at Duke Hospital and one at the VA.

Because doctors who had completed their internship were eligible for the military draft, many young doctors had their residency interrupted by two years of military service. As a result, few doctors progressed through the sequence of internship and residency in lock-step formation; instead, there was a great mixture of individuals, some of whom had just finished medical school and others who had substantial life (and death) experiences.

Dr. Robert Whalen:

> The transition from intern to junior resident at Duke was the biggest and most difficult change because it meant going from handling immediate critical problems to being an administrator and teacher. I was responsible for being sure that the medical students knew what they needed to know about a patient, and being sure that the interns had evaluated each patient appropriately and were taking good care of them. I had to interact with the nurses to be sure that they were relatively happy and doing what I thought they should be doing. During my first few weeks as a junior resident I stood in the middle of a ward and watched the two new interns, whom I thought were absolutely incompetent, scurrying about in confusion, doing nothing that they were supposed to do. There were 40 patients on the ward, and I said to myself, "I'm going to send these two dopes home. I can run this whole show better by myself than I can with them around." And then I realized that was not the goal. The real challenge of the junior residency was to get everybody doing what they could do best so that the whole system worked well. It might take an intern an hour to work up a patient and another hour to do lab work, all of which I could have done in 30 minutes. I had to realize that the interns were just learning how to do all these things, just as I had done the year

before, but it pained me to have the whole system slowed up so. We might just be getting started with new patients at 11:00 or 12:00 o'clock at night when I thought we should have had them all worked up and tucked in by 8:00 or 10:00. I had to stand back and let the interns learn the hard way, but letting go and giving someone new a chance is a hard lesson to learn.

Stead was such a good teacher because he was able to let young people take charge and do things from which they would learn. If I had been more aware of that at the time, I might have learned from his example. As it was, though, the lessons of the Chief's example far exceeded those of the textbooks and conventional education.

Most of the medical students who came into the system were primarily fact-oriented. Whatever degree of human kindness they had before going to medical school had pretty well been wrung out of them by the time they were through. Stead, however, saw compassion as an integral part of the care of patients. He dealt with patients in a professional and caring manner, and he nourished the re-establishment of humane qualities in young doctors. He didn't get us to perform by preaching; he coaxed us into conformity by following his own rules. As a result of his example, many of us remolded our image of what a doctor ought to be. He most affected us by always insisting, in attitude and performance, on the dignity of the patient. You would never, never hear the word "crock" applied to a so-called psychoneurotic patient on the Medical Service. It might be used on other services at other hospitals, but not on Stead's. It was a proscribed term and a proscribed concept. That was not the way to think about people and it was not the way to take care of people. Dr. Stead's emphasis on the patient's world, and the patient's response to his world, were the most lasting of his lessons for the housestaff. As with most of the lessons I learned in medicine, though, this one, too, came hard won through experience.

I remember a young patient we had on Osler Ward. She had 18 separate admissions to Duke Hospital over the preceding two years. It appeared to us that she had a series of psychoneurotic complaints, although we never used the term out loud. One of Stead's theses was that each person's central nervous system was unique and therefore interpreted input from the outside world, as well as its own inner world, uniquely. But as residents we wanted to treat "real" diseases, not neurotic complaints. In our opinion Mrs. A was floridly "psychoneurotic" and there was nothing we could do for her. We knew, though, that we would be in high hot water if Stead ever got to round on this woman. He would spend all day asking us questions about her and her life, which we wouldn't be able to answer because no one had taken the time to really go over her case. We hid her on the back porch of the old Osler Ward, hoping he'd never find her, and for a short time we deluded ourselves into thinking we could get away with it. He had a nose for trouble though, and on gallop rounds, which were apt to last for 4 to 5 hours as he checked on every patient, he found her. He spent an hour and a half at the bedside of this lady as all of us developed varicose veins trying to answer his questions. Thereafter he made a point of stopping by everyday to check on her. "How's Mrs. A" and "What's new with Mrs. A?" He became so interested in her case that he even stopped by Osler Ward during his vacation when he came in to pick up his mail. When it was time for her release, I held my breath as Stead asked, "Now who's going to follow Mrs. A in the clinic?" Obviously, there were no volunteers, but since I was the resident, Stead gave me the honor, though I would have dearly loved for her to sink into the sea somewhere. At the time I really couldn't understand why he thought this patient's case was so important. In fact, it puzzled me that he would make such an effort to see that she got the best care at a time when we had patients with much more serious illnesses. Dr. Stead's teaching was remarkable that way. He often didn't explain why he thought something was important for you to know; he presumed you'd figure it out somewhere along the line. And while that was usually true, I could never quite get a grip on his reason for spending so much time on Mrs. A.

Four or five years later, after I finished my residency, I asked Dr. Stead why he insisted that we be so involved with Mrs. A. He told me he figured this woman had a large family structure that would have been destroyed if she became really incapacitated. She had a child who suffered from diabetes insipidus and had to have her fluids carefully regulated with pituitary hormone, and her husband was working at graduating from school at the time. If she were completely unable to function, her daughter and husband would have suffered severely as well. As it turned out, I did follow her and have for over 30 years. True, she has had a lot of ups and downs, but she has managed to remain functional, which clearly made a critical difference in all their lives. Her husband earned a degree in political science and went on to become Chairman of the Department of Political Science at a university. Stead never said, "If you can keep this woman going for 25 or 30 years, you're going to keep her daughter going and her husband functional." He never spelled things out that clearly, but usually the lesson eventually came home—some of us were just slow learners.

Many patients go from doctor to doctor thinking that they are sick, and are never told that they are really well in a way they can understand. If a hundred people listen to a Beethoven symphony, some will be in ecstasy and some will be bored. These are not good and bad people, but people with different central nervous systems. Some people interpret almost all signals coming in to their central nervous systems as signs of sickness. They are not sick, but just have sensitive brains.

The junior residency on Osler Ward was a difficult experience, though I wouldn't necessarily call it hard. All year long, Dr. Stead served as one of the two attending (senior) physicians. For the housestaff, it was considered both the plum and the pits of rotations, depending on how it went on a given day. I wanted to show "The Professor" that I could run a perfect ward, even when it was sorely obvious that I couldn't. When you're dealing so many beginners, it doesn't matter how smart you are or what you want done or how you want it done, it's not going to be done the right way all the time. There were moments when I thought, "Man, we screwed up badly, and it wouldn't have happened if I had been the one who was doing this or that, or making decisions this way or that way." I'm sure Stead was well aware of the pitfalls, but the junior resident looking in the mirror was hoping to see the reflection of somebody who was absolutely perfect, and nobody was.

As I finished my time on Osler Ward with Stead, I looked back on all the things we did wrong. When I started out, I'd thought I was smarter and better than the record showed. During one of my particularly low moments I stopped in to see the Chief Resident and told him quite frankly that I was a little disappointed with my rotation on Osler Ward. Despite exerting a maximum effort, I felt that really never got very close to perfection. In response he told me very reassuringly, and very honestly, not to think that I was different from anybody else they brought through the system. He said that everybody who made rounds with Stead found him or herself sorely lacking at times. The Chief always showed us how much more there was to learn that we could never rest on our laurels. All who rounded with Stead exerted themselves to the utmost of their capabilities. It wasn't that you didn't put out what you felt was a maximum effort on teaching rounds with other senior staff, but on Stead's service you tried to put out a super-maximum effort, something above and beyond whatever you could do. It imbued us with a sense of doing things the right way. We established very high standards for ourselves and, in turn, expected the same from others working with us.

One of the ways in which Stead infused *esprit* and enthusiasm into his house staff (and senior faculty) was through their group teaching and learning interactions. The most famous of these was his "Sunday School," a weekly conference that he had begun at Emory and continued at Duke.

Dr. Robert Whalen:

Sunday School convened on Sunday mornings at 9:30. Each house officer in rotation reviewed a state-of-the-art topic having to do with a particular disease, a medical problem or medical breakthrough. Sunday School created a great deal of stress because we were expected to do a really good job, and in preparation we reviewed the world's literature on our chosen topic. One of the worst misfortunes I recall involved Charlie Rackley, who later became Chairman of the Department of Medicine at Georgetown. He spent months reviewing his Sunday School topic and making very extensive notes. Well, one day he forgot his notes in the library and when he went back for them, they were gone; three or four months of work down the tubes and poor Charlie disconsolate, trying to reconstruct all of that work. One of the most interesting Sunday Schools was prepared by Bill Harlan, who at that time was a Junior Resident. Bill had become interested in the biochemical basis for schizophrenia and had actually taken LSD the weekend before to see if it mimicked the described delusions and hallucinations of schizophrenic patients. He vividly described the effects of taking LSD, long before it was used as a recreational drug.

House officers prepared so hard for their Sunday School that they probably could get up and deliver a spontaneous lecture on that topic many years later. Mine was on thrombotic thrombocytopenic purpura. How I ever got to that one, I don't know. But getting up there to give it was nerve-wracking. I had the ultimate case of stage fright. Sunday School was like a grand performance because every house officer knew that he was being judged by Stead in a variety of ways. And on top of it, we were also performing for our peers, and we had a very competitive housestaff. We were all bright and had done well in school, so going up there, we had the dual problem of appearing bright in front of Stead and fostering our careers, and also being bright in front of our colleagues. In the long run, I guess it was sort of a rehearsal for many other kinds of performances we'd have to make, academically and otherwise.

Dr. Stead really didn't have much to do with the senior assistant residents, those in the third year of training, and they really didn't have much to do with him. The Senior Residents had four three-month rotations on the medical specialties—gastroenterology, cardiology, neurology, etc. I often thought that working in sub-specialty areas as a senior resident was like being a voyeur; we watched over everything, but never really were vital to the whole process. It was a time to see specialty medicine in practice; time to make a career choice, if you hadn't done that earlier. The people who provided most of the consultation services were the post-doctoral fellows in the specialty. The Senior Assistant Residency provided free-floating time; we really didn't have that much responsibility. It was a time for reflection and study after two clinical years that were so intense and practical and demanding that you didn't have a lot of time to sit back and look at diseases or patients with a broad overview, and there was very little time to understand what the rest of the world knew about a particular disease. Senior residents were only on call one night out of three, so they had a lot of time for the library to see what we had missed while we had been so busy "doing."

I first began to really enjoy learning when I was an intern. It was so important to learn because you needed to know how to take care of people the right way—the ultimate test of being successful. Once I started having fun learning the practical things, I began to get intellectually involved. The junior residency whetted my appetite, and the senior residency let me begin satisfying that appetite. There is a romance to medicine; every disease has a wonderful past history of discovery and description and then treatment. By the time I finished my senior residency, I was much more of a scholar than ever I had been in college.

During my junior residency, Stead had called me in and asked me what I wanted to do, but I really didn't know at the time. Primarily I wanted to practice medicine, and he suggested that I get some basic background and knowledge. He thought that the best way to prepare for the medicine of the future would be by learning some biochemistry. The last thing in the world I wanted to be was a biochemist. I didn't like chemistry in college, had hated biochemistry in medical school, and couldn't conceive of working with those damn test tubes and laboratory models. On the other hand, Stead was such a strong influence that I didn't turn down his suggestions lightly. By that time everybody in our program was imbued with the idea of going into academic medicine in some capacity; it was just the blueprint we had. One didn't turn down Stead's hints about what you ought to do if you wanted to go into academic medicine, so I talked with Phil Handler, Chairman of Biochemistry, but I wasn't happy about it.

John Hickam was in charge of the housestaff program, so I went to see him. I told him about Dr. Stead's suggestion, but that quite frankly I hated biochemistry. Hickam thought for a moment, then suggested that I put off making a decision. He thought Stead might be needing a Chief Resident, and if so, I could consider that instead. I asked him what he meant, knowing that Stead had scheduled Stu Bondurant to be Chief Resident. Stu was a former Assistant Resident who had gone to the Peter Bent Brigham Hospital for a last year of residency. As it turned out, he went on to have a distinguished career, and become Dean of the School of Medicine at the University of North Carolina, but at the time he was slated to return to Duke as Chief Resident. Hickam implied that we couldn't be certain about Stu, and advised me to see him about the matter in six months, before making a decision about the biochemistry business. Unknown to me, John Hickam was planning to go to the University of Indiana as Chief of Medicine, and he intended to take Stu Bondurant to help him run the department there. Six months later, I went back to see John and he asked me if I'd like the Chief Resident job. I said "Of course." I wanted another year of training before I took my board examinations in Internal Medicine, and I was enough of an egotist to want to head up the show. I said I'd wait to hear from Stead, but Hickam threw me a curve ball. "Oh no," he said, "you've got to go ask him for it." "What? I have to go to Stead and ask to be Chief Resident?" I couldn't believe what I was hearing. It just didn't seem appropriate. I just assumed he would anoint the person he deemed most desirable and that would be it. "I can't tell Dr. Stead I want to be his Chief Resident." Hickam responded, "If you want to be a Chief Resident, you're going to have to ask Stead for the position." "OK," I replied, and went to see Dr. Stead. He described how he conceived of the Chief Residency so I'd know what I was getting into, and told me he thought it would be fun to have me as his Chief Resident. I was a little perplexed, because the interview wasn't nearly as traumatic as I had anticipated, it fact, it was almost pleasant.

The best thing Dr. Stead ever taught me occurred as I was just starting the Chief Residency. On the first day in my new position he said, "Bob, I want you to know and understand something that will help you this year: most people do not really want what they say they want." I didn't really understand what he was talking about, but that wasn't unusual. He said, "There will be a lot of things that people will ask you to do or change, that in reality they don't want done or changed at all; they're thinking about something different or they're reacting at that moment in time. Think twice before you make big changes because you'll be sorry later when you find out that the very people who asked for the changes will be the most unhappy with them." And as I look back on my career in medicine, having watched how people did evolve in their careers, he was right. The very people who screamed for change were the most unhappy when they got the change that they screamed for. For instance, a faculty member spending most of his time in research would whine about making less income than one who spent all day seeing patients. When the researcher changed his career around to spend full time in clinical medicine, he would yearn for the good old days of laboratory research.

As it turned out, the Chief Residency at Duke was the icing on my cake. In a sense, I had license to walk about the medical center and look at anything. If I had seen a patient the night before, and there was some disagreement about whether or not he had leukemia, I could walk into the hematology area, where I had previously been the senior resident, and examine the blood slides. I knew enough hematology to be able to interpret the findings without someone else's help. I was equipped with all the tools. I could walk anywhere and look at any interesting problem, picking and choosing what I wanted to learn more about. In that sense, it was a year of total freedom. It was also a very good year because for the first time I was responsible for most of the things that happened on the Medical Service. It was like a super junior residency because I was responsible for the education of all the medical students coming through, and responsible for the housestaff and their education and their health. It was then that I learned that some house officers become so depressed that they can't perform, they literally become paralyzed. They work so hard and yet never finish all the work they want to complete. They become over-tired, depressed and inefficient. I rapidly learned that the Chief Resident's most important job was to identify problems before they became really serious. I strove to appear the wise and bright man and capable leader in front of Stead, who was still my standard. I tried to perform perfectly for him, even though he didn't impose many demands. He was a very benign chief; he never raised hell with me when I was Chief Resident. Occasionally he would bring problems to me, and point out that they needed some thought, but he was really more a colleague, and he had a great sense of humor about problems as they evolved.

As Chief Resident, my contacts broadened not only in the medical center, but in the community, as well. I had to deal with referring physicians in the area, which also meant I was responsible for the referred patients as they came through. Stead let the Chief Resident run the service. Because Duke was dependent upon referring physicians for its financial livelihood, there was precious little criticism, even on a subliminal basis, of what those referring physicians had done or not done in their care of the patient. Very rarely did I ever hear a house officer comment that a community physician had missed an obvious diagnosis or had screwed up the patient's care; the system didn't allow for it. It was a no-no; you didn't call a patient a crock, and you did not criticize an outside physician's performance. When a referring physician wasn't pleased with our work, however, he would send a note to Dr. Stead explaining his dissatisfaction. Then we got a note or a visit from Dr. Stead asking about the patient and explaining why the physician at home was upset.

One particular doctor in the state was very efficient, very compulsive and extremely demanding of the housestaff: let's call him Abner Thompson (not his real name). I don't think he particularly liked Duke, but in the long run, Duke was a valuable resource for his patients who needed complicated procedures like bone marrow tests, cardiac catheterization, or kidney dialysis. On one occasion, Abner sent us a patient with a peculiar illness that he couldn't diagnose; it seemed the man had transient paralysis in his hands and feet. After a thorough work-up we finally decided that the patient was suffering from arsenic poisoning. I was Chief Resident at the time and, aware that the man was Abner Thompson's patient, I said, "We're not going to have any mix-ups with this." Since the patient was ready to be released on a Friday afternoon, I told the junior resident to dictate the discharge summary immediately so we could get it in the mail to Dr. Thompson right away. Our secretary gave the letter top priority, and once it was signed and sealed, we put it in the outgoing mail. The following Monday I got a phone call from Abner Thompson. He was never the most diplomatic person, and when I said hello, he greeted me with, "How dumb are you?" "What do you mean?" I innocently asked. "Well," he went on to explain, "you know that patient I sent over two weeks ago the one you discharged?" "Yes," I replied, "you should be receiving a summary of our final records in a day or two." "I have the records," he assured me, before continuing on. "I see, in retrospect, that he had arsenic poisoning. In fact, I'm sitting in my office with him right now. He's here with his wife and the local sheriff." "Why?" I asked, still confused, "What's the matter?" "Well, his wife tried to poison him again this weekend." Then he let me have it. "Aren't you smart enough to realize that, if a man has come out of an environment where he was poisoned, you shouldn't send him back there? Why didn't you call me up and tell me he'd been poisoned?" I thought to myself, "My god, he's right." And then I had to laugh at myself for this gross oversight. By that point I was confident enough that Stead wouldn't be inflamed about the situation, so I told him the story. He just laughed and said, "Old Abner isn't so dumb, is he?" I had to agree.

Dr. Stead allowed all his Chief Residents to undergo psychoanalysis, and I was no exception. Three times a week I met with Dr. Bingham Dai as part of my advanced training. In the beginning, it wasn't terribly clear to me that it would be valuable, and so I asked Dr. Stead why he wanted me to go. Surprisingly, his answer was a very simple one. "People who are very sick or psychotic don't really benefit much from psychoanalysis," he said. "On the other hand, I've been impressed with the progress that can be made by relatively healthy, productive people. It can make them more productive once they understand themselves."

Working with Dr. Dai turned out to be the most important single item in my housestaff training. We spent most of each session going over what I did every day, and why I reacted to certain stimuli the way I did. Eventually, Dr. Dai built a character analysis for me so that I could see how my behavior was structured. He did this for all of the Chief Residents, and most of the people who underwent analysis agreed that it was the most revealing experience they'd ever had. Each session lasted an hour, during which I would sit back in a lounge chair and talk about myself. I spent the first session giving an autobiographical account of who my parents were, where I was born and where I went to school. From there, the conversation was free floating; I could talk about whatever I wanted to talk about. Dai would ask a few questions here and there to get things going sometimes, but lots of times he didn't do anything. He'd ask me how things were and the rest was up to me.

For six months, Dr. Dai collected data from me, making notes on "5x8" cards as I talked. Then, over the next six months, as I described how my day was and what problems I might have had either running the service or at home, he began to pull out the little bits of information that I had given him and to weave them all together. He drew connections between the background information I had given him and the problems of my current life, and ask if I thought one had anything to do with the other. He was a master at recalling things; he would point out how my family background or past educational experience had, in a sense, positioned me to react in a particular way to a given situation. It took the mystery out of my behavior.

I was extremely compulsive when I was Chief Resident, and expected the housestaff under me to be, too. However, we had our share of lackadaisical residents who weren't as concerned with taking a complete history as I wanted them to be. Gaps in needed information would come out at the history meetings, and, although I didn't consider it a reflection on me personally, it bothered me terribly that I couldn't have a perfect history meeting. Dr. Dai and I discussed this over and over again. He asked me why perfection was so important to me. The patient was alive, he was home and everything was all right; what difference did checking the stool for blood make? And the more I tried to explain my reaction, the more inane it sounded. Eventually I began to wonder why I was getting so upset, which ultimately lessened my demands on other people. But it was harder to ease up on my expectations for myself.

I slept in the hospital five nights out of seven, not because I had to but because I wanted to know everything that was happening every minute of every day. I not only wanted to be a good Chief Resident, I wanted the housestaff to know that their Chief Resident was there, to inspire them to perform well. And I loved being in the hospital; it was a tremendously exciting place to be. I also loved golf and I played whenever I could, but I decided that I was not going to play golf while I was Chief Resident. For me it was like putting on sackcloth. Dr. Dai was extremely interested in why I had given up something so important to me. In fact, golf was not the only enjoyment I had relinquished during my Chief Residency. I hadn't thought that much about it, but Dai was persistent in wanting to know why I was sacrificing everything to be Chief Resident. I argued that I didn't have the time, but that wasn't true; I could have played golf every afternoon because I was "off" and it wouldn't have mattered. In fact, I had an inner standard I felt I had to live up to, one that I believed was the yardstick Dr. Stead used to measure my performance. Stead was the source of all my anxiety and all my satisfaction at that time. My mind and feelings were really intertwined with how I thought he viewed my performance. I couldn't allow myself to do something that didn't support the standards I believed Stead expected from me. In retrospect, I realize they were not Dr. Stead's standards at all, but an unachievable goal that I had internalized. As Dr. Dai was able to show me, very little went on internally without a reason.

Dr. Stead was relatively mellow by the time I came along (at least compared to the rumors about his first years at Duke), but he still was capable of acting quickly on an issue. And it did not always result in the best or even the fairest decision. In my junior year, Dr. Stead fired a junior resident despite having previously appointed him to become a senior resident. Since I was close to the situation, it made a lasting impression on me. The event had to do with golf. I was playing with three other residents, one of whom was on call on Nott Ward. It was a beautiful spring day, and he asked a colleague working on another ward to cover any problems that might arise while he was out. This is commonplace nowadays, but then, if you were on, you were on. None of this signing-out-to-a-colleague. You didn't even get a haircut without permission. As it happened, a patient with meningitis was admitted to Nott Ward, but the covering resident got the situation under control and by the time we returned from the golf course, the patient was being treated appropriately. Everything had worked out smoothly and we didn't give it another thought. But Dr. Stead learned that the resident had gone out and left someone else to cover, and quite a scene ensued. In the end, the resident was asked to leave. From the resident's perspective, it was difficult to understand what the fuss was all about. The patient had been treated correctly, and was going to recover without any complications. But we were imbued with a sense that the patient was our responsibility, and that there was no excuse for shirking that responsibility; the patient was the bottom-line; the patient was the reason we were here. When you're young, you often don't know the possible effects of lackadaisical decisions; if young and inexperienced doctors were allowed to make ill-informed decisions, not every patient would be well cared for. The system is more forgiving now, but I think we have lost something in the training of young doctors. Still, if I were Chief Resident today, I think I would be out on the green every afternoon. After all, we were in the hospital late every night.

The Chief Residency was, in a sense, a three-year tour of duty. The actual year of service as Chief Resident might come at the start of the tour, or it might be the 3rd year; the other two years were to be used to do whatever we wanted. It was like a laboratory scholarship that allowed us to decide what kind of work we wanted to do. I started my three-year stint as the Chief Resident and then I spent two years in the cardiac catheterization lab. It was a busy and exciting time. Cineangiography, making radiographic movies to visualize the valves and chambers of the living heart, had just come along, and Henry McIntosh was very excited about this. We acquired a good cineangiograph and, fortunately for us, the radiologists at Duke didn't know enough to buy one of these machines, so we didn't have any real competition. Elsewhere, these units were set up in Radiology, so the cardiologists had less chance to work with them. We got to look at all the interesting cardiac cases and it was a productive time for research because almost everything we did was new.

Stead was always interested in what we were doing. After the first year, Stead asked me how things were going and what I wanted to do; I told him I was interested in staying in academic medicine. He said he thought I could probably make it in academic medicine, but that I ought to recognize that there would be no place for me at Duke after I finished up my fellowship. He told me very succinctly that my skills were too similar to those of Henry McIntosh, and that, while I was good at my job, Duke didn't need two people with the same skills. That was tough coming from the Chief, but I understood, and I fully expected to be looking for a job somewhere at the end of my fellowship. In the meantime, we really did very well with cineangiography, and our reputation rapidly spread. We got a very large grant for a brand new cineangiograph and then a large program project grant to look at some important questions with our new equipment. All of a sudden, Duke went from having too many people in the cardiac cath lab to needing more hands. Henry McIntosh asked me to stay. He'd talked to Stead who wanted to keep me on at a salary of $7,500 per year. This was a large increase over the $3,000 I earned as Chief Resident, but I still thought it was low because I knew that a full faculty member would have gotten $9,600. I told Stead so. We went around and around on the issue until he closed the discussion by telling me to think about it. It seemed, however, that Dr. Stead was the one who took his own advice because the next day his secretary, Bess Cebe, called and said, "Dr. Stead thinks your argument has some merit." I

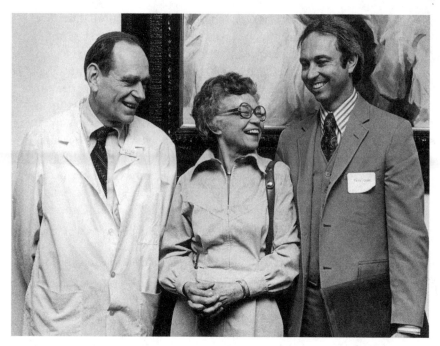

Dr. Stead with his long-time and ever-important secretary, Bess Cebe, and her son, Pete Cebe.

said, "Bess, just tell me is he going to give me $9,600?" and she said, "That's basically what he means." I don't think he wanted to admit that he had to give in, but I'm glad he did. I stayed in the lab for 8 years and had a lot of fun.

As I look at Stead's career, the most interesting thing to me is how much he's changed. I came along in the late 1950s, at the tail-end of his really vituperative period. He had done some very difficult things to get the Department of Medicine turned around, and while he certainly didn't endear himself to everyone in the process, he was respected and even feared. By the time I arrived, he was more of a senior statesman and he cared more about people. I didn't meet many doctors who dealt with him in the late 1940s who thought he gave a damn about anybody. But once he had the department under control, he loosened the reins a little.

Stead's methods evolved over the years. In the beginning, he was what I would call a hard-ball politician. He over-prepared for meetings and for negotiations with hospital administrators, and he won because he had the guns. Later, when he had assembled his team, he won because he had the people. The former Chief of Pediatrics, never a friend of Stead's, observed that Stead got everything he wanted because he always had a young faculty person to plug in the spot that was to be created. He always had a young person to put up for every new appointment or a new project or new grant. And so he won all the battles.

As Stead's time as Chairman neared an end, he had to develop new tactics. He knew that, if he was to accomplish his goals without the leverage of being department chair, everybody had to get something out of the deal. His very original ideas about the use of computers in medicine were a major contribution to the Medical Center, but he wasn't going to persuade people to give up their old methods unless they were going to get something in return. There had to be a significant payoff in patient care, research and education—and the scheme had to be self-supporting. It's like the old baseball adage: it isn't a good trade unless both teams gain from it! Knowing how to manage that requires good political skills. And he was extremely skillful.

On the other hand, he could still revert to his old form sometimes, even after retiring as chairman. He would play hardball, if he thought it would help him win. He would cajole or coerce, threaten or do whatever was necessary to accomplish what he thought was right. I still have a letter he wrote me about a project on which he wanted my help. He wanted all the cardiologists to get computer-generated "prognostigrams" on all patients who were admitted with chest pain. The computer generated these prognostigrams by comparing certain key data elements (symptoms, ECG and cardiac cath findings) to a large database of patients with chest pain due to different types of coronary artery disease. The computer would list the outcomes in all similar patients so we could predict how the new patient would respond to treatment. The idea was to predict how coronary bypass surgery or heart medicine would work in a new patient, based on how similar patients had done in the past. We were a little hesitant about this because each patient would be charged (and Stead would collect) $43 for information that, while useful, did not seem to be anything we didn't already know because we had analyzed the data. But Stead was adamant. He was to chair a grant review session for the Prudential Insurance company and he wanted very much to be able to tell Prudential that every cardiologist at Duke used this tool every day with every patient in the hospital.

One of our independent clinicians said, "The hell with that. I am not going to use it on every patient. It's a waste of the patient's money and it isn't warranted." I was stuck in the middle and Stead wrote me one of his succinct letters:

Dear Bob,

I understand Dr. Smith is unwilling to say he'll use the prognostigram with every patient. Unless he changes his mind by next Tuesday, when Prudential is coming down for their visit, you'll be running the visit.

Gene

That's hardball!

CHAPTER 17

A Second Career as Editor

For better or worse, editing is what editors are for; and editing is
selection and choice of material.
> Warren E. Burger, Chief Justice, US Supreme Court

During his long career in and beyond academic medicine, Eugene Stead
served as Editor of three journals: *Medical Times*, *Circulation*, and the *North Carolina Medical Journal*. His tenure at each of these positions was in adjunction to
his continuing activities in medical education and health care. Still, each of these
jobs gave him an opportunity to articulate his vision of modern medicine and
to leave his distinctive imprint on the organizations that sponsored the journals.

The first stint was at *Medical Times*, which published articles of general medical interest to family doctors, and was made available *gratis* because advertis-
ing revenues supported its printing and distribution. In December of 1965, Per-
rin H. Long, the incumbent Editor, died unexpectedly; it is not clear why the
publishers of this "throwaway" journal turned to Stead, or why he would be interested in doing something he had not tried before. However, never one to hide
his light under a bushel ("I have to say, looking back over it, Gene Stead always
had a pretty good notion of himself. I was never very humble."), he doubtless
relished the thoughts of a public forum from which to set out his views on medical education and health care in general. Furthermore, the opportunity came
at a propitious time: Stead had already declared his intention to resign leadership of the department at Duke in 1967, and the job would allow him to try his
wings in a new venture as well as to supplement his retirement income.

Beginning in March of 1966 and for the next 53 months, his name appeared at the top of the masthead and on the editorial pages of each monthly
issue of *Medical Times*. Each issue carried a column, entitled "Read in Good
Stead," which consisted of capsule summaries of several papers or books recently read by the Editor and which he considered of enough general importance to share with his readership. A perusal of the 250 or more papers cited
shows the breadth and range of his reading: cardiology, of course, but endocrinology and metabolism often, along with infectious diseases, pediatrics,

and a smattering of legal and ethical topics. Often Stead inserted some comment from his personal experience, and usually some wry twist was applied to the summary, either in the text or in the title. The subjects chosen give us a glimpse of Stead the scholar and thinker, the visionary and man of practicality, always with a sense that the subject reviewed would (or *should*) be of interest to all his readers. Like reading someone else's mail, these very brief summaries give us a window into the personal side of a professional mind.

Even more revealing are the editorials prepared by Stead for the Journal. Each issue had an entry on what soon came to be titled the "Editor's Page," and Stead provided 9 or 10 a year (the others were contributed by guest editorialists, usually his associate editor, Charles A. Ragan Jr.). Stead was pleased with the opportunity to put his ideas on display in the public arena, and remained proud of what he did to the end ("some of the best things I wrote"). The titles (see Table) again open a window onto who Stead was and how he looked at the world. The topics ranged from recollections of his time as a young man at the Thorndike Lab to his vision of how health care might be financed and what doctors should do and think about in their day-to-day work with patients.

Dr. Stead:

> Frequently I paid a small fee [to a contributor] if I wanted a particular article from a particular person; I bought a few of the lead articles, which provided the journal with a number of well-known physicians as authors. It gave the illusion that all kinds of doctors liked to submit journal articles to the *Medical Times*. I didn't spend a whole lot of money, and what I did spend was carefully thought about, because the management of *Medical Times* was very good. You see, we kept the general level of the journal sufficiently high that many people simply sent articles to us. In other words, I used what money I spent as a trap to make the unwary send manuscripts to us.
>
> Of course, I was the sole determinant of whether papers sent to us got published or not. And I kept in mind that that *Medical Times* was a throw-away journal, but with a standing that other throw-away journals didn't have. And we were highly successful in that. I wrote editorials, and I enjoyed writing them—some of them are pretty good still. I enjoyed the whole enterprise, kept at it until 1970. I'd have to say that, in the early days, the people publishing *Medical Times* were pretty good. Eventually they began to die off, and when I became Distinguished Physician at the VA, I said, "I'm not sure that this journal is not past its prime, and I think that I'm going to have

Titles of Editorials by Eugene A. Stead Jr., in *Medical Times*, 1966–1970

Challenges And Opportunities
Your National Library Of Medicine
The Many Facets Of Asbestosis
Hypertension—Highways And By-
 ways
Looking At The Heart In 1966
Intern And Residency Training
Hyperbaria
On Bacterial Endocarditis
Reversible "Madness"
"Good Will Towards Men"
Health Manpower
The Lung
Quality Of Medical Care
Traps And Stratagems of Diagnosis
Thinking Ward Rounds
Patients That Recover
Prevention Of Myocardial Infarction
Postural Hypotension
The Rights Of The Foetus
The Birth Of A New Educational
 Venture— The Association Of
 Schools Of Allied Health Profes-
 sionals
The Delivery Of Health Care
More Knowledge About The Renal
 Factors Influencing Sodium Re-
 tention
Myocardial Infarction—The First
 Fifteen Minutes

Health And Illness
A College-Based Physician's Assis-
 tant Program
Cost Conscious Doctors
The Need For A Machine Process-
 able Medical Data Base
Words Make Pictures
The Assets Of A Community Hospital
Picking Other Peoples' Brains
To Manage Or Not To Manage
A National Academy Of Medicine
Space Biology And Medicine—An
 Unmet Challenge
The Physician's Assistant—Job De-
 scription And Licensing
Public Assistance And Society
The White Bear Syndrome
Why Moon Walking Is Simpler Than
 Social Progress
"Clinical Trials" For Proposed Legis-
 lation
Congestive Failure Revisited
Angina Pectoris Teaches
"Origin Of The Species"
Dialogue In California
Universal Service—A Necessity And
 An Opportunity
"If I Become Ill And Unable To
 Manage My Own Affairs"
Up The Health Staircase

enough money and enough to do, and I think I'll just stop editing."
So I resigned from *Medical Times*, and I think I probably did it at just
the right time.

The Editor's pen lay idle for a few years until the American Heart Association's
journal, *Circulation*, began looking for a new Editor. By the start of 1973 the
committee had made its decision and the journal announced on its cover that
potential contributors should send their manuscripts to Stead.

Dr. Stead:

Well, the Editorial Board approached me about the job, and I told them that *Circulation* was potentially the leading cardiovascular journal, but it had a very long turnaround time. By the time you had anything published in it, you know, it was already out of date. I told the committee: "I don't really know whether you want me as an editor or not. First, you must remember I'm not a card-carrying cardiologist. I've done quite a lot of research in the cardiovascular field, but I'm really not a practicing cardiologist. And you've got to appreciate the fact that my interests are broader than yours, and I will publish, if I'm the editor, things that will amaze you, that you just never would have thought of publishing. And the only thing you will be able to say is 'Well, we've got a kind of crazy editor, so don't worry about it.'

"Secondly, I will set up a system in which every manuscript that comes into this office will be attached to a reviewer on the day it arrives, and I'll have the shortest turnaround time between acceptance and publication of any major journal. That will be possible because I will have an editorial assistant who knows that no manuscript will sit unmailed, and we will have a careful record of who actually wants to review articles and do it well. People who say they'll do it will never get another chance if they don't do it well the first time."

Thirdly, I told them that, like any other editor, if I got a paper with a brand new idea that broke the common mould, "I'd reject it like any other editor. I'm not God, I'm just Gene Stead!" I said, "If you want to put up with these problems, I'll take the job for five years." And they did, and I enjoyed it.

Stead set about assembling a team of Associate Editors (Drs. Victor S. Behar, Richard G. Lester, Patrick A. McKee, and Harold C. Strauss, all at Duke), but the all-important position was that of Assistant Editor, who would oversee the day-to-day management of the journal. For this position Stead selected Patricia K. (Penny) Hodgson.

Dr. Stead:

Well, it was perfectly clear that I had to have people that knew something about manuscripts. I called up UNC and talked to the head of the University Press. And he said, "I've got a wife I've trained carefully. She takes no initiative, she just does what I ask her to do, but she does it very well. She's available, if you want to offer her a job." So I called up Penny, and I knew perfectly well that her husband wasn't going to like what I did, because the general notion that she would do only what I told her to do seemed absurd to me. If that's all she was going to do, I didn't need anybody! So, without telling him that I was going to tear his system apart, I got Penny to come over. She liked me, I liked her, and we took over *Circulation*.

Stead soon set about to deliver his promise of a rapid turnaround in submitted manuscripts. Volume 48, the first volume edited by Stead, contains 119 Original Articles and lists the names of 288 individuals who served as reviewers during that six-month period. Toward the end of his tenure, Volume 56, with fewer pages than Vol 48, contains 143 Original Articles and names 452 reviewers, many of whom read 2–4 articles each. Clearly Stead had attracted and kept a cadre of reviewers who vied for the honor to work for him under his rules. Clearly, too, he had attracted many more submitted manuscripts from which to select.

Dr. Stead:

> All medical journals have a long delay between submission of the manuscript and publication, but we just chopped the time off of that. The manuscript went out for review the day it came in, and reviewers knew that, unless the review was done quickly and done well, they would never be asked to review again. I kept a record, so I knew how long they took, and I knew the quality of each review; I was not hesitant to simply say: "He'll never get another manuscript."
>
> If I didn't want but one review, I didn't have to have two. But in general we tried to have two reviews. We valued the reviewers' opinions, but every now and again I made a decision against my reviewer, because my frame of reference was frequently better. When it came to decisions about publishing, you know, I was the chief editor. Don't forget that! We became the most desirable cardiovascular publication in the world.

In contrast to his visible presence on the pages of *Medical Times*, Stead's name is conspicuously absent from *Circulation*. In fact, his name is only listed three times in the indexes of the 10 volumes he edited. He was content to put his stamp on the mechanics of running the journal office and let the product speak for itself. That changed once again when he took over the editorship of the *North Carolina Medical Journal*.

After a five-year hiatus in editing, Stead was approached in 1982 by Dr. Charles Styron, a Raleigh-based practitioner and former president of the North Carolina Medical Society, who was chair of the *Journal's* Editorial Board. The *Journal* was in dire straits. A large percentage of Society members were indifferent about its publication and a vocal minority was clamoring for its dissolution. Manuscripts were in short supply, and those that were in hand were dull and repetitious. Would Dr. Stead, Styron wanted to know, be willing to take over the Journal and breathe some life into it? Stead agreed, but with several provisos: the editorial office would have to be based in Durham not Raleigh; he would be allowed to appoint a Managing Editor who would report directly to him, not to the executive director of the Medical Society; they would have to pay him more than they thought an editor deserved; and, finally, the name was to be changed to read "*North Carolina Medical Journal: for Doctors and Their Patients.*" Styron enthusiastically agreed, and took on the Herculean task of negotiating the agreement through the political minefield of the Medical Society. This he did successfully, and in 1982, Stead became Editor with Penny Hodgson as Managing Editor.

Stead's inaugural editorial outlined the five "objectives" that comprised his vision for the *Journal*. As a manifesto for a true medical journal, these seem as valid today as they did then:

> 1. Presentation of interesting clinical material by young authors who need to try their wings and develop skills in communication. I hope this material will be crisp and to the point. I want each report to highlight a single nugget of learning derived from clinical practice.
>
> 2. Presentation of new and old ways developed by North Carolina doctors to enhance services to patients.
>
> 3. Presentation of socioeconomic issues pertinent to the North Carolina scene.
>
> 4. Preservation of North Carolina medical history, past and present. The *Journal* is available in libraries throughout the country and is the only place where historical material can be placed with assurance that it will always be available.
>
> 5. Presentation of material of interest to our patients and the large number of persons in doctors' offices and in hospitals who make possible the delivery of care by doctors. This section will appear in the center of the *Journal* and will be printed on blue paper.

In addition the those five points, the editorial outlined the fiscal steps taken by Dr. Stead to improve the solvency of the *Journal*: a contract with a new printer who promised more rapid and less costly turnaround times, and the use of less costly paper stock on which to print the journal. Finally, he pointed out his need for unsolicited manuscripts of sufficient quality to warrant publication. He was sure that he did not want to run a "journal of last resort," where local authors sent only their most mediocre papers, ones that had failed publication everywhere else. Stead was well known throughout the state of North Carolina and his name still had a cachet, but he pointed out to his readers that because "of my long association with Duke and the fact that I still have a number of 'green stamps' outstanding, I can garner material from Duke with little difficulty. I need your help to balance out the Duke Mafia."

Styron's gambit was successful. He and Stead resuscitated the *Journal*, and Stead served as Editor until 1992.

Dr. Stead:

> You see, what had finally happened [before I took over] was that the content of the *NC Medical Journal* was being written by the staff, which is not a good way to produce any journal. And of course it became less and less relevant to any of the practicing physicians. But Charlie Styron thought that discontinuance of the *Journal* would be a sign that organized medicine was taking a setback. So Charlie Styron went to the editorial board and said that he would like to take one last crack at finding a different editor. Since he was pretty good in the organized medical world, they said, okay, we'll give you a year, and if you change that journal it'll be remarkable. He said, okay, let me look around. So he called me and said what his problem was, and I said, well, you know, Gene Stead just might take the challenge if you wanted him to do it.
>
> I proposed that we designate the *Journal* as being "for doctors and their patients." The Society said, "Patients shouldn't be reading the *Journal*." I said, "That's crazy, you know. You can't practice medicine without those patients, and patients need doctors, so the *Journal* ought to be for doctors and their patients. They finally came around and said "Okay, it seems a little crazy to us but if you insist we'll do it."
>
> And we did pretty well, but when Charlie Styron died, that made a difference. Charlie really was a very helpful man. He was just smarter than most of the Medical Society. Otherwise I never would have been involved with the *Journal*. Well, I enjoyed that, too.

Stead stepped down as Editor in 1992. He had completed nearly 20 years in charge of three remarkably different journals. He made his mark at each.

CHAPTER 18

ELECTRONIC TEXTBOOK OF MEDICINE

The technological revolution will come only when doctors or groups of doctors using computer technology have a clear advantage in practice over doctors who maintain the status quo. There is need for a careful delineation of an important problem that has no solution other than computerization.

E. A. Stead Jr.

Dr. Stead was one of the foremost advocates of using computers in medicine, particularly cardiology. His early grasp of the importance of prognosis (identifying the characteristics that would, for instance, predict who would do well after a heart attack and who would not) brought home the need to relate massive quantities of data. But how could a physician crack the computer world, where funding was controlled by computer scientists? Could such a system, once developed, be self-sustaining? The ideas came rapidly; the opportunities came more slowly—but when they came, Gene Stead was ready.

Dr. Robert Grant graduated from Cornell Medical School and interned at the Brigham with Jim Warren. As a student, he became interested in electrocardiography and worked with a Dr. Stuart, who was in charge of electrocardiography at Cornell's New York Hospital. Like most young doctors, Bob had a long stint in the military during World War II and afterwards went back to Cornell, but he had a falling out with Stuart who didn't like Bob's view of electrocardiography. One day, Gene Stead returned home from a short trip to find Bob Grant in his laboratory at Grady Hospital. He'd always liked Bob, and they got caught up with each other's news. Afterwards Stead said, "You're welcome to stay around a while if you want to but I've got work to do," and he left. A few weeks later it dawned on him that Bob Grant was still there. So he approached him saying, "Bob, what are you going to do? You must need some kind of job," and Grant said, "I've got a job, I work for you." It turned out that Warren and his colleagues had hired Bob while Stead was away. So Bob Grant

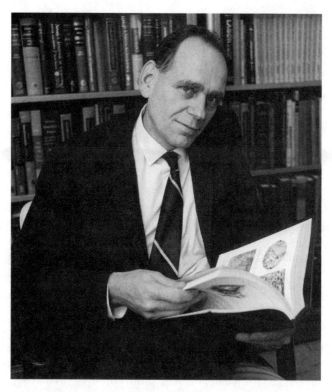

Eugene Stead, photographed while visiting the University of Florida.

stayed at Grady, and he and Harvey Estes, who was just beginning his career in cardiology, wrote a classic book on electrocardiography.

Stead had special respect for Grant because he was the first person to figure out that not every change in the ECG indicated damaged heart muscle. The system that conducts the electrical impulse through the heart could alone be damaged and produce changes ordinarily associated with severe heart attack. Bob Grant became a leader in electrocardiography and, eventually, Director of the National Heart Institute where he and Stead were to meet again.

At the National Heart Institute, Grant became interested in the care of patients with myocardial infarction. It seemed to him that there were no really meaningful treatments for heart attacks; patients were simply admitted to an institution, put to bed and told not to move while somebody fed them and helped with the bedpan, and they either lived or died. The system was at a standstill, with no investigation at all into whether specific treatments could make any difference in the outcome of infarction. Patients were diagnosed with an infarct, ECG changes documented the fact, and that was it. Grant thought it was time to try to find out what really went on, and if anything could be done. In the mid-1960s, when the first Coronary Care Units were just emerging, he persuaded the NIH to set up study groups in the USA and in England to observe the results of treatment for myocardial infarction. Gene Stead was asked to head the survey team and to come up with recommendations about active treatment of heart attack victims. The survey team would comprise a small group of cardiologists and a cardiovascular surgeon; Bob Grant and a young cardiologist would serve as NIH staff representatives. Unfortunately, Bob Grant died, and Stuart Bondurant took over his role in co-ordinating the study.

Dr. Stead:

> We found out that there were some things that clearly could be done to learn more about heart attacks and their management. We had the feeling that if the NIH supported a clinical staff to actually do some research in these areas, the system would get off dead center, and we would move forward in the field of heart attacks. So Bob Grant had been right.
>
> We were beginning to see that patients could be studied and that meaningful observations could be made and that the field could be opened, primarily by young investigators—if funding was available. Myocardial Infarction Research Units (MIRU) grew out of our survey; teams were assembled to carry out innovative research on the subject. A MIRU unit was formed at Duke with Andy Wallace as its Director. The NIH gave us a lot of money over many years to study heart attacks.
>
> From the beginning I was interested in the record keeping system. It seemed to me that, in general, we were tied to a process analysis, and if you wanted to know whether an institution was practicing good medicine in a particular specialty area, you went to the chart and looked to see if they took a history, recorded the physical exam, and made progress notes about the laboratory and x-ray findings. But nobody really knew how to handle a large amount of data so that it could be stored and coordinated over time. It seemed to me, that if we were going to start a new clinical research endeavor in heart disease, we should pay much more attention to how the information was collated and handled and stored so that it wouldn't be lost, as was otherwise bound to happen. I had a gut feeling that this was a serious deficiency in most clinical activities, but we weren't very smart about how to do this at first. Since nobody was making observations

in that area, it gave us the opportunity to develop a different kind of data system.

At Duke, we were able to get what we wanted for our MIRU; my leadership role in the overall national study probably helped in this regard. But we had trouble breaking into computer-oriented activities, because it took a fair amount of money. We needed a special air-conditioned room to house the equipment and the machinery was not only big but it required a lot of maintenance. At that time, doctors knew very little about computers so you had to have a separate staff to operate them. And the computer scientists who had gotten in on this activity early on had cornered all the money so there was none for the late-comers. A track record of achievement ordinarily would be needed to justify a grant application for a study to use the computer. However, the NIH agreed to pay for computer activities and expertise at participating institutions that expressed a strong interest in using computers to study infarcts, regardless of whether they had a track record of past accomplishments. Essentially we qualified for a computer facility just because we were willing to have people devote their time and effort to making observations in this area, even before we had established investigators. The NIH also was willing to make some equipment available before we had proved that we knew how to use the equipment. And so Duke ended up with a fairly sophisticated computer operation.

Following the conventional wisdom of the time, the first thing we did was to automate the Cardiac Intensive Care Unit. And we discovered that we could produce reams of data, but that it was an extraordinarily expensive operation because all the data had to be handled, collated, charted and interpreted by personnel. We generated far more data than we needed, but could not reduce the heavy personnel demands of a traditional medical unit. This was not an efficient service and once we discovered it wasn't profitable, we quit. But then we had the computer system and the question was how to use it efficiently. I looked around to see what we could do with the computer that would be useful, an activity we couldn't do without. Once we could determine that, we would get out of the argument of cost-effectiveness and start dealing with what we wanted to learn.

The first thing I could think of was the need to predict patient outcomes, or to identify the factors that relate to survival in infarcts. Medicine, as practiced in Duke Hospital, gave you outcomes on a short-term basis—whether or not your patients recovered enough to go home from the hospital—but never gave you long-term outcomes. Therefore, to determine whether we were practicing medicine correctly, we depended on whether we were doing the correct procedures, not on whether we got better results. I thought that the computer could act as a slow motion camera, following a patient for eight or ten years and then compressing and manipulating the data, using the same analysis that you ordinarily use to follow the person with acute illness for a week. That was my hope for a method of studying procedures and treatments of myocardial infarcts.

Most people in the medical computing business were going one of two ways: toward the automation of intensive care units (which we didn't want to do) or toward using the computer to make diagnoses and leave the doctor out of the system. That didn't appeal to us either because there were relatively few diagnoses that even the medical student hadn't made by the end of 48 hours. It's amazing how few possibilities are left that haven't already been thought of in the course of working up the patient. Obviously there are some situations where the analysis is wrong and the diagnosis is missed, but that's a minute part of clinical practice. If you look at the total picture in geological time, it doesn't make a difference whether you make those rarely missed diagnoses or not. I felt we should tackle something that the doctor couldn't do—carry long-term information that would allow us to sort patients into groups with similar characteristics and determine the kinds of treatment they had, and whether over many years anything we did to them affected the outcomes.

Rather than going the route Jack Myers went in Pittsburgh (using computers in diagnosis), I thought long-term tracking of patients would be more profitable. But it was a judgment call on my part and the verdicts are not in. There are more people who think like Jack did than who think like I do. I may still turn out to be on the wrong side of the equation, but I really thought it would be most useful to get information that you wanted but couldn't get from any other source. If you wanted to write a textbook about any illness, you found yourself with more questions than answers, and in the end, textbooks contain a remarkable amount of guesswork. We were willing to put our eggs into the basket of belief that good clinicians will make sufficiently accurate diagnoses most of the time. As long as we are talking about serious disease, from an overall point of view, the errors are irrelevant, and the error margin becomes less as the effort put into solving a problem becomes greater. We planned to focus on common diseases, like heart attacks, which were expensive to the individual and society; it seemed crazy to set up a system to monitor people over time if it would not be cost-effective, and equally crazy to study illnesses from which people recover on their own, like infections. But it seemed sensible to examine areas where large sums of money were being spent to see if they were being spent wisely and to determine what was being accomplished by the expenditure. We accepted as fact that diagnoses were being made by humans who liked to make them, and we began to work instead on the problem of prognosis, to try to predict the outcomes of different kinds of treatments given to different kinds of patients.

In my experience with the housestaff and students, the question of how you care for the patients depended, to a tremendous degree, on the patient's socio-economic and cultural background. That always seemed rather obvious to me, but most doctors did not recognize how their treatment decisions were influenced by non-scientific factors. My decision to concentrate on prognosis also depended on the fact that a diagnosis has an extraordinarily broad range. Within any given diagnostic category, say myocardial infarction, there are people who will die within a minute and people who live thirty years. Therefore the notion that the correct diagnosis would help you predict the future for an individual patient seemed foolish. In order to benefit from such information, you had to break the diagnosis down into more finite categories than you could ever get from standard diagnostic groupings, and the only way to tell whether you had broken them down correctly was to see what happened to patients in those separate categories. In general, if you group people who are alike, there ought to be some commonality of outcome. If you think they're alike at first and then they turn out to behave very differently, it's clear you didn't know how to determine like and unlike kinds of patients.

It seemed to us that the medicine of the future would give up diagnostic categories, and focus instead on how many patient characteristics to collect. The process would depend upon a judgment call of the doctor, who would subsequently be able to modify the amount of data he needed to know and what tests to order. If he decided a patient had a common cold, and later the patient got a chill and a bad headache and couldn't stretch his neck, then the initial data were not sufficient; the doctor would need to collect more data from additional tests. But I really thought eventually, instead of having diseases characterized the way we label them today, each disease would be listed individually. A young man who suffers a myocardial infarction with little impairment of heart muscle function and no disturbance of heart rhythm has a totally different prognosis than a fragile diabetic whose infarct caused marked rhythm and muscle disturbance. There is no point in saying both patients have the same disease (myocardial infarction), because it doesn't describe their individual illnesses. Collecting only a few characteristics from a very large group of people in whom lots of things might happen allows for too much variation to predict outcome. But as we begin to collect more and more characteristics on our patients, we have to consider how many markers to collect because each costs money. There are a considerable number of variables that need to be determined in order to find common outcomes. Once we know the important ones then it would be very simple to identify who has these markers and what happens to them.

The potential for savings was first realized on a study of patients with myocardial infarction who shared certain characteristics. We looked at people who were kept in the hospital for a period of time after their infarcts, and determined the number who suffered complications for which hospital care was useful. After we had entered information on a lot of patients into the data bank, we picked another group of patients with myocardial infarcts and tested the mathematical formula we derived from the first group to see if the formula we established predicted their subsequent complications or recovery. Eventually, we gained confidence in our ability to tell which patients would do well and then we studied the effect of early discharge of those patients. Prior to that time, every patient who had suffered an infarct was kept in the hospital for several weeks, but we discovered that people with certain characteristics would do just as well if they were sent home days earlier. It saved the patients a lot of money and curiously, also made Duke a lot of money because the more rapid the turnover of beds, the greater the profit.

All the effort being put into making more and more precise diagnosis of heart attack is going to be wasted at some point because the benefits really stop at diagnosis. Prognosis, although more useful, is infinitely more difficult to accomplish than diagnosis. It's harder to set up the system to monitor patients over time and to collect data in a systematic fashion. And until enough patients have been followed for enough years to get answers, this system suffers from the tremendous disadvantage of having no gain in it. These are costly programs and are not systems to be set up lightly. I understood from the beginning that the data system could not be built as a research endeavor. In our society, research grants are awarded by research committees, which decide what is exciting, novel and well-designed. And while you never know what a committee will consider worthy of funding, you can be absolutely certain that they aren't going to want to fund what they had funded before. They might fund it once, but probably not repeatedly. So a long-term project like a data bank needed stable rather than sporadic or unpredictable funding.

One of the great advantages of an ongoing data system to document clinical practice is that it captures the changes that occur in practice over time. The nature of the clientele can change and so can the treatment. Our coronary care population, for example, is undergoing dramatic changes. We admit more patients earlier after infarction because they are flown by helicopter for special tests that are not available in community hospitals, and which had not been developed when our computer project began. A static system would not be very useful to us because our medical world is changing so rapidly. An extensive program will be required to train individuals who work with the computer project, and it will be ten years before the first products of such a training program reach a position of authority within the hierarchy and can really change the system. Because this is necessarily a slow process and you can't fund it totally as research, the money for the program has to come from the patient care system, and the practice has to have enough private patients to yield meaningful data, including the important years of follow-up information. A city hospital patient population wouldn't be appropriate because you are not likely to see the patients again once they leave the hospital. It would need to be done in a place like Duke, which has sufficient numbers of private patients. I do believe that this is going to be the medicine of the future. It will permit doctors to tailor treatment to the individual patient and not treat everyone alike, just because they have the same diagnosis.

Furthermore, I think that office practice is going to change and computers will be needed to keep track of patients and treatments. There's a tremendous amount of pressure in keeping up with all that a doctor has to keep up with. The average doctor today has got to serve five times as many patients as he had to serve ten years ago in order to stay economically even. That means he's got to remember five times as many routine mammograms, he's got five times as many patients to follow to find out whether they are complying with his prescribed treatments. The profit margin is roughly a fifth of what it was, due to changes in Medicare and insurance reimbursement for medical services. The private practice of medicine is being pinched on the community level because of restricted payment by insurance companies, and because increasing numbers of patients are going to large medical centers for their care. Large hospitals like Duke will be pinched as Medicare and other reimbursement programs tighten up the criteria of what they will pay for and further limit how much they will pay.

The Electronic Textbook of Medicine got its start because I saw it as a vital tool for justifying the care that we give to patients, and for measuring the quantity and cost of procedures and medical decisions. The fact that we were able to begin the project depended on my having the clout to raise the money. I couldn't do it today, and shouldn't be able to because I am no longer in a position of power and authority. Everybody has his day; I'm not fussing about that. The problem with financing a unit like that was that we were always over-financed, which meant that we had no secure line item budget source. If you have a secure source of money, even a small source, you can use it very intelligently. If you don't have a secure source you have to cover yourself from every which way, requesting money from many different sources, and that leads to waste. We would have been a better unit if we'd had less money and more stability. With less money that you are certain of getting, you can make long range plans and wait for the data to mature before writing preliminary papers to help justify a grant renewal. You can also be more selective in recruiting because you can offer a more stable job, which is always attractive.

I do believe that, in the future, clinical information will be stored in the electronic textbook. It is easily formatted and accessible, making it possible to generate a record for a given patient and to analyze the records and outcomes of other patients with histories like the one in your office at the moment. This is a powerful source of information, one that can become invaluable. I think it will be stored in a central library with a series of regional centers for collecting and processing the available information for everybody to use. But I think that kind of a system is probably 25 years away. It can't really become widely available until the generation that developed the system begins to use it.

The use of computers is foreign to doctors who learned to practice in the absence of a good record keeping system. One of the peculiar obstacles to the use of computers is that medical practice is doing well, even though the doctor hasn't the foggiest notion of what he's doing. People come to him and he does what he's always done; he makes notes, but if he wants to know something about what really happened to patients with a specific problem, he doesn't obtain the information from factual records. Instead, he calls one of his colleagues and asks, "What do you remember about this," and his colleague replies, "I've seen two people like that in the last 20 years and both of them lived." If you take the trouble to check it out, you discover that in fact he hasn't seen anybody like your patient, and that everyone with similar problems seen at Duke Hospital died. Misinformation doesn't trouble the doctor, he's just happy with the information he's received—an incorrect but hopeful prognosis.

CHAPTER 19

RETIREMENT

My life's work has been accomplished. I did all that I could.

Mikhail Gorbachev

As Dr. Stead planned his retirement from the chair at Duke, he wrote to the Dean:

I would like for the new chairman of the department to have the same freedom to bring in new people and to make needed changes, which I have had. For this reason, this projected change requires some careful financial planning. For the 10-year period from June 1968 to June 1978, the budget of the department will need to be increased by the amount of my salary. I am paid equally from University and departmental funds. By 1968, sufficient department funds will have accumulated during my tenure to cover my salary for a 10-year period. The University needs to make plans in advance for the portion of my salary carried by the university.

The progress of the Medical Center can be greatly limited by intellectual failure of one of its major departmental heads. The best way for the University to insure itself against this potential hazard to its intellectual and financial security is to have the decisions in regard to long-range policy and in regard to new appointments to the staff in the hands of young men. If my health remains good, I will simply continue to work at whatever tasks I seem best suited for, and the University suffers no loss. If I become unable to function well and my colleagues wish to give me less work, the University does lose something. Its loss under this arrangement is small compared to the loss if I should remain as chairman under these conditions.

I therefore present this program to the University as a form of insurance, which will assure the continued excellence of that area in the medical school which has been entrusted to my care. (*E. A. Stead, Jr.: What This Patient Needs Is A Doctor*, p 170)

Dr. Stead:

My decision to retire at the age of 60 was really unrelated to my father's mental impairment as he aged. Usually when a chairman retires from a medical school, he stays on the payroll, so the new chairman has fewer resources because he has to pay his predecessors' high salary. In order to free the new chairman of that responsibility, an early retirement plan is important. So I went to the Dean when I was about 50, and offered to retire as Department Chairman at the age of 60. I proposed to underspend the budget of the Department of Medicine by an amount equal to half of what I was paid for ten years if he would agree to increase the budget of the Department of Medicine by the same amount for ten years. That would provide me a full salary for ten years (until age 70) without any drain on the resources of the new Chairman. If my head continued to work after the age of 60, I had no doubt that I would bring in more than enough money to make up my salary and then the department would gain all that extra money. If my head stopped working, then the University would have a tremendous bargain. They wouldn't have to start talking about it's being time for Stead to retire and how they could bring that about because they already had a letter guaranteeing my resignation. I thought this was in the best interest of the school and that's what I told the Dean.

The Dean was interested in my plan for a different reason. He thought that if I retired at 60, it might put pressure on the other department chairmen to do the same. So we worked out the arrangement and I signed the necessary papers. I put my half of the money aside in a separate fund, and I presumed they did the same. Consequently, when Dr. Wyngaarden took over, he had no obligation to pay my salary. He could simply spend his current budget. It is a dangerous thing to have department chairs retire without planning in advance because it's a real drain on the budget, as I indicated. I always underspent my budget anyway, and put any free funds that we had into a separate account used for capitalization.

Dr. Henry McIntosh:

One night, when I was just a young fellow, Gene and Madison Spach, a fellow in pediatric cardiology, and the famous cardiologist Tinsley Harrison and I drove back to Durham from an American Heart Association Program in Lumberton, NC. I was driving and Harrison was sitting in the back seat with Gene Stead; Harrison said, "Gene, I'm going to retire next year." Gene replied, "Retire? Why are you going to retire? You are a young fellow, only 60 or so." Harrison said, "Yes, but I never saw a chairman of a department do anything really productive after his 60th birthday." Gene said, "Now I don't know about that." Harrison said, "Well, let's look at it. There's Barr (at Cornell). How old is Barr? Has he done anything recently?" And they went on naming all the great men of American medicine around the country. Matty Spach and I just sat there listening; I was awestruck— so much so that I didn't pay much attention to driving or the car. When I pulled up in front of Stead's house and let him and Harrison out, I started up the car and after one block, discovered that I was out of gas (it could as easily have happened on the road because I was so absorbed in their discussion). Three weeks later Stead dropped by the laboratory and said, "Remember that conversation I had with Tinsley Harrison? I've just made arrangements to retire as Chairman on my 60th birthday. I've arranged to have the money put aside, so it won't cost the incoming chairman anything for me to stay around until the regular age of retirement."

Subsequently, at the Association of University Cardiologists meeting in Chicago, Gene said, "We're going out with George Burch, how about joining us?" So I did, and Gene told Burch that night about his plans to retire at age 60. Burch, a well-known Chairman of Medicine in New Orleans, was about 60 or so and he said it was the craziest thing he'd ever heard and he sure wasn't going to do that. So George hung on as Chairman and wore out his welcome at Tulane; Gene didn't persuade him, but it was a very impressive conversation.

Dr. Jack Myers:

Gene held that a person should be Chairman of Medicine for only so long and then move over and let someone else take over because you get a bit tired if you've been Chairman too long. He violated his own principle in that he told me he was going to retire at age 55, but he didn't quite stick to that.

Well, at Pittsburgh we had a large efflux of faculty in the late 1960s, and by 1970 I had been Chairman for 15 years. I thought that was long enough, and I was confronted with the fact that, if I wanted to build a new team, I'd have to stay on as chairman another 5, 7 or 10 years. I decided not to. You can argue with that one way or another, but that was my decision. Another thing that happens in academic medicine—and I don't know how often this is recognized—the longer you're in a position of major administrative responsibility, the more enemies you make, because you have to take positions that are bound to be unpopular to some, and of course that builds up and pushes you to retirement.

Many people make arrangements to retire when they're young, and then, as the designated age approaches, they change their minds. That happened to Harvey Cushing. In 1913, or maybe 1912, Cushing and Henry Christian moved from Hopkins to be the first Professors of Surgery and Medicine, respectively, at the Peter Bent Brigham Hospital. They were both young men (Cushing was 43), and they said: "You know, one of the troubles of academic medicine is that people stay in these chairs too long. Harvard's official retirement age for a chairman is age 65, but we're going to move that down to 60." So they went to see the Dean, who didn't agree with them, and they compromised on 63. Well, in the early 1930s, when Cushing turned 63, he thought, "You know, I'm just as capable as I ever was, I'm not ready to retire." So he went over to the Dean and said, "Look, I'm supposed to retire next year, but I think I'm good enough to stay on. I'm a world famous neurosurgeon." But the Dean said, "How old are you Dr. Cushing?" Cushing said "63," and the Dean asked, "And who made this arrangement to retire at 63?" The Dean wouldn't budge. That's when Cushing got mad and he took his library to Yale and so forth. He thought Harvard had done him dirt, but he had made the original agreement.

CHAPTER 20

A GOLDEN MARRIAGE

Life is the succession of generations, with heaven on earth as its goal.
Dr. Rhoades

Dr. John Laszlo:

They called it a freak storm—a ferocious February ice storm that deposited six to eight inches of freezing rain on the North Carolina countryside. "Freak" is the weatherman's way of explaining why his predictions for "clear and sunny" conditions must not be ascribed to meteorological incompetence. The storm was just beginning as I left Durham at 8:00 A.M. for the one-hour drive to Kerr Lake, to the house Gene Stead and his family built by hand. Freezing rain coated the road and the windshield with such intensity that the defroster could not keep a granular mass from caking on the windshield; every five to ten minutes I had to stop, scrape it off, and hurry on. No gloves made can keep the fingers warm in such work.

At first, cars moved slowly, making dramatic rushes up seemingly minor hills that looked to me like Alpine passes under the glaze, or unceremoniously sliding backwards in agonized angular positions. I made my way north towards Oxford, Bullock and Kerr Lake; near the Virginia border, the road became totally devoid of cars. Many had skidded off the road, others had simply been abandoned. That made driving much less risky.

My twelve-year-old Chevy Blazer had always been something of a white elephant, poorly engineered and expensive to repair. But the four-wheel drive and wide track tires moved me along despite the ice. Visibility became an increasing problem, and the Stead driveway was not clearly marked, so I drove past it, turned around, drove past it again. It had to be nearby. All the other houses on the lake were unoccupied, so there was no one to ask for directions. Finally I found the high gate that formed the main-road entrance to a very long

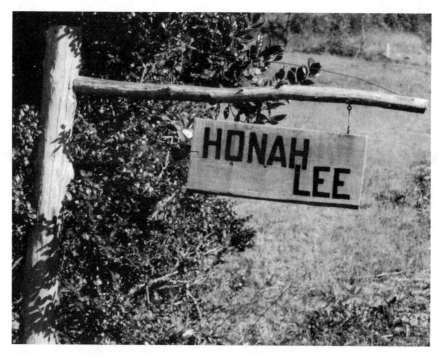

Entrance sign at Honah Lee, the Stead house at Kerr Lake, in Bullock, NC.

driveway—and the gate was locked! No visitors were expected in this weather! In the country, addresses are rural box numbers, and there are no bells or intercoms by which unexpected visitors can announce their arrival. Perhaps the high fence did not extend all the way around the property to the lake. Unbeknownst to me, the Stead house and the neighboring houses had been burglarized on one or more occasions and the high fence *did* extend all the way around to discourage this from happening again. I made my way through the frozen underbrush until the house was visible, perhaps 150 feet away. My shouts were muffled by wind and hail; no response from people or dogs inside the house, but the steel-wire fence was not difficult to scale. A knock on the front door brought the two large dogs to a high state of attention, their loud barking augmented perhaps by the indignity of having been caught unawares.

Gene and Evelyn had battened down the house for the storm; the stove kept the main part of the house cozy warm, and they were surprised and delighted by my visit. The living room-dining room is a large open area with sliding glass doors facing the lake. There is a tiny kitchen, and bedrooms and bathroom in back of the house. Gene and I worked in the glassed-in solarium, which provided comfortable space for two chairs and a view of the lake (when viewing the lake was possible). Gene reminded me that we were sitting in the site occupied by the original entrance to the house. I had visited there almost thirty years earlier, when the concrete was freshly poured and the door hung slightly crooked on its hinges. The flawed early work had been repaired once the house was closed in to the elements and they could take the time and develop the skills to make everything come out right. Then, they had closed off the entryway and created the solarium in its place.

Dr. Stead:

We wanted a house that belonged to us, but we thought that we really couldn't build a Durham residence and also build a place in the country. We decided that Kerr Lake would be both our vacation and our retirement home. We bought the land at Kerr Lake, about an hour north of Durham in the Spring of 1953, and started building our house a year later. (Kerr Lake was built by the Army Corps of Engineers for flood control, and the lake level fluctuates considerably between the rainy and dry seasons.)

Originally we owned only one lot but ended up buying the piece of land next door from a colleague who had originally owned it. We had to fill the land before we could build, as a precaution against flooding when the lake rose. I think it took us close to 25 years to build our house; we did it ourselves and it was a labor of love for the family. In August of 1953 my son, Bill, had his fifth birthday party up here, but we had only a lean-to at that time. We broke ground in April of '54."

Evelyn Stead:

Gene tried to persuade a builder to build us one room but he wouldn't do it because he said, "By the time I get through, it will seem very expensive to you for such a little area. It's not reasonable." Gene's approach to doing anything was to learn about it first, so we bought some books on building. Adams' Concrete Company in Durham was really just getting going, and they were evangelistic about the merits of concrete blocks. I wasn't terribly enthusiastic, but I did know that up here in the woods there were going to be lots of bugs and concrete would provide the most permanent kind of structure. I used to pick Bill up when he was going to school in the morning, and we'd go have

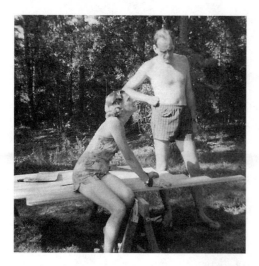

Evelyn and Gene Stead consider the next step in building their house at Kerr Lake in August 1959.

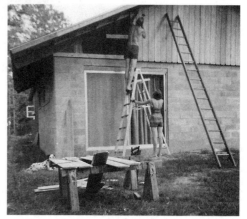

Closing in the house that Stead built. Gene and Evelyn Stead working at Kerr Lake in August 1959.

lunch and then go up and see Mr. Adams at Adams' Concrete. He would tell us what we ought to do on a particular weekend and we'd do it; we learned as we went along. We would travel up to the lake on Saturday afternoon, go back to Durham for Gene's Sunday School, then back to the lake and work Sunday afternoon. We traveled back and forth a great deal with three young, tired children. The first door that we had built had a frame that never looked right, ever, and it took us thirty-odd years to rebuild it. When we did, we finally got a decent looking doorway.

It was a job to pack up on Saturday at noon and go to the lake, and then drive back to Durham, and do it all over again on Sunday, but it always seemed worthwhile, and so we just did it. One year, when Bill was about five, we decided traveling had gotten so hard that we would stay for a week, and we struck a deal at a little motel in the town of Oxford. We rented a bedroom with two beds and a cot. Gene and I had one bed, the girls had the other bed, and Bill slept on the cot, which we had to walk over to get to the bed. We also had a beagle, and Bill had a pet turtle—the dog slept in the car and the turtle slept in the bathroom. We spent a week there for seven dollars a night. We would come up to the lake house in the morning and work all day and go back to the motel to sleep. It was much easier than picking ticks off of three little children, and going back and forth to Durham day after day with them. Oxford is about a half hour away from our lake house. That motel eventually didn't make it, and I can see why if we could rent a room for seven dollars a day for five people, a dog and a turtle.

It was a long time before we could stay in the house. We finally managed to sleep up here when we built the living room and got the strips of wood for the ceiling up and put up insulation. Then we built a wall that cut the living room off from the kitchen area. After that we built the bathroom and then the area which is presently the kitchen and study. That allowed us to stay in warm weather, but to stay here in cold weather we had to have a closed-in place. So we closed in the living room and bought our first electric blanket, and Gene and I slept in a bed with the electric blanket. We had four cots (because Bill always had a friend with him), and our daughters and Bill and friend slept on cots in front of the fire. We started staying up at the lake for New Year's quite early on.

Building the house on the lake really gave us a "family project," something we did together. At one point Bill decided that he really wanted to paint the outside of the house. We honestly didn't have time to do it, so I made a deal with him—if he would paint the mass, I would paint the trim and all the tricky places. So he stayed up here at the lake by himself and went to Clarksville by boat to get what supplies he needed. He had a case of shingles at the time and I never understood how he managed to paint when he was hurting so, but he did. And we picked the color, a very soft shade of green, which Gene always thinks is white, but it really is a very soft green. When we were trying to decide what color the trim and wooden door should be, Bill's friend, Riddy, brought us a piece of driftwood colored a dark, dark brown (it's still out on the doorstep), and Bill thought that would be a nice color for the trim. So I took the driftwood to Claude May, a big paint dealer, to mix the paint; as long as I saved enough liquid paint, they could always mix it up again. It's called Special Brown.

Deciding to use concrete blocks made planning fairly simple because everything was a multiple of four. I used graph paper with squares that equaled four inches, and drew in walls, not forgetting to allow for the fact that the wall had thickness and was not a straight line. We bought a concrete mixer from Sears. It was advertised as a "trailer,'" so we thought we'd hitch it to the back of the car and haul it up here, but it was a very strange little concrete mixer and had no intention of riding behind the car right-side up. It was all we could do to get out of the Sears parking lot with it trailing behind, and an elderly lady scolded us on our way out. Anyway, we got it home to Durham, took it apart and rented a trailer to take it to our building site. Even before we got that concrete mixer we built the bathroom with Gene mixing the concrete for the footings in a tray he had built. We had a Dalmatian at the time and the neighbors had a boxer. This led to a terrible struggle with the strings we put up to mark where to dig the trench and so on. As soon as we got the strings tight, the dogs would run through them and ruin our markings.

It took us close to 25 years to finish our house. We built the main house and the tool house and Bill and Gene built what was meant to be a boathouse, but we now have our cars in it. The art studio was a gift to Gene in 1968 from his confreres. Then we built a second house because we thought we might use it as an antique shop when Gene retired. We thought at one time that we would go into business, and that we could be open certain days. We installed a kitchen before we knew we were going to turn it into a residence, and a bathroom because we thought that since we were out in the country, if people came, it would be nice to offer them tea or coffee and a place to freshen up. And we got fairly far with the idea. We had a dealer's number and planned to call the business *Sassafras Fork Antiques*, because the house is in Sassafras Fork township. We didn't think we'd make a very great living, but thought we could add to our existing income. It was really an extension of a hobby.

We had become interested in early lighting when we bought two little lamps from an old bachelor in Clarksville who lived by himself with about twenty cats. He had all kinds of odds and ends and antiques, but we just bought two little lamps. We meant to collect miniature lamps, but now we have a pretty good collection of lamps that reflect the development of lighting. We belong to a society called

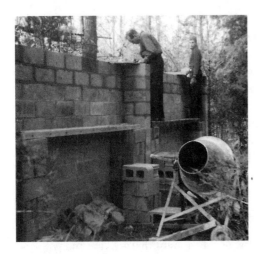

Gene Stead and his son Bill constructing the wall of the "boat house"
at Kerr Lake, January 1965.

the Rush Light Club, which is a club for collectors of lighting. We
have between 450 and 500 lamps. Some of them are quite valuable
and some not so. I have catalogued them, explaining what we know
about each lamp and the price we paid for each, and we have a picture of each lamp. When Gene kept on working, however, it became
clear that we couldn't run a business, although we got all the way to
the point of printing up our cards. So we simply turned the building
into a second house, which we use when our family visits.

Gene had hoped to do some pottery. The year after he retired as
Chairman, we lived in New York, and he took pottery lessons at the
West Side YMCA. One of his sisters was an excellent potter. Gene has
a wheel and a kiln, but somehow we always kept building things so
he never really got around to taking the time to pot. When we went
to the University of Florida for a month in the Fall of '67, we were
given living quarters in the Student Union, and in the basement there
was a craft shop. Gene was busy from 7:00 in the morning until
nighttime, and the only thing you could take that particular month
was batik. Since I'm not choosy, I took batik. It's an interesting craft.
It's very hard to find good dyes, but at a craft show in New York we
met a woman from Canada who sold dyes, so I did that for a while.
I sold a few of my pieces through a store called Cedar Creek but I
never produced enough to be a reliable supplier.

Our children always went to the lake with us. I don't think Lucy's
first husband particularly liked us and he especially didn't like coming to the lake, which made it difficult. But her children came, par-

ticularly Patrick, who has been here ever since he was a little fellow. We have movies of him when he was too little to walk, crawling around out here. Bill always was very fond of the lake, and before he was married he said, "I won't marry anybody who won't ride in my jeep and go to the lake," and he stuck to it.

We moved to the Lake permanently in January of 1977, though Gene might spend part of the week in Durham or elsewhere. We'd been in our Durham house for 30 years, staying on even after Gene retired as Chairman, but by 1977 we were ready to move. Nancy had come back from her medical training in Boston, and bought a house; Lucy was married and living in the Washington area. Our house at the lake was finished and it was a lot of work to take care of two houses. While we were still using both houses, I discovered one day that I was responsible for eight bathrooms, and I thought that was too many.

Dr. Stead:

Two of my children are in medicine, but I'm not sure how much influence I had in that. I never felt that they should be like Evelyn and myself, and I never felt they should be like each other. From the very beginning, we knew they were highly individualistic and we never tried to compare them to each other or to us. On the other hand, I clearly enjoyed medicine and got a great deal of fun and satisfaction out of it, so if all three of my children had not been interested at all in medicine, I would have felt maybe I was kidding myself, maybe I'd come home and said, "Life is so hard," though I didn't think I was doing that.

I was pleased when Nancy and Bill went into medicine because it seemed to make me an honest man. It meant that they had seen me do what gave me the greatest satisfaction and it still appealed to them. They hadn't felt cheated by the time I gave to the profession because they chose a similar path. If they had had talents in music, dance, literature or business or something, and had wanted to go those ways, we certainly would not have objected. I made no attempt at all to influence what they did. I believed we should support the children in a reasonable way, until they were capable of earning their own living. Like my parents, I never believed we should support our children in school if they were non-performers, but they knew from the beginning that the way they took, and the direction they went, was completely open. They only had to demonstrate that they weren't throwing Evelyn's and my money away.

Neither Bill or Nancy said anything at all about medicine until their senior year in college, and then they both said they were going to apply to medical school. Nancy has had a perfectly conventional career. She's done what a bright, compulsive young lady might be expected to do. From the very beginning of making his career decision Bill said, "I think I want to be a doctor." But Bill also wanted to have a second profession. He said, "I'm going to be a doctor and I'm going to be good at it, but I don't want to be economically dependent on being a doctor." And so, even before he entered medical school, he intended to diversify his interests so that he could either support himself as a physician, or have the option of a second pathway. And he picked the computer as a second pursuit.

Children don't do what their parents tell them to, but one of the successes I did have was in persuading my daughter Nancy to take a medical school rotation with Dr. Billy Peete, a Senior Professor of Surgery, who spent most of his time caring for patients in the Surgical PDC. Billy is not only a fine surgeon, but also a wise man and most of the senior doctors wanted him to care for them if they needed surgery. I thought that she would see what the overall practice of surgery, including diagnosis, operating skills and post-operative care really were, and she did profit tremendously by the experience. She never would have done it if I hadn't encouraged her. Billy wasn't thought of as a person whom you really ought to take a senior rotation with because he wasn't flashy, didn't do research, or give a lot of conferences.

My daughter, Lucy, had no scholastic ambition. She was a giddy-headed little girl who was meant to get married, which she did. She is a very non giddy-headed little girl now. She rapidly discovered those things that seemed so alluring as a sophomore in college weren't very alluring in real life. Lucy was the worst scholastic performer because she had the least interest, but she performed well enough to get accepted to Duke without any difficulties. Lucy didn't want to go to Duke, but I didn't think the prep school had pushed her in any way, and so I decided that she should go to Duke for two years. At the end of two years, if she performed well, we would support her at any school she chose. So that was our agreement. But before she had finished her second year, she had Patrick, and was married when her sophomore year was over, though she did eventually graduate from Duke. Lucy had very clear ideas about the world. When she married Claude she thought that he was going to be a second lieutenant, but he only scraped through by the skin of his teeth. She thought she could support Claude while he went to law school or something, and so they went to Norfolk and Claude discovered that the best he could do was the Five and Ten. So Lucy decided education had its uses after all. She went to school, at whatever the local college was, and did acceptable work there, and then when Claude went to Vietnam, she came back to Duke and turned in an entirely different academic record and graduated with her class.

Lucy knew she had to make a living because they clearly weren't going to be able to live on Claude's income. She had a high aptitude in mathematics and had always done well in it, so I persuaded her to take most of her classes at Duke in mathematics when she returned. The most amusing thing about that episode was that when she went to the math department, they told her, "You're so far behind, we don't think you can make it." But after thinking about it, Lucy said she knew there was a graduate student who worked as a tutor and guaranteed D students a final B average if they worked with him. She said, "That's my man," and employed him for three months and she did just fine.

Evelyn Stead:

I think it's a compliment to Gene that two of our children, Nancy and Bill, went into medicine. Some doctor's children won't have anything to do with it because they don't like the way their parents lived. Gene really wasn't too busy. Sometimes Gene is forgetful, absentminded. But he's never absentminded about anything truly important. He can tell you the last detail about a patient he saw ten years ago, though he may drop his mail on the way down the road. He's been a very thoughtful person to live with, he tries to do his share.

Dr. John Laszlo:

The craft house was a gift from the medical staff at the time when Dr. Stead retired as Chairman. I remember the ceremonies honoring Dr. Stead, with most of his former colleagues in attendance. One of the medical research buildings at Duke was named in his honor and a nice bronze bust of Dr. Stead rests there. He gave a moving talk at the end of the ceremonies, acknowledging his good fortune, the help of his wife and that of his outstanding secretary-assistant for all of his years as Chairman, Ms. Bess Cebe. With regard to the building dedication he allowed as how this occasion meant a great deal to his children and grandchildren, but that in perhaps 15 to 20 years the school should re-dedicate the building to someone else and give that family the pleasure. He figured that by then the Steads would have gotten their enjoyment from it and he thought this should be shared on a

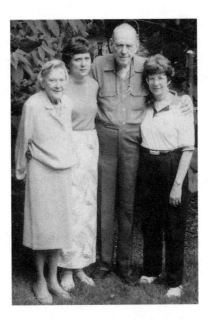

The Steads—Evelyn, Nancy, Eugene and Lucy—at Kerr Lake on Father's Day, 2003.

rotational basis. That suggestion might have seemed ungrateful had it come from someone else, but Stead has always been modest and exceedingly pragmatic. Coming from him it only seemed like a good idea that should be examined for its general utility.

Gene and I worked together for a time; Evelyn worked on her own, and then prepared for us all just the right lunch for the occasion. The bowl of hot soup was delicious, followed by a Scandinavian-style cheese fondue with a salad on the side. Gene loves fondue, but they eat it rarely because it is hardly a low-fat dish, though lower fat cheeses are used. "This is my only vice," he smiles. A tasty tort and tea rounded out the meal. Gene did the dishes before the work resumed.

The warmth of the Steads' relationship together is easily felt but difficult to describe. Usually articulate on other topics, they are either reticent or lack the vocabulary to describe aloud their close personal feelings for each other. It doesn't seem important or necessary to do so, because it is only important to them. After all of these years they continue as the best of friends; all feelings are shared, and yet each respects and admires the integrity, rights and interests of the other. In showing a visitor around it is evident that Gene prefers to talk about what Evelyn has done in the house, and vice versa.

I ended the working day early in order to make the trip back in daylight. With Dr. Stead dressed in high boots and winter gear, and carrying a pot of hot water to thaw the ice from the windshield, we hiked up the driveway, beyond the gate, to where the car was parked. There were no tracks on the paved road. The car was covered with 6 inches of solid ice and it took time to pry open a door so that the engine and heater could be turned on. Dr. Stead helped hack away at the ice casing, urging the visitor not to travel until conditions were safer. It was tempting to stay, but regular business called back in New York. There was barely time to get to the airport to catch the last plane out, if the airport were not yet closed. I promised to report in when the return journey was safely concluded. Dr. Stead turned back to lock the large swinging gate that commands the driveway.

CHAPTER 21

THE PURPOSE OF LIFE

Emotional debts are much harder to collect than other debts.

E. A. Stead Jr.

The essay printed here was entitled "Paid in full by the satisfactions of each day" when it first appeared in a 1973 volume entitled *Hippocrates Revisited: a search for meaning,* edited by Roger J. Bulger, MD. This slightly edited version is included because it accurately portrays the unvarying characteristics of Stead's vision of medicine and the world.

The past is gone; the future may never be attained. The present is real, tangible, and waits to be enjoyed. In my professional life, I have never spent a year with any other purpose than to enjoy the year. If the year advanced my career, that was an additional bonus; if it did not, I had lost nothing because I had been paid in full by the satisfactions of each day.

Each person must sooner or later face up to the question, "What is the purpose of life?" The answer will have a great deal to do with the way one lives and one's relationship to others. I have never had a clear understanding of the purpose of life. I have, however, defined certain limits within which I think the answer must lie and, in this way, excluded a number of possible answers that lie outside these limits. The purpose of life can hardly lie in the past. That period of time is over and will never recur. The purpose of life can hardly be to achieve something in the future, because the future has too little reality. In some way, the purpose of life must relate to the present. The present is real and tangible. It belongs to you; it cannot be taken away from you.

The realization that the returns from living are collected each day does modify one's behavior. One is unwilling to sacrifice everything in the present for something in the future. As a doctor, I have taken care of many parents who, over the years, gave everything to their children with the expectation that the children, when grown, would return this devotion. In fact, as the children matured they developed their own worlds, had their own lives to live, and their own children to care for. They resented their parents' dependence on them and

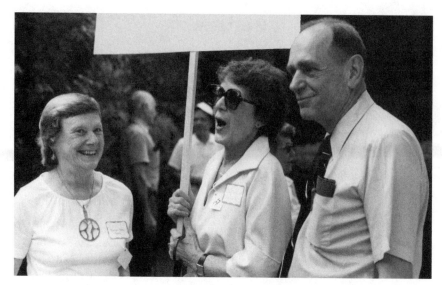

Evelyn Stead with her good friend and classmate, Polly Fendrick, and Gene Stead at Mount Holyoke College reunion in May 1980.

wished the parents had developed interests to supply pleasure from living independently of them. My wife and I, because of our belief in the present, did not give up everything for our children. We kept some time for ourselves and always spent some part of each year away from the children. What resources we had we shared. We had our share of the free money; the children had theirs. We enjoyed our children each day and, when we put them to bed each night, the books were balanced. We had cared for them and we had enjoyed them. They owed us nothing. As the children grew older, we made it clear that we would support them until they were able to support themselves. After that, we would expect to see them and their children, if all of us enjoyed the venture. When they were capable of independence, we owed them nothing and they owed us nothing. We had collected our pleasures as we went, and there were no debts.

Balancing the books each day was an idea that grew out of my medical activities but it relates to parenting. I was impressed that many parents, as they got older, made a tremendous effort not to become financially dependent on their children. Yet many of these same parents became emotionally dependent on their kids. If I had to pick one or the other, I'd rather be financially dependent on my children than emotionally dependent on them. I watched the kinds of troubles that mothers, fathers and children got into. It seemed to result from the idea that the children owed their parents some kind of debt, the kind of debt I didn't want to accumulate and urged others not to. That fits the only personal philosophy I have, which is that life has to be lived. Therefore I will get from each day the fun that's in that day, and my children should pay me currently so that, at the end of the day, I have what I want and I hope that they have some of what they want. I was perfectly aware that if I had financial needs as I got older, the children would step in. That never worried me because it's part of the societal pressure. However, the children were free to choose to go their own way if they wanted to, or to be with us if they wanted to, and we would be delighted. If they elected to do something else, the bonds were cut, they were free. I never looked at it from the perspective that we had taken care of them and so, when their turn came, they would look after us. It seemed to me that if we got satisfaction from our children each day while they were young, that was kind of money in the bank.

Many young people have talked with me about their plans for the next year or years. My answers have always reflected my belief in the importance of the present. If the young person is contemplating a position that he may wish he had not taken unless he achieves a particular rank in some hierarchy, I advise against it. If the program pays dividends in satisfaction and pleasure while it is being pursued, he cannot lose. No matter what happens in the future, the fun of the present belongs forever to him. I have been surprised at how rarely young doctors, engaged in planning their careers, ask the question that I judge to be of the greatest importance: "How do I plan my educational program to help me gain the greatest satisfaction out of each day of my life?" The greatest concern is usually to become technically competent, with the assumption that out of this happiness will flow. Experience shows that this may be too simple an assessment.

A doctor cannot treat disease. He must care for the patient who has the disease. The doctor who wakes each morning with zest for the adventures of the day is at peace with his patients. He knows the limits that the structure of the nervous system put on the behavior of people. He does not expect all things from all men. He can comfortably make many demands on persons capable of rising to these demands; he can comfortably make fewer demands on persons who, because of genetic background, unfavorable environment, ignorance, fear, or prejudice, have ceilings on their performance. The doctor who enjoys the day develops a high degree of tolerance for the frailties of man, and enjoys to the fullest the triumph of individuals. The educational program chosen by the young doctor should be one that teaches him to enjoy the people who have the illnesses he is learning to treat. That is the only way to assure that the work of each day will bring true satisfaction.

To keep one's perspective on the problems of living, one needs to have some sense of the geological time scale. The most famous men of recorded history occupy only very few moments in our thoughts. How few of us spend any time thinking about Alexander the Great or Julius Caesar! Within a few million years, all traces of them could disappear from the thoughts of any living man. The purpose of life can hardly be to obtain fame, because it is too impermanent. Events that add to the enjoyment of the day may bring distinction and fame, but the achievement of fame and distinction at the expense of the enjoyment of the day does not bring happiness.

Knowledge of the uncertainty of the future does influence the direction of one's life. A doctor knows that he, or anyone else, may die before a new day dawns. The wise man is not disturbed by this. He does each day what he wants to do and, even if his impending death were known, he would not need to change his plans. He has planned his life with the knowledge of its impermanence. It's not exactly living each day as if it were the first—or the last—day of his life, but by living in the present, he need have no fear of the future.

A doctor's philosophy does have an effect on his practice. I believe that young people can become "insurance poor" and give up too much of the present by worrying about the future. I am not enthusiastic about burdening my patients with too many don'ts when I have no way of knowing what will remove them from this earth. All preventive measures are wasted when the patient dies from another cause before the diseases that were being prevented could have interfered with his way of life.

Many persons complain to doctors of certain ailments for which the doctor, despite much testing, cannot find disturbances of function great enough to account for the complaining. He will often find asymptomatic diseases that might at some future time cause symptoms—obesity, hypertension, abnormal blood lipids, elevated uric acid, and an abnormal glucose tolerance test are common. In his search for a solution to the patient's complaints, the doctor may institute a costly regimen of preventive medicine in a person who sought medical help in the first place because he was barely able to keep his nose above water. The preventive measures extract money and energy from the patient, but in no way relieve the situation that drove him to the doctor. A doctor with an eye to the present would never initiate programs aimed at the future until the patient was back on an even keel. Which preventive measures to initiate and when is a matter of judgment—mine was sometimes different from Dr. Kempner's on this, for example.

I have had little enthusiasm for the annual physical examination, which is strongly test and x-ray oriented. It is a kind of negative medicine, which puts me to sleep. On the other hand, I am keenly aware that our bodies are undergoing continual change, and that our behavior and our interaction with our environment change with the years. It is worthwhile for one to have an evaluation of his body and how he is using it to determine whether he is getting as much as possible out of each day's living.

Department heads should work harder to devise social systems that recognize certain biologic facts. They do not appreciate fully that all manifestations of behavior derive from the structure of the nervous system. The structure is a mixture of modifiable and non-modifiable units. The number of modifiable units decreases with age. Every five years, enough change occurs in each of us that, from the viewpoint of the body-environment interaction, we can be considered to be a new person. This new person has different perspectives, different aptitudes, a different interaction with the environment. The returns from the day will decrease unless we can change our activities as our bodies change. No one knows the direction or the magnitude of the changes that will occur in a young faculty member as he grows older. All we know is that change will occur, and we should structure our affairs to profit by the change.

Many times the social structure is so tight that only penalties accrue as change occurs. A young man starting his career may be able to offer many contributions before he retires. He may begin as an excellent bioscientist. Later, as clinical interest becomes stronger, he becomes an increasingly important clinician; he now gives up a large part of his laboratory space to a younger person and takes a more prominent role in advanced graduate training. In due time he becomes an outstanding leader in his area of clinical specialization and devotes more time to national affairs. This evolution requires a flexible system of funding so that the person can be supported from different sources as his functions change. In time, the teaching and research dollars are replaced by patient care and administrative dollars.

Each intern, resident, or fellow has some particular environment with which he interacts best. The head of a large educational program is responsible for identifying that circumstance. He must guide young people to recognize their potentialities and limitations so that they can live comfortably with these realities. False notions that one kind of work is more honorable than another must be stripped away. Young doctors must be persuaded to determine the personal satisfactions—the returns of each day—that will come from different careers. Each career, however different, must be seen as equally honorable, even if the returns in satisfaction to different persons may be widely different. The career that has been completely satisfying to a mentor may be a disaster for his pupil. An instructor interested in the joy of the present will not try to mold in his own image the young people whom he encounters.

CHAPTER 22

COLLEGIAL REFLECTIONS

Talent hits a target no one else can hit; Genius hits a target no one else can see.

Arthur Schopenhauer

Dr. Stead was often reticent in describing his personal life and friendships. The recollections of Dr. James Warren, probably his closest friend, while respecting his friend's privacy on many issues, still provide insights into the man and a separate perspective of some critical developments that changed them both.

The thoughts of three other notable colleagues, Drs. John B. Hickam, Paul B. Beeson, and Michael E. De Bakey, are included here, along with recorded recollections of his doctor brother, William Stead and his doctor son, William W. Stead. Hickam and Beeson served as chairs of medicine departments (at Indiana and Yale Universities, respectively); their papers originally comprised part of a *festschrift* for Dr. Stead, collected on the occasion of his retirement as Chairman of Medicine at Duke in 1967, and published in the Annals of Internal Medicine in 1968; De Bakey is the renowned cardiac surgeon and guiding spirit behind Baylor College of Medicine in Houston. William Stead, a notable authority on tuberculosis, was professor of medicine at the University of Arkansas; William W. Stead is Professor of Medicine and Biomedical Informatics, Director of the Informatics Center, and Associate Vice Chancellor for Health Affairs at Vanderbilt University Medical Center. Over the years, many house officers referred to Eugene Stead as "Big Daddy," but Dr. William W. Stead was in the unique position (with his two sisters) of being able to call him just "Daddy."

Dr. James Warren:

I can't tell you the instant I met Gene, whereas I can tell you that for Paul Beeson or Soma Weiss. As a student at the Harvard Medical School, I undertook the so-called tutorial program, which allowed for several months of research as part of the curriculum. I elected to work with Dr. Soma Weiss. That, in turn, threw me together with

Louis Dexter (later a famous cardiologist at Harvard) who was also at the Thorndike Lab at the Boston City Hospital. Some of our work on toxemia of pregnancy was tangential to the research that Gene was doing. I had a little bit of contact with him during those last few years of my medical school training at the Boston City Hospital. Then, in the summer of 1939, Dr. Weiss became Chairman of Medicine at the Brigham and Gene, one of his three major lieutenants. Internships at the Brigham during that time were staggered, and I was on a rotation that started in December, which meant I was unemployed from my graduation in May until December. Gene was starting up what they called the Physiology Laboratory at the Brigham—a fairly large room with a tilt-table and the bare minimum of equipment in it. Gene was working on some cardiovascular problems with Dick Ebert, thinking about how shock, infectious diseases, and pneumonia altered blood flow in the arms and legs and throughout the cardiovascular system. I was enlisted as the junior assistant, which meant that, at times, I was the subject. That was when I really began to work with Gene, and we accomplished a lot in those few months. Two or three papers came out of that period, all authored by Stead, Ebert and Warren, even though I was a lowly lab assistant. We were interested in congestive heart failure and in treating acute pulmonary edema by causing blood to pool in the extremities with tourniquets. There was a question about how much blood you actually can pool in the periphery using tourniquets in a normal subject. Well, if you look back in the *Journal of Clinical Investigation* in 1941 or '42, there's a paper by Ebert and Stead or Stead and Ebert on this very topic, and a nice chart showing how much blood was pooled in a subject. If you look down in the fine print, it says the subject was Jim Warren.

In one of the few dog or animal experiments I ever did with Gene, we measured albumin production by the liver during shock. Dick Ebert made the determinations in the lab of the Harvard Medical School, which was near the Brigham. Right from the beginning, Gene was very gracious and kind to me as the greenest of green, and I found it a very rewarding experience. I became an author on a paper when I should have been an author, and not when I shouldn't have been. The point is that everything we touched in that period was successful, and we got to be pretty much of a factory of papers for a while. If you look at his bibliography and you look at mine, we have many common papers. We were both involved in them and on his suggestion we rotated authorship. In certain instances it didn't come out very fair, but I think he felt, and I certainly agreed, that this system was better than debating whose name would appear first. On one of our best papers, the one on fluid dynamics in congestive heart failure, my name was listed first. We both worked hard on that paper, as we did on a lot of others, but he never made a claim to his name first because he was the senior authority, and that is unusual in science.

One day, I shocked everybody when I took a patient up to the male medical ward. I can't remember what the problem was, but it was a very puzzling thing, and in front of a group of students and faculty, I said to Dr. Stead, "If you're so smart, what's wrong with this guy?" I could tell right away that I caused some of the people in attendance there to think I was an impertinent upstart. Yet in our relationship it didn't mean anything of the sort to him or to me, even though at that time he was building up the legend around his clinical presence. Of course, at the Brigham, Dr. Weiss was a similarly overwhelming person—his presence was keenly felt by everybody in the room. It may be that he overshadowed Gene at that time, and Gene came out into his own after he moved to Atlanta.

The Brigham internship at the time was very peculiar because it lasted for 21 months. The third year was called an assistant residency, but it was more like a fellowship in that you consulted on assigned wards. You were a resident, yet you also functioned in a laboratory. When I was approaching the end of my second year I asked the Chief Resident, Jack Myers, "What do you suppose I ought to do next?" Well, Dick Ebert, as I mentioned, was still working with Gene as Gene's only fellow. I knew that when I was finished with my 21 months of internship, Dick would finish his fellowship and that job would be opened, but I also knew that Dick had more training than just two years, and I felt that Dr. Stead was going to pick somebody who had three or four years out of medical school. And Jack said, "Well, I'd get another good solid year of clinical training." This made very good sense to me; Jack was very influential for me at that time. He said, "Why don't you go out to my old school, Stanford." I'd always liked California, so I wrote to a professor out there and asked if he had any vacancies for a residency beginning next July. He wrote me a nice letter back saying he didn't have any vacancies, but he'd put my letter in his file and would let me know if anything did turn up. One fine morning Soma asked me to stay behind after morning report was over. He said he'd heard from the man I'd written to at Stanford, and he said, "If I will recommend you, he'll accept you next year as an assistant resident out there." Then Soma looked me squarely in the eye and said, "Is that what you want to do?" And I said, "Well, yes, it's my second choice, I'd like to stay here and work as an Assistant Resident with Dr. Stead, but I realize I only have two years of postdoctoral training and I feel like he probably wants somebody with more experience than that." Soma said, "Well, I'll have to talk with Dr. Stead about that." But then he said, "If you don't do that, you'd like to go out to Stanford?" And I said, "Yes, I'd do that." That afternoon, right after lunch, I went by my mailbox and found a nice little note from Dr. Weiss and it said, "Dear Dr. Warren: With great pleasure I offer you the position with Dr. Stead beginning July 1." Well, of course, that was just great. I waited a polite few minutes and I went up to Dr. Weiss's office, which was in the balcony of the lobby at the Brigham. Dr. Weiss' secretary, Evelyn Selby (later Evelyn Stead) was there, and I told her I'd gotten this letter and that I really was excited and wanted to do that and accepted. In those days everybody sent telegrams, so I said, I suppose we ought to send a telegram to Stanford to say that I'm not coming out there. Evelyn looked me straight in the eye and said, "Oh, don't worry about that, we've already told them you're not coming."

I had an appointment at Harvard as a Research Fellow to work on problems with blood volume, and at MIT to use radioactively labeled cells, which was a new thing. I was all excited about that. But at the end of January, after Pearl Harbor, Soma died and that sort of knocked the bottom out of that project. After Pearl Harbor all the young people who thought they were draft eligible tried to get into the Harvard Red Cross Hospital Unit, as I did. But Eliot Cutler, a surgeon, told me it would be a long wait before we got mobilized. Gene had actually accepted the Emory position prior to Soma's death. John Hickam was going to be Chief Resident and I was to be a special fellow, working on a war-time cardiovascular project. The pull of Dr. Stead going down to Atlanta was so great that it was a very natural decision to make; it didn't seem like a major sacrifice because of Soma's death. Although I liked Boston and I liked the Brigham, the challenge of doing the other thing seemed much more exciting.

I was fortunate enough to have had a car. So in May of 1942, when the annual Atlantic City medical meetings were being held, I packed up my limited belongings and drove to Atlantic City. Gene rode with me, then he went on down to Atlanta and I went to Columbus to deposit some things before I dropped down to Atlanta in the next couple of weeks. So I really walked into Grady Hospital around the same time Gene did. That was when John Hickam was supposed to become Chief Resident, but he had been ill, so at first I was the Chief Resident. After he came back, I continued to live in the hospital so that I could always be there for the shock patients who came in for our cardiovascular studies, and I sort of roamed the wards. I knew what was happening on every ward.

At Emory, we were very short-handed. Gene was starting literally from nothing. Most of the clinical teaching had been done by voluntary faculty from the community. There was virtually no full-time faculty; the hospital people didn't know what it was to be well staffed; and the housestaff literally ran the Grady Hospital. But we did pretty well. The major teaching exercise of the week was like a Grand Rounds, held on Sunday morning and affectionately known as Sunday School. It was pretty heavily attended by community physicians and particularly by a group of doctors from the various military establishments. Gene, Paul Beeson, John Hickam, and a few others put on all the presentations. It was very good for my medical education because I presented things that I never would have thought of talking about at Grand Rounds.

The Grady Hospitals were divided into Black Grady and White Grady, and the Black Grady had been run almost totally by the housestaff. There were a few faculty people around Grady Hospital, particularly in the surgery department, so through his own personal power and ability Gene came in with a few lieutenants like myself and took over. There was no major upheaval at all. Maybe I'm looking at it through rose-colored glasses, but I never heard much dissent. Gene was strong then about protocol and discipline. For example, if doctors made ward rounds carrying a bottle of Coke with them, boy, that didn't wash well at all! This carried over to the Duke days. Once one of the senior professors of psychiatry, Stead's good friend, Dr. Leslie Hohman, came into Grand Rounds with a Coke and after he finished it off he put the bottle down by his feet. I had a meeting with Gene after Grand Rounds and as we walked toward his office, he went over and picked up the Coke bottle and said, "Just a minute, we have to do an errand on the way." We went to Dr. Hohman's office where Dr. Stead gave the bottle to Dr. Hohman's secretary and said, "Give this to Dr. Hohman; he left it in the auditorium."

The situation on the White side of Grady was somewhat different. When he went down to Emory Gene believed he was going to be chief of both sides of the street, but it took a period of time and political persuasion for him to become chief of the White Grady. There were a certain number of situations there that were always a little uneasy. The difference between the Black and White hospitals could be seen on various levels—race was only one manifestation. There was a lot of trauma at Grady Hospital; the "inside joke" in the medical community was that Atlanta was a stabbing town and Birmingham, a shooting town. I looked the statistics up once for Grady Hospital and found that 365 patients with stab wounds to the chest had been seen in the emergency room that year. I saw a lot of healthy young Black men die in that place. It was tragic, but while waiting for of these trauma victims to come in, we studied some heart failure patients. Interestingly enough, that time may have been our most productive in terms of scientific progress. While we waited for the next emergency to arrive, we talked about congestive heart failure. Once we got started, we used human serum albumin in the treatment of shock and found out how well it worked.

I was not at Emory when Gene decided to go to Duke. I was at Yale for a year, and so I left my spy, John Hickam, behind. I think Gene felt a little bit trapped at Emory. Besides being Chairman of Medicine, he'd become Dean, and too many things were dropped in his lap. Dr. Bernard C. Holland, a student or a first year intern who had the nickname Crip, talked to me one time and said, "It's just magical the way this place has changed since Dr. Stead and you people have come to Grady." But there were still problems at Emory. The divide between Emory and Grady Hospitals had always been salt in the wound. The powers that be when I was at Emory never really understood the difference between a good medical clinic—a Mayo Clinic—and a good academic medical center; they got them mixed up. I think Gene looked at Duke as being not quite as good as Emory on January 1, 1947, when he first went there. But I think he felt that the stage was bigger, that the play could be larger (which indeed it was), and freer. It had economic freedom, which he used to the hilt in building the department. Grady Hospital never had any money, because the money was always out at Emory. And I think it probably was the practical ability to manipulate dollars to good ends that tilted the scale. The first word I got was a telegram in New Haven from John Hickam in the fall. It said, "He'll be smoking Lucky Strikes from now on." He didn't smoke much, but that was the tip-off that Gene was moving.

Gene went to Duke on January 1, 1947, and I went back to Emory in July. I was there for five more years with Paul Beeson as Professor of

Physiology. When Paul finally decided to leave Emory, I was a little upset with the administration there. I could have stayed on in physiology, but it didn't look too exciting. At the same time, Gene came to me and said, "Look, they're just finishing a big red brick building up here called the Veterans Hospital, why don't you start it?" That was my first assignment. Indeed, I was the first employee at the VA I didn't have a title, but I had my own morning report and it was a very pleasant situation for me. I enjoyed the beginning of my appointment at Duke, but then later on, when we wanted to do more research, the VA seemed a little constraining. I had done my job of assembling the medical team, and yet Gene wanted to keep me over at the VA.

My wife, Gloria, had been Chief of Therapeutic Dietetics at Duke, but she quit her job after we got married, and spent a lot of time working with Evelyn Stead on a cookbook. It was the first book of its kind, and it went through numerous editions. Gloria did most of the technicalities and Evelyn was proficient as a writer and typist. It was very much a joint project. They worked together a great deal without problems; Gene and I looked at the overall book, but we wrote only the first chapter, which wasn't a big deal for us because we'd written so many papers together. It never hit me as a traumatic or difficult project, but it did cement our family relationship.

Evelyn Stead:

In 1954 Gene and I started writing a low-fat cookbook (*Low Fat Cookery*) with Gloria and Jim Warren, and it was published in 1955. The project was Gene's idea. He thought there might be some way to assemble the information, which he thought was needed. We'd known Jim from the Boston days, and Gloria was a therapeutic dietician who knew where to look for information. Gene thought I'd had quite a lot of manuscript experience, and we certainly had experience feeding a family. Gloria and I worked together three mornings a week, and two mornings I worked by myself. Then I usually worked at night, when the children went to bed and Gene had gone back to the hospital. We got it out in just about a year, which we discovered too late was a financial error, because we made the most money early on, and if we had gone over the year we could have prorated the income over two years for taxes. My share of the earnings sent Nancy to Medical School.

Low Fat Cookery sold more than 100,000 copies over time. There have been three hardback editions, the last in 1975, and three paperback editions. Now, of course, there are many diet books, and ours has been forgotten, but I think the reason our book was useful is that I look on myself as a lay person. I majored in English and Art, and so Gloria and I wrote the book as lay people for lay people; Gene and Jim told us they wanted a practical cookbook, and they wrote the introduction. Many books get so technical that they mix people up, but we really did manage to write a practical book with the idea that if you understood what we were doing, then you could take your own favorite recipes and modify them. We gave complete information about the fat content. Now that's on every can and every box, but when we were doing this we had to write to each individual manufacturer to find out how much there was. And we had reams of correspondence. The Department of Agriculture also publishes a bulletin, which has the fat content of many generic foods, but if we were going to give a name brand, we couldn't use average figures. The manufacturers were amazingly helpful—we wrote on stationary from the Department of Medicine at Duke, so that we appeared to be legitimate—but it really did take a great deal of correspondence

I think the fact that people have become interested in diet is a fine thing. When Bill and Nancy were in Medical School they complained about the fact that they really did not learn anything about diet and nutrition. When they asked Gloria Warren what they might read, Gloria had trouble knowing what to advise at that level, but they had learned about low fat cooking because they were raised on it. Gloria and I incorporated the diet into our lives, though Jim never wanted to. He really loved steak and baked potato and chocolate mousse and all those things. Nancy became interested in low sodium cooking because her husband was somewhat sensitive to salt, and so she watched that.

Dr. James Warren:

I have no siblings and Gene isn't all that much older than I am. Since I first worked with him I would have to say he's been my friend, not my boss. I've always felt that way about him. Every time I've had medical problems, he's been the first person I call. When I had my splenectomy for leukemia, now over 15 years ago, the Steads were the first people on the scene. There are a lot of demonstrations like that of their friendship.

The group dynamic in the Stead family always puzzled me a little bit. I knew Gene's brother, Bill, pretty well, first as a student and later as a resident. He and Gene seemed to have a reasonably close relationship. I never had a feeling for his relationships with his sisters; they were not as I would have viewed a relationship to a sister, and yet I can't put my finger on anything that was specifically different. As far as friends were concerned, Gene had a friend named Bailey who went to Emory with him. Gene said he went into medical school because he got into an argument with Bailey who said he could not get straight "As" in Anatomy. Gene took that as a challenge. I don't think he did have a lot of friends, though. He started working with Paul Beeson at the same time he started working with me, and he's very good friends with Paul too.

Gloria and I had no children, so on Christmas Eve we always went over and had Christmas Eve dinner with the Steads. Dr. Kempner gave us a smoked turkey and after dinner we'd decorate the Christmas tree for the children. In more recent years Gene's son, Bill, has had a Christmas party up at their place on Kerr Lake and the Warrens are part of the celebration.

When I considered leaving Duke, the jobs I looked at weren't all that many, but I did talk to Gene in great depth about it, and he was very helpful to me. I left initially for the University of Texas, Galveston, as Chairman of Medicine. I was there only three years when the opportunity came to move to Ohio State. My family was from Ohio.

If you take a set of facts and give them to ten smart people, nine of them will see the data the same way and come to the same conclusions. But there's always the tenth person, and that was Gene's role—that's one of his very stimulating powers. He's able to look at things from a different viewpoint and that stimulates the other person to think and consider the matter more deeply. I find him so educationally powerful. He's an unusually smart person. He's not the kind of a person who wins television quiz shows or has a remarkable computer-like brain that's able to handle more facts than anybody else. But he uses the facts differently, and he has the ability to generate thought. He gets to work every morning and generates new thought; if that's genius, then he's a genius.

John B. Hickam, MD:

The Grady Hospital of 25 years ago [the 1940's] was not a likely place to start raising a family of medical scholars, and the fact that it was done there shows the extraordinary talent of the man who did the job.

How did Eugene Stead go about doing this job and others like it in later years? In the first place, this teacher had, even in the early years, reasonably good material to work with, and this was no accident. He drew good people to him. Later on, good people were attracted in part by seeing that things went well for those who had worked with Stead, but in the beginning they had to be attracted largely by their own estimate of the man. Some of the qualities that proved so attractive to critical, ambitious, young people, even in the days when the professor himself was very young, are precisely that he was, and is, himself critical, ambitious and competitive, (although now more urbane in the display of these characteristics than he was 25 years ago). He was even then an outstandingly competent clinician, and this always commands the respect of pupils young and old. He was a skilled clinical investigator who was doing exciting and imaginative work in the field of cardiovascular disease, but such an attribute mainly draws people who know already that they want to do the same kind of work, and most of us had no such definite ideas in mind when we first joined Stead.

He was hard-working and demanded that others work hard too, but this trait by itself has only a limited power to attract pupils. He demanded excellence in all professional activities. He believed in himself, had faith in his own judgment, and enjoyed watching his own head work on a problem. These are attractive and interesting traits if the judgment and the head are good enough, which they were.

While all these comments are true, they do not begin to explain the peculiarly compelling effect that Stead exerted on the young men around him. They wanted very much to deserve his good opinion and not to merit his disapproval. When he first moved to Duke there was a sinister character in the comic strips called "Influence" who bent people to his will by a hypnotic stare from his prominent green eyes. We who remained at Emory were soon charmed with the news that medical students—and others—at Duke had begun to call Dr. Stead "Influence". How could he have such an effect on tough-minded, independent young people? We too were critical, ambitious, competitive and, in our own private judgments, fine clinicians, skilled investigators either actually or potentially, and hard-working men dedicated to excellence. How did he get to us?

This is one of the crucial questions in trying to understand a great teacher. What does he show that alerts people to his special presence? This probably has different answers for different pupils. For many of us, the most attractive and compelling intellectual feature of Dr. Stead has always been his tremendous ability to analyze a complicated problem, reduce it to essentials, and express it with clarity. When one puts this ability together with a strong and determined character, a gift for colorful statement, and an insistence on meticulous excellence in all phases of medical care, then a picture does begin to emerge of a teacher, a service chief, a senior research partner, and an administrator who commanded deep respect and whose good opinion was earnestly desired.

The skill and the response have depended in large part on the consistent devoted use of his talents to enhance the understanding and development of pupils.

Stead students know the phrase, "Life is hard." It became famous from situations in which a complex medical problem of the night before would be described, with a detailed account of herculean diagnostic and therapeutic efforts. After Dr. Stead had heard about the problem for a while, he would ask for additional data as, for instance, "What did the spinal fluid show?" The unfortunate house officer, who now perceived that it would indeed have been useful to know about the spinal fluid but did not have the information, would still be anxious to defend his position. "Dr. Stead", he would say, "we were up until four o'clock with this patient, and it was a very confusing picture at the time, and we did all these other tests, and so on." This was the point at which the axe would fall: "What you're telling me is that life is hard. I already know that. What I want to know is, what did the spinal fluid show?"

Bedside medicine provided rich opportunities to show the value of clearly identifying and examining the basic findings and assumptions that were being used to understand and manage a puzzling illness. Many a pupil's embarrassment began with the words, "I think this patient is trying to tell us something"; or the harsher criticism that came when the professor was convinced that nobody was getting an effective message from the sick man: "What this patient needs is a doctor!"

Stead's remarkable ability to think clearly and freshly helped pupils to deal successfully with many different kinds of problems. Years ago one of his young professors who was a new department chairman elsewhere complained of his frustration and unhappiness because the administration of his school seemed indecisive, aimless, and slow to move. Gene could have simply said, "Life is hard." What he did say was, "A strong, decisive administration is helpful to you only if their ideas happen to coincide with yours. Otherwise, it's much better to have an administration that will leave you alone, and then you can work things out for yourself."

He paid close attention to his pupils and so came to understand them individually very well. He was determined to make them grow. To this end he often gave jobs to people who needed to grow when others could have done the work better. He removed his name from many scientific papers written by pupils who were working out his ideas. For those who did not respond to his efforts, he had little time because there were many pupils. In those who did respond, he built confidence, self-respect, a conviction of being on the first team, and a need to live up to that position that carried them where they otherwise would not have gone.

He has helped us to understand, to grow up, and to do what we can do. We bear some scars, but we are grateful. (Ann Intern Med. 1968;89:993–5)

Paul Beeson was one of the great leaders of internal medicine in the latter half of the 20th century. A major contributor to our knowledge of infectious disease, he was a prolific writer and extolled teacher. He worked with Dr. Stead during his early professional years and succeeded him at Emory; thereafter, he assumed distinguished chairmanships in medicine at Yale and at Oxford Universities. His memoir nicely summarizes Stead's career and their long professional association and friendship up to 1967. Truly they formed a mutual admiration society.

Paul B. Beeson, MD:

I first became acquainted with Gene Stead in 1939 at the Peter Bent Brigham Hospital in Boston where he was a research fellow in medicine. Before that, he had spent his boyhood in Atlanta and had studied medicine at Emory. After internships in both medicine and surgery at the Brigham he had gone to the Thorndike Laboratories as a research fellow, then to the Cincinnati General Hospital where he was Chief Resident in Medicine. He had returned to the Thorndike for a year; then moved to the Brigham when his chief, Soma Weiss, at age 39, became Hersey Professor of the Theory and Practice of Medicine at Harvard and Physician-in-Chief to the Brigham Hospital. Weiss liked young people and gave them scope. One of my first impressions on taking up my residency there was to note with some surprise that comparatively young doctors were pushed to the fore and that they could be stimulating and exciting teachers. Weiss gave such men as Stead and Charles Janeway, both research fellows, regular turns as attending physicians on the medical wards. The word soon got around among students and house officers that their rounds were among the best.

I visited the ward where Stead was attending one day and can recall the scene with great clarity. He had been shown a man just ad-

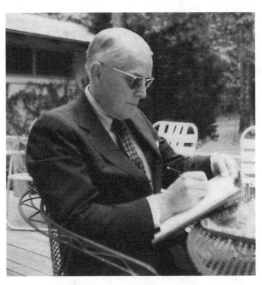

Dr. Paul Beeson, Stead's assistant at Emory and later professor of medicine at Emory, Yale and Oxford Universities, inscribes a book for Stead at Kerr Lake in October 1975.

mitted with hemiplegia after a cerebrovascular accident. In examining the patient Stead noted that he had edema that was unilateral in distribution. He turned to the group accompanying him and for about half an hour led a discussion of the probable mechanism of this phenomenon. Subsequently, I saw him do that sort of thing many times. He was truly fascinated by the mechanism of pathologic events. In addition, he enjoyed the challenge of having to find some noteworthy aspect of a case that others might have passed off as a common and rather uninteresting clinical problem.

In 1942, at the age of 33, Stead was invited to return to Emory as its first full-time Professor of Medicine. It was my good fortune to be invited to go along in the only other full-time post in the department. He also took with him, from Harvard, James Warren as research fellow and John Hickam as resident in Medicine. In Atlanta we shared the teaching and patient care with a group of able physicians in practice there, and for the next four years at Grady Hospital, all of us experienced a truly exciting adventure in medicine. Those years saw the first clinical trials of penicillin; in research, there was the introduction of the flame photometer and the cardiac catheter. Our Grand Rounds on Sunday mornings drew packed audiences: students, house officers, local physicians and medical officers from nearby military hospitals.

In research Stead forged a remarkably effective partnership with Warren. They were invited by the Office of Scientific Research and Development to undertake a study of shock, using the "new" technique of cardiac catheterization. Warren spent some time at Bellevue Hospital learning the methods from Drs. Cournand and Richards, then he and Stead set up their own laboratory adjacent to the emergency department at Grady. They used this special laboratory to the full, not only in the study of shock but to obtain information about many other cardiovascular matters. Their laboratory, together with that of McMichael in London, did much to define normal values and to measure the effects of anxiety and postural changes. Their work on the influence of anemia on circulatory dynamics is still referred to. They explored the use of the catheter in other parts of the circulatory system, finding that they could obtain samples from the pulmonary arteries as well as the hepatic and renal veins. Their brief notes announcing these were the first in the field. This team was also the first to make use of the technique of cardiac catheterization as an aid to diagnosis of congenital heart disease.

While waiting in the emergency department of the hospital for shock patients to come in at night, Stead, Warren and their colleagues, Arthur Merrill and Emmett Brannon, held long discussions of the physiology of the cardiovascular system and of the sequence of pathologic events in circulatory disorders. Stead and Warren tested some of this thinking with careful observations of patients in heart failure and eventually formulated a "forward failure" hypothesis. The hypothesis, supported by comparatively little in the way of tabular information, was published in their celebrated "fluid dynamics" paper. This aroused great interest and no little controversy, centering on the stark opening sentence in the conclusions: "Edema develops in chronic congestive (heart) failure because the kidneys do not excrete salt and water in a normal manner."

In 1946 Stead was invited to take the chairmanship of the Department of Medicine at Duke. To those of us associated with him at Emory, things were going so well that the thought of his leaving was almost inconceivable; nevertheless, he did decide to move. Undoubtedly a factor was that he had found the additional administrative burden irksome. Another was that he saw the immense advantages in the situation at Duke, where the hospital was under university control and where there was a completely flexible system of faculty appointments, ranging from full-time private practice to full-time academic work. As I have struggled with such matters subsequently in other places, I have often recalled how quickly he appreciated, and later made good use of, the possibilities presented at Duke. So off he went.

In the next 20 years at Duke, Stead built up a large and outstanding Department of Medicine, making the fullest use of the flow of public and private benefactions into medical research and teaching. A Veterans Hospital was constructed on the campus, and he smoothly moved people back and forth between that and the University Hospital. He preferred to put young people into positions of responsibility and somehow managed to help them bear responsibility ably. With all the growth, the recruitment and the necessary traveling, he gradually found it necessary to give up personal participation in research but continued to be in close touch with what the other members of his department were doing, frequently displaying that characteristic knack of recognizing something of interest in the findings that others had overlooked. One portion of a professor's work that he never allowed to shrink was active participation in teaching and patient care. Never was there a doubt that the man at the top was a good doctor or that he placed a high value on clinical performance.

Stead is relinquishing the chairmanship of his department several years before the statutory retirement age. He will continue to work there and will of course go on with the teaching of clinical medicine, not only at home but in many other schools, because he is justly recognized as the unmatchable visiting professor. I predict that he will develop a new career activity, plunging into that as if a second stage rocket had ignited, putting him in a different orbit. Of late he has become increasingly concerned about problems of delivering good medical services to all the people, and this may be the area to which he will give his major attention. That would be everyone's good fortune, because he is a wise man. (Ann Intern Med. 1968;89:986–9)

Dr. Michael De Bakey:

I've known and admired Gene Stead for many years, and we are good friends. I'm especially grateful for the help he gave me when I became Vice President for Medical Affairs at Baylor College of Medicine in 1968. At the time, the situation at the College was critical, and I accepted the vice-presidency at the urging of the senior faculty who were concerned that the school might go downhill. We had a deficit of several million dollars and no new funds available in the immediate future. Seven departmental chairs had left, and the morale of the faculty was quite low. The unrest had been brewing for some time: the Chairman of the Board had run off two deans and thereby created a state of near-crisis. When I accepted the position, I realized that we desperately needed outside help if we were going to save the school. So I called Gene. He had recently retired from the Department of Medicine at Duke, but was still very active. I explained the situation and told him that I'd really be indebted if he would come here on a sabbatical to serve as an Associate Dean and perhaps even head the Department of Medicine, which was in a crisis. He accepted, and was a tremendous help to us.

He had a way of getting right to the heart of a problem. You would sketch out a complex problem and he would cut right to the core. And of course, his medical competence, judgment, and clinical ability immediately raised the academic spirit of the school. I was as busy as I could be because I was also Chairman of the Surgery Department and had a heavy daily operating schedule. So Gene played an important role in helping me turn the school around. He spent nearly a year with me during that sabbatical, and together we reversed the direction of the school. We had many discussions about what we needed to do; we recruited some highly qualified faculty, and after he left, he kept in touch with me about people we should recruit, including several good people from Duke. Gene's academic analysis of our programs and our people was a tremendous help in determining the direction we had to take to build the school's academic standing. It led ultimately to the development of a truly excellent school. We had ongoing meetings to decide the competence of the existing chairmen and whether we should keep the present staff or let them go. Many changes resulted.

Besides the new faculty, one other factor changed the direction of the College: it was a plan that I formulated, with Gene's help, to separate the College of Medicine from Baylor University. We needed financial help that we couldn't get as long as we were affiliated with the University, all of whose trustees had to be Baptist. We needed more flexibility to appeal to our sources of support. I succeeded in separating the medical school from the University, and obtained a charter to make it into an independent college. This enabled us to select members for our Board of Trustees who had financial resources.

Gene does have a higher standard than most in everything he does, whether it's writing a letter or a sentence, or making rounds, or anything else. If he thinks that people are not meeting his high standards, he has no hesitancy in making that point clear. If he has some responsibility for it, he will tell the person involved. But he will do this in a way that is not directly harmful or hurtful to that person.

The quality that I admired about Gene right from the early days, when he was active in clinical investigative work in cardiology, is that he had a very strong interest in learning the cause of things and in trying to get a better understanding of them. This applied not only to medical problems but to all problems. Once he understood the problem, then he could start working on the solution. And that's what he did with us at Baylor. He immediately started making rounds on a regular basis at our VA hospital, then at our city-county hospital, and then at our private hospital. He'd make rounds with me, and then he'd make rounds on his own. And he assessed the people we had and what we needed to do. We had a very different situation than existed at Duke. At Duke, the faculty had authority not only at the school but in the hospital, but we did not have, and never had had, a university hospital. And so our medical school faculty had to relate to two different authorities while trying to control our destiny. Gene understood and appreciated that problem.

I wanted a Professor of Medicine to be in charge of the program, someone who had a broad base, and it seemed to me that medicine was the discipline in which we were weakest, except for the basic sciences. Among the people I have known in medicine, Gene Stead stood out in my mind as the leader who came closer to being a Sir William Osler than anybody I ever knew. I needed someone who was wise as well as medically competent. And here was a man whom I'd known and admired so much over the years because he had built one of the best departments of medicine in the country. He was a tremendous influence in making Duke one of the truly great schools in this country.

Dr. William Stead:

The advantages of being Gene's brother always outweighed the disadvantages, and I figured out how to cope with the situation. I've always said that the reason I've lived 1000 miles from Durham is that his shadow is 900 miles long. I've avoided walking in his shadow when I could help it, but once or twice I couldn't, and found myself winning or losing because I was Gene's brother. This happened when I went to Cincinnati. It was at an odd time because I had been in military service for 15 months. When I was discharged in September,

1946, all the housestaff places were filled; Dr. Blankenhorn had created some extra jobs called senior interns and all the junior resident slots and senior resident slots were filled. It literally was chock-a-block. So Dr. Blankenhorn said, "I'll take care of you. You'll have a job, I just don't know what it will be." The next morning he came to visit and said, "How would you like to be assistant to the Chief Resident?" Well, I had one nine-month period of internship and one period of junior residency at the "Gradys" before going off and sitting on a ship for 15 months, doing nothing. I felt very uncomfortable about this. Dr. Blankenhorn was certain I could handle it, but I was uncomfortable for the full year. After that he wanted me to be Chief Resident. Well, this was pushing me along faster than my training would justify. You see, Gene had been his Chief Resident in 1937, and so he was pushing me along fast but I just didn't feel up to it. So I took a fellowship in cardiology with Gene Ferris, and then went to Minneapolis to work with Dick Ebert (from Boston), where I was a junior resident again. But that was what I wanted to do—I wanted to start my training and get a good foundation. Dick Ebert took me on as junior resident and I went on from there. I needed to be back on the ward for "hands-on" medicine.

The many people who know Gene fall into two groups: those who love him and those who hate him. I found this out when I made a mistake: I moved from Minneapolis to Gainesville, Florida, and Gainesville is not 900 miles from Durham. Most everybody in Gainesville was trained by Gene. Florida really didn't have a medical school—the University of Miami had started up, but not long before, and the medical school at the University of Florida was in its first year of existence when I got there. Some of the faculty were from the University of Georgia and such, but the predominant group had been trained by Gene at Emory or at Duke. The people there either expected too much of me, because they admired Gene greatly, or took it out on me because they hated his guts. I was in Gainesville in the late 1950s and being there was really too close. Some of the people who admired him expected me to be as good as he was, and Gene and I are different. I hadn't lived as long and wasn't as wise and all of those things. Some people were very easy on me, easier than they should have been because they admired Gene; others were unduly hard on me because they didn't like him. Among those who didn't like Gene were some who were very devious about it, and would do or say things as a way of getting revenge on Gene without ever having to face him.

Let me give an example of how we are different. Gene integrated the Blood Bank at Grady Hospital. It was rigorously segregated and Gene said that was foolish because blood's blood. That was in the 1940s while there were still two hospitals. The Blood Bank was the first thing integrated at Grady Hospital. When you're brought up in a situation, you accept it. I look out and I see green leaves. I've always thought leaves were green, that's just the way they are. And when I was growing up in the South, the way in which Blacks were treated was very much like the color of leaves: it just didn't stand out. I never thought about it. Gene knew about it before I did. But I caught on in the '40s when Gene and I both lived in Decatur, and we often rode the trolley to Grady together when I was a junior and senior medical student. And he said, "You know before long now there are going to be a lot of Negroes coming home. Having been off to fight for the freedom of this country, they are going to expect some freedom of their own. And so there's going to be some changing times." This was one of the first times I had ever stopped and thought about it. Gene would say something to me, things I'm sure he has now forgotten because the things people remember are different, and this would trigger something I never had thought about. It would give me some insight. He could give me more insight with one sentence than anybody else could with a whole book. So when he said this, I began to think. With one sentence he opened up a whole new view of things for me, which never stopped. I very quickly changed and developed a somewhat unusual degree of tolerance, I think. I voted for Jesse Jackson in the presidential primary because I thought he said more of the right things than anyone who was running. Whether he'd be capable of carrying them out is another question, but as far as the primary campaign was concerned, I felt that he deserved really to be heard. So I changed a lot because of one conversation with Gene.

When Gene got to Grady Hospital as the Professor, the Blacks carried what they called "sick and accident" insurance. They all had an insurance policy at 25 cents a week. A man in the hospital went around collecting the money from people in the community. And whenever they came in the hospital, they had some modest amount, $5 a day or something of the sort, from this insurance policy. For them to collect, someone on the housestaff had to fill out a form and would be paid a small amount per form. Gene figured that this was a big enough business that he should be involved with it. The Chief Resident had been doing it all and had been collecting all the money.

Gene took a page out of Karl Marx and had all the housestaff and residents do a share of the forms. It took a lot of time and the Chief Resident spent too much time doing it, but of course he liked the money and so he kept doing it. But Gene took it away from him and spread it around, so an intern, rather than getting nothing, got $10 a month. We got something when previously we had gotten absolutely nothing but room and board.

Gene and I arrived at Grady Hospital within one week of each other, he as the Professor and Chairman of the Department of Medicine and I as a brand new junior medical student going on the wards for the first time. We had an understanding that we were brothers on the weekend, but we didn't act like brothers in the hospital. I was going to do what I was going to do anyway, which was study hard as I was supposed to do. It really didn't bother me because I'd been with Gene all those years. My classmates were tolerant. They could see that I really wasn't asking for or getting any favors. I did my job. I got in there early and worked a number of holidays and so on. I hit the ball pretty hard. I didn't ask for any soft treatment.

Gene told me at the beginning "Bill, you're going to hear me called a son of a bitch on every corner of Grady Hospital, but don't let that bother you. It doesn't have anything to do with Mother, it's just me." He knew he was going to be making changes that weren't going to make him popular. I always thought Gene's leadership was phenomenal, but I know that I saw it from a different perspective. The housestaff really revered him and worked hard. Gene was doing research during the war and was determined that those who remained behind were not going to goof off. So he worked doubly hard all through that period, and I'm sure part of that was because he knew he wasn't off in the trenches. He had a little bit of guilt about not going. One could say he shouldn't have, but when you're inside yourself you just have to think of it. He really was up many a midnight, or at 3:00 A.M., working on somebody with a stab wound to the heart.

Gene Stead's only son recorded his thoughts about growing up in the Stead household and then choosing a life career that intersected and at times collided with his father's.

Dr. William W. Stead:

In the early years, most of us were unaware that Daddy was any more special to the outside world than any other father. Because nobody told us that he was special, we didn't feel we were growing up in the house of somebody who was important. He worked hard, but he always managed to spend some time with us because we lived near the hospital and because he wanted to. He would come home almost like clockwork at 6:00 P.M., and we would walk together over to the chapel and back. As a rule, he spent close to an hour with us at that time of day. Then he might well end up going back to work, but there was some contact virtually on a daily basis and usually in a fun setting. He didn't sit down and do things like our homework with us; that really fell to Mother.

The other thing that clearly was important to us all was the house at Kerr Lake, which we build with our own hands. The free time that Daddy might have used to go to the country club and play golf or whatever, he devoted to what was, in effect, a cooperative family project. It's really unbelievable what he and Mother did. Daddy used to come home around 3:00 on Saturday and spend time chopping wood and so forth, and then he would have Sunday School with the housestaff on Sunday. The way I decided who were good Chief Residents and who weren't was that the "good" ones didn't have conference on Sunday, and we could go skin diving at the lake. If he did have Sunday School, we would get up in the morning and he would go to the hospital while mother took us children to another kind of Sunday school, and thereafter we all went to the Lake. We'd get there around 11:00, maniacally mix a load of mortar, lay one mixer load's worth of blocks—a full day's work—and then come back home. Getting home at 9 or 10 P.M. with three rather dirty, picky children had to be awfully hard, but somehow my father would get up and go back to work on Monday morning.

The amount of energy he had available for the family was somehow always quite high, and therefore I think of myself as having grown up with a fairly normal situation. We'd make dams in what's now the natural part of the garden and run the hose down into the gully and have a lake. He made a little concrete lake in back of the house in Durham, and we always had sort of creative gadgets—he put energy into fun at home so that in that regard, I think we were fairly normal.

There was certainly no expectation that we children should go into medicine or even anything related to it, though we were clearly unpopular at home when we did not perform at whatever we were doing, no matter the reason. At such times he would set up a plan to give us more work to be sure that such dereliction would not happen again. It wasn't by yelling, it wasn't by spanking, it wasn't by restricting privileges, but it was quite clear when you did something sub-optimal that a plan would then be jointly put together that usually involved efforts on both people's parts. And again, this responsibility fell more to Mother than Daddy. But clearly my father was concerned with maximum achievement. Only in recent years, has it sunk in that he would love us just as much no matter what we did. I always assumed that I was supposed to perform. Exactly how that was transmitted, I don't know. I never felt that I had to conform to other people, but I had to perform well; perhaps it would have been helpful to know that there was some play in the system and that performance was not always absolutely critical. I still have a tendency to take everything much too seriously and I'm sure that somehow came from that background.

I'm only now beginning to learn that if I just decided not to go to work for a day, it probably won't matter. I remember one Sunday when I was getting ready for a working trip that would take me away from home for three weeks to San Francisco, then Philadelphia, and then to Amsterdam. I was supposed to leave on Wednesday and I was worrying about how I was going to make rounds at Duke when I got a call from Daddy saying he wanted me to come up to the Lake Monday morning and walk over a new piece of land we were thinking about buying and sort of figure out what we ought to do. When he first called me I thought it was crazy. I thought that I couldn't possibly fit it in. After about an hour I called him back to tell him I would be up in the morning. We spent a very pleasant couple of hours walking around in the woods and then working for an hour and a half before I came home. It's been hard to learn that work is often not as important as time in the woods with family. Clearly, there was sort of a pressure put into the system that I still do not understand.

When my sister Nancy and I started at Duke Medical School, Daddy was superb in staying out of our way. When I came along, Daddy was no longer Chairman, so he never had control over either grades or dollars. Personally, I think that would have been very difficult if he had. My performance in medical school was somewhat checkered, depending as it did upon where my interest lay at the moment. I essentially flunked the Physical Diagnosis course and then went on to get honors in Second Year Medicine. I got involved with a very dynamic group of house officers who were able to keep me out of the computer center, which was my hobby, and at the bedside. They changed my career more than most other factors have. Daddy stayed totally out of my life during that time. I asked him to come over and round with us one night at the VA during my second year medicine rotation, but that was at my own and the housestaff's request, otherwise he would not have done it. The medical school years were a time when I was sort of socially rebelling, and I moved away from home. Daddy obviously could have come to the Medical Center and found me without any trouble, but he never did. Our lives were always insulated and I think that's to his great credit. He must have been curious and I suspect that he occasionally manipulated things in the background in ways I didn't know.

The first time I caught him manipulating anything occurred one summer when it was clear that I was overworked. I had gone from running a department service at the VA, which had sort of become routine like clockwork, to taking over responsibility for information systems; I had not been able to untangle myself from all of my previous responsibilities. Daddy went to Joe Greenfield (then Chairman of Medicine) and made it quite clear that it was not in my or Duke's interest for me to continue running the housestaff selection process, and he thereby freed me up. I figured out I was in trouble when I had walked into Joe's office and said I was having problems, and Joe suggested that I get out from under it. I called up Daddy and said, "That man's a lot smarter than I thought he was," and he said, "Well, he had some help." But how much of that kind of thing went on in the background, I don't know.

I know there are individuals who have looked on me as my father's son, but I've viewed myself quite differently. It always seemed to me to be somebody else's problem and not mine when they approached me that way. If decisions were not being made the way I wanted them, I never brought the problem to my father, so both of us insulated our relationship with each other as father and son. The advantages of having grown up in the Medical Center are obvious, especially in doing what I want to do, but they're due less to being Daddy's son than from just having lived my life here. Although, if he hadn't gotten me a job early on within the computer projects in Cardiology and those kinds of things, I wouldn't have known all the people I know and wouldn't have known as much where people are coming from. So that was an advantage. One of the disadvantages of growing up in the place was that I was very naive about people's motives. I am just beginning to grow out from under that. I assumed all the faculty were intelligent and well-meaning, but when I went to my first Nephrology Division staff meeting and found that the only things that seemed to matter were issues related to who got a secretary and who had parking privileges, I began to get disillusioned.

Daddy and I had different approaches to some computer issues at Duke, and rather publicly took opposite approaches for close to 10 years before things eventually came back together. I was not only not following directly in his footsteps, but I was actually doing things in a way that he thought made no sense on the national scene. I think he's since changed his mind; he simply didn't think I would be persistent enough to make my ideas work.

Daddy has given me a series of specific statements that have proven true, so I've learned things faster than other people, even when I didn't accept the statement at first. When I started my Second Year Medicine course, we took a little walk to the Chapel and on the way back he told me, "Nobody is going to remember what you know, they're simply going to remember whether you made their day better or worse." And even though I might not have agreed with that at the time, having such an idea in the back of my mind meant that I figured things out faster. He had a specific approach to earning money, and he made it very clear to me when I first joined the faculty that Duke would never fully support me. Doctors on the faculty who thought that Duke would support them well enough to raise a family and so forth were wrong. You had to do a certain number of things that produced extra money, and so he involved me in some consulting activities. He showed me early what most of my colleagues are just beginning to learn. The things that he suggested I do to earn additional income were never things directly related to my Duke job, but things that would complement it and still provide supplemental funds. Growing up we didn't have a lot of free money. We were never poor, but mother really did count pennies. The proceeds of the cookbook she wrote introduced the first extra money into the system. Daddy spent a fair amount of time helping with the concepts behind the cookbook, but Mother did most of the work. It allowed her to earn money while staying in the home.

The second thing that introduced free money was when he took over editing Medical Times. That's not much different than Jim Wyngaarden's editing the *Textbook of Medicine* when he was Chairman. In our case, Daddy set up a management consulting group:

computer experts Frank Starmer and Ed Hammond, medical administrators Jim Mau and Ralph Hawkins, and me. I was the last addition. We would go into medical centers that were having economic or administrative problems and study them for a couple of days; then suggest how they should redo their medical practice plans and a variety of other things. It was a way of producing some income, but Daddy was also smart enough to know that if he could remove Jim Mau, Ralph Hawkins, me, Ed and Frank from Duke Medical Center and its politics, and allow us to think about somebody else's problems, we were likely to come back with a fresher approach to our own problems.

Daddy had a unique way of teaching, though I really only had one medical teaching experience with him (when I was an intern on Long Ward). When he thought I should begin to look at buying stock, he found the first investment for me, and paid for half of it. Then he dropped out of business to see whether the seed grew or not. And the consulting endeavor was the same kind of thing; he pointed it out. And that's been a tremendous advantage. He doesn't teach by lecture, he does it by example. When we were growing up, he would pay half of anything we wanted, provided we paid the other half. We were never given anything big without paying half. It's a terribly useful lesson. It enabled us to not become depressed about not getting things, and yet made us darn sure that we wanted what we got. It makes you think of budgeting and, again, that's the way he taught us. We benefited from his general ability as a teacher.

Looking at the people in the medical center, I find that there are different kinds of individuals. There are those who learn to do something well and then continue to do it forever. As a rule, those individuals get very stale. One of my role-model doctors and the reason I went into Nephrology, really doesn't have much fun in the Medical Center anymore and that's wrong. I think the difference between him and Daddy is that every ten or twenty years Daddy has done a totally different thing. He had a period of administrative responsibility, and then he had the period after he retired as Chairman and before he became a Distinguished Professor for the VA when he really put a lot of energy into his ideas about the computerized data bank as a way of keeping and using medical records to make decisions, and at the Regenstrief Foundation project for John Hickam. He started a variety of new kinds of things and then got involved with the VA and with geriatrics at the Methodist Retirement Home and elsewhere.

But I didn't see his head change despite the changes in interest and activities. Right now he puts a significant amount of effort into the stock market and he doesn't understand why I can't keep up with the latest change in interest rates. When he was Chairman of the Department of Medicine, he kept up about as well as I do now, but at present it's a major focus of his. These days he watches a whole hour of the business news, and I think he's done as well as any amateur does on the stock market. His drive and intensity, his approach to how he does anything, is all the same; he just applies it to different projects. He's clearly changed physically, especially over the last couple of years. But he still gets out of bed at 5:00 in the morning, often drives to the airport and flies off for a day to lecture or consult, flies back and drives to the Lake that night.

The advice that he gives me usually turns out to be right five years later, in terms of where I am. He's watched the whole spectrum of his career and is able to reflect on what had impact; he may think that he should have spent some of his early time differently, and therefore thinks that I should. It's much like when he told his brother (my Uncle Bill) that he would pay Bill's way through medical school, provided Bill did not get above a "C" in anatomy because he had gotten an "A" in anatomy and learned that it was useless to spend that much time on the subject. I suspect that some of the feedback I'm getting now comes from things he would have done differently when he was running the Department 20 years ago. But I find his approach very much the same, I just think he remembers it differently.

His tolerance has not changed. He doesn't round on the medical wards now because he simply doesn't like the way the service is run. He doesn't like the way the students and housestaff spend their time. I don't know that he necessarily has an idea of how to fix it, but it's no longer fun, and it doesn't lend itself to the kinds of things that he wants to do on the ward, so rather than getting mad about it like Dean Davison did, he simply says I'm going to spend my time some other way. He thinks students don't go into medicine now because they don't have fun there.

Daddy told me to be careful about whom I respected because he said it was going to change. The people I respected the most when I was an intern were those whose knowledge left me in awe; the people who drove me crazy as an intern—those who knew that things were variable and therefore didn't give me precise answers—are the people I now recognize as being great. He said to watch for that phenomenon and boy was he right. Jim Wyngaarden was one of the people I was frustrated with because he didn't put the energy into the clinical service that I thought it needed. He's one of the people whose value I've really begun to understand through subsequent dealings with him. It's been fun to watch the fact that I've become a Wyngaarden supporter. I wish I had been smart enough to do that earlier.

If you look at Daddy's *curriculum vitae*, you see that during his entire productive period there were very few papers. A lot of papers were being written, but the young people working with him got the glory. He didn't need the credit and the young people did. He was smart enough to understand that once he took over responsibility for the Department, his success was going to be measured by the fame of the people under him, and not by his own. Remarkably few current faculty understand that.

I do not believe that a careful physical exam and an accurate history are any less important today than they used to be. This gave him a tool that was translatable across the different specialities. It wasn't a catheter, it wasn't a bone marrow test, it wasn't a gastroscope—it was the ability to examine and talk to a patient. Then he had the ability to stimulate and propel young people. Professors, teachers who came after him, have had impact on the institution, but less impact on individuals. He's terribly correct about the fleeting nature of fame; most of present day people at the Medical Center don't know who he is. That is unbelievable to me and yet so it is. So to worry about fame is crazy. Yet if you influence a certain number of people, who then go off and promote your ideas, you've managed to affect a larger circle of people. And that's what he did. He basically produced copies of himself. I think he did this superbly, teaching by example. It's exactly how he dealt with us at home.

My father is remarkably realistic about what can and what can't be achieved. He may not try to solve all the problems of humanity, because he knows they not all can be solved, but he does recognize certain things. A doctor ought to be intelligent, but 95% of what a practicing doctor needs to know is how to have a sympathetic ear for the patient. So he concentrates on that when he's taking care of a patient. Anybody who's a good doctor enjoys human contact, enjoys trying to sit down and understand a patient and help him. I think Daddy was an early holistic doctor. He views medicine as an extremely flexible career. It's a ticket that will let you do anything. I don't think he knew that when he started.

Both Daddy and I feel that the recent Medicare laws are the broadest piece of legislation that we've managed to get from this country in a long time. But somewhere we've got to back off. When I went to college I was the best political liberal I could be. I took part in what was known at Duke as "The Vigil" after Martin Luther King was assassinated. But father's generation was raised in a world where decision-making was fundamentally done by the family unit, based on the family's resources. The extended family took care of grandma, and grandma babysat. We've now changed and the responsibility for care has been put on the back of society; we have eliminated decision-making based on what people can pay, but haven't relooked at the decisions we are making. We would be much better off taking all the money we spend on any health care for anybody over a particular age and spending it on education for children. Society would clearly be better off, but the change would need to be dealt with in some sort of humane way.

I think the best thing you can say about Daddy is that he applies his rules to himself and to his family—and to the great benefit of the individual. My mother's mother died at close to the age of 90, and she spent the last year of her life in a little five-person nursing set up where Daddy and I took care of her without ever sending her to the hospital. It's quite clear that the first admission to a hospital would have killed her. She had significant chronic lung disease, and we did little simple things—a touch of diuretic here and a little of something else. Although the nurses were not totally comfortable with this, when she eventually got to where she couldn't eat, we said, well, put the food in front of her and if she's not able to eat it, she's not able to eat it. But we backed the nurses up with three visits a day from us as emotional support, and rather than being institutionalized, grandmother ultimately died peacefully "at home." Whenever I went to see her, her only statement was, "Bill, please don't put me in the hospital." There's no question that she knew this wasn't in her interest.

For years my father has had written instructions specifying that, if he ends up sick, we've got two weeks to cure him or get him out of the hospital. He understands the limits of what hospital care can do. He understands that you've got to die sometime, and that merely prolonging life usually isn't in anyone's interest. When you can cure something, fine; when you can make people comfortable, fine; but he understands what the choices are. Unfortunately, Congress and the non-medical people don't understand that. They think we can solve everything. I got really interested in this because of my work on the Dialysis Unit. I was known as "Dr. No" at the VA, but I had a very good track-record for keeping people off of kidney dialysis when that was only the prolonging of the inevitable. I didn't start out that way; I learned it the hard way. When I was a Fellow in Nephrology, I consulted on a 23-year-old mother of a four-month-old child who was in Duke hospital with total kidney shutdown and an advanced form of connective tissue disease. She was a medical disaster because all of her organs were failing, not just her kidneys. I persuaded Dr. Caulie Gunnells to let me dialyze her to keep her alive. He said, "You can dialyze her on one condition: you follow her from now until the day she dies," which happened six months later. I believed there was every reason we should try to save this woman, but he saw that it wasn't going to happen. And so what I did was kill that lady off over a period of six months instead of two weeks. And on top of wasting costly resources, I effectively tortured somebody. Most of the non-medical community doesn't understand that. I'm presumably a reasonably intelligent person and I'd already had some experience with terminal illness, but it took me a long time to really understand the implications. When Daddy went to work at the Methodist Home, he discovered individuals who were unable to take care of themselves because their thyroid glands were not working, and a number of things like that, which could be corrected relatively simply and without pain or danger. There are things that you can do that really will help, and I think Daddy totally supports that. But he doesn't support pumping money into terminal care. It's a waste of resources, like paying for elaborate funerals; it doesn't make good sense.

One measure of the man is probably the way that he handled John Hickam's death. They had been good friends during their years in Boston, Atlanta and Durham. John suffered a fatal cerebral hemorrhage just after he had really begun to get things moving as Department Chairman at Indiana. John had established something called the Regenstrief Foundation, a special health care initiative. Despite all the other things he had to do, after John's death, Daddy commuted to Indiana, two days a week for a year, to implement things that John had started at the Foundation. My father went to pick up the pieces and make some of John's dreams work. There are not a lot of people who could do that and so I think that is probably a measure of his commitment.

Eugene Stead claimed that he never had very many friends. He talked about people who were "very close to him," but he said he wasn't really sure what friends were. At the same time, he almost never mentioned any enemies. Yet, from the outside it seems his professional associates either loved or hated him—there seemed to be no neutral ground. His son, Bill, shared his perceptions from hearing his father talk at the dinner table.

Dr. William W. Stead:

> My wife, Janet, is slowly developing a collection of friends who are people she spends time with. I spend time either at work with associates or with Janet. We don't have a lot of friends in Durham. We go to the lake and lock all the gates; we don't run around and visit everybody. I'm discovering that I'm building a group of national associates, people I am very close with, who I think will be my version of my father's Warrens and Hickams, and so forth. When Janet and I moved into our first house, our next-door neighbors were also newly arrived, none of us had children, and we all had a lot of time. We would go sleigh riding together, mow our lawns and garden together. We were friends in the classic sense. None of us yet had responsibilities. We get together once every year now, and still thoroughly enjoy each other, but we don't have time to build those kinds of relationships anymore. People who come home at five o'clock on Friday afternoon and stay there all weekend need something to do with their evenings, so they build traditional friendships. We don't have time for that. It would be different if we took every Wednesday afternoon off and played golf or socialized with other people, but we went to the Lake and built a house.
>
> I think Daddy's always been a bit of a loner. He told us that when he was young he liked to go out with a kite or hike through the woods. He had caches of water bottles here and there, for use on hikes. There are gregarious people who appear to like everybody, but I don't think that's his nature. The way he chose to spend his time at work was more of a factor in building—or not building—friendships than being chairman. Daddy was in leadership roles when the people like the Hickams and Warrens, who clearly became his friends, first knew him, and that didn't prevent the relationship from developing. I really think how he spent his time was a factor in determining his friends and associates.
>
> Daddy was hard-nosed when he was convinced of something—he would push and push, though not in a personal way. Take me and

the computer business. Daddy and I had a mutual interest in new ways of handling medical information, but there were two different approaches to this: his group's and Ed Hammond's (where I worked). Daddy felt that having what he viewed as redundant efforts made us look silly on the national scene, and made it difficult for any of us to get funding. He had actually provided some of Ed Hammond's salary at one time, and so he went to Ed and said, "I recognize that I've supported you and I recognize that you and Bill have elected to work together. I simply want you to know that I'm going to put my full energy against you now, because we have two competing systems." Thereafter we not only had to generate money from somewhere else, but he really did try to put us out of business!

In the 1970s, when the split took place, I tried to explain to him (but never succeeded) that we were building a clinical data base that would be the front-end of a later system and his cardiology team was building a research back-end; if we could all survive long enough, we could merge the two together and have quite a system. In fact, that's actually what we did get after 1981 when our programs merged, but as equals rather than one taking over the other. He had wanted to unify things early, but I was committed to building the clinical front-end and was not going to change. We had some serious problems because, before I really got hold of the finances and sorted things out, I managed to get us many thousands of dollars in the hole. It was a fairly tense situation for a while, but as long as the word computer was not mentioned, Daddy and I got along fine. We could row in the boat together and cut down trees and do anything else. The Lake was always a haven, something we could sit down and talk about with interest. It was a glue, a subject we could go back to on common ground.

Daddy doesn't waste time or energy dithering over a decision. Once he decides, he watches the results and puts his full energy into trying to make sure that his decision was the right one. He may eventually change his mind, so I don't think he puts his ego into it, but he sure puts energy into it. If he then turns out to be wrong, he backs off. The thing he really protects himself from is wasting time by pretending that the decision-making process itself is so important. What he really says is he doesn't care if it was right or wrong; he makes a decision, he puts his full energy into making it work, and if it turns out not to be right, then he makes another decision.

I think the real essence of what he has contributed lies in his ability to teach, and in his having developed a value system that has some chance of lasting over time. Very few people who have had the kind of reputation he has had can be as human and normal as he is. One of my professional colleagues from another institution once came to look at our program here. When we got through watching the television news, Dad wandered in, sat down in a rocking chair and talked a little bit in a very human way, just like anybody else. I think if people kept their distance from him because he was Chairman, it was their problem, not his. It's almost the same thing as if people worry about me being his son.

His ability to teach by example, to provide opportunity together with a value system, is something that stands out. He and Mother and now Janet are my best friends. Whether that means that none of us can make other friends or not, I don't know. Once we got to be friends, once it was quite clear that I was supporting myself, he and I could offer each other advice and then accept or reject it. There was a transition point in our relationship and it is remarkable that he was able to make that transition with me, his son. Faculty members have the same problem in dealing with somebody as a student and then later as a colleague. That transition had to take place in order for us to be friends. We're able to be friends and still appreciate being father and son, which we probably could not have done without having become friends.

CHAPTER 23

CARING FOR THE ELDERLY

One needs to appreciate the fact that growing old and dependent are not things that make life joyful. But as far as I've been able to tell, unhappiness is totally drug-resistant. Joy is a thing created within yourself, and if you can't create it within yourself there's no doctor or drug that can create it for you. I've always been skeptical of the ease with which psychiatrists can diagnose depression in the elderly because for me it's a much more complicated situation.

E. A. Stead Jr.

When Eugene Stead stepped down as Chairman of Medicine at Duke, he did not fade into a retirement of golf-communities and travel. Instead, he assumed the position of Physician-in-Chief of the Methodist Retirement Home in Durham. It was located within walking distance (for Stead) of the hospital, and he divided his time between both locations. In order to convey the flavor of his work, we offer a "reconstructed" view of his activities there. Although the names and incidents of much of what is recorded here are fictional, they are based on extensive interviews and conversations with Stead, and accurately represent his attitudes and activities at the Methodist Retirement Home:

The Case of Bessie Greene: *At 82, Mrs. Greene went to live at the Methodist Retirement Home in Durham, North Carolina. After a relatively healthy life, in her eighth decade she became frail and had difficulty remembering; her husband had died almost two years before, and it was impossible for her to live any longer alone in her large house. She was lonely, but even more she feared that something might happen with no one around to help her. What if she were to become paralyzed and unable to call for help? She had treasured her independence, but now she dreaded solitude more. Her two children had moved north years before: Jim Jr. to Washington, and Elizabeth to Boston. Their closeness was unchanged by distance, but day-to-day Bessie was alone. She did not want to be a burden to her children, but she had no intention of ever leaving North Carolina, where her roots were sunk deep and she found comfort in the news of old friends. Both Elizabeth and*

Jim knew that, when their mother's mind was set, there was no persuading her otherwise. Jim Sr, was buried in the old churchyard beside his family, and Bessie intended to take her place next to him when the Lord called her. Until then, she would live out her days on the same stage she had occupied for more than 80 years. Of the options open, Bessie reluctantly agreed that the best, perhaps the only, solution was a nursing home. She hated the idea of forsaking her lovely home with its cherished memories, but it seemed to be the only way.

Always the realist, Bessie was grateful that the Home's Medical Director, Eugene Stead, was someone with whom she could talk freely. He was mature, down-to-earth, and seemed to understand people her age, not some young upstart who knew Bessie's interests better than she did herself. She was not a fussy woman and didn't need to be waited on, but she liked knowing that help was there for the asking. When she met Dr. Stead, she told him she needed to discuss something very important. She adjusted herself a little, smoothing her dress in her lap as she spoke. "If the occasion should arise," she started, uncertainly, "what I mean is, if I should suffer a stroke like my husband, or something like that," she paused briefly, "I don't wish to be hooked up to any of those contraptions. I've read that doctors can keep patients alive that way and that worries me. I've had a good long life but if I can't make it on my own, I would rather not have it that way." Bessie looked up at Dr. Stead and was relieved when he assured her that he would have no problem honoring her wishes.

Jim and Elizabeth listened quietly as Bessie outlined her instructions, but later Jim pulled Dr. Stead aside and whispered confidentially to him, "You're not really going to let her die if something happens, are you? We want her to have the best of everything, regardless of the cost."

"I've agreed to follow your mother's wishes, and so I will," he replied.

"Mother's always been a little queer in her notions," Jim tried to explain.

"There's nothing queer about dying," Stead replied candidly, "people do it every day."

Jim was taken aback by the blunt, almost insensitive, statement. Where was he leaving his mother? A wave of guilt flooded over him and he turned a deep crimson. Dr. Stead had seen such reactions before, however, and he realized that the family needed to understand the patient's wishes and, to the extent possible, accept them. After Jim and Elizabeth got their mother settled in her room, Dr. Stead invited them back to his office to discuss more fully the kind of care Bessie could expect to receive at the Home.

Motioning the family to sit, Dr. Stead leaned back in his chair and looked at each of the three people before him. Elizabeth was biting her thumbnail, and Jim drummed on the arms of the chair he occupied. Only Bessie seemed relaxed. After about a minute, Dr. Stead broke the silence: "Jim and I had a little chat earlier," he began, "and I have learned that he is not comfortable with your request to die naturally, Bessie." Jim was embarrassed, and flushed again.

Bessie looked at her son tenderly and reached over to pat his hand. "I guess we never really did talk to you children about it, but your father and I reached this decision a long time ago. When your father was taken with his seizure the day before he died, I only called the doctor because I couldn't go through it alone. But we had promised each other no medical hocus-pocus, and I can't see that it was wrong. I couldn't bear to see him a shadow of who he was, and I don't ever want to become just a shadow either. I've had a good life. Why stay past my welcome?"

Jim was beginning to relax as he listened to his mother.

"People often think they're not being good family members unless they do 'everything medically possible' for a loved one," Dr. Stead explained, "but that isn't always the best solution. That doesn't mean that everyone has to agree with my professional view; if you don't, why blessings on you, and we'll help you locate another facility that meets your needs. But we don't perform cardiopulmonary resuscitation here, and most of the patients agree that it seems like the kindest way to go."

Jim smiled self-consciously. "If only we lived nearer to Mother. I hate the idea of being so far away from you. What if something happens?"

"We'll call you and Elizabeth if anything happens," Dr. Stead assured him, "In the meanwhile, visit Mother as often as possible—you can be sure she will be looking forward to each visit. She's well and can enjoy you fully. And, if it feels comfortable to you, say your good-byes like each is the final one. It's a good practice anyway, and if turns out to have been necessary, you said your good-byes; if not, you have gotten yourself an extra gift."

When Jim and Elizabeth took their leave, they felt somewhat more comfortable about leaving mother in the care of Dr. Stead and the staff. The nurses and staff members seemed cheerful and helpful, and the elderly residents were much more active than in other nursing homes they had visited, with a busy calendar of activities to stretch both mind and body. As time passed and they saw that mother really was well cared for, guilt and worry subsided. When they talked to friends about other nursing homes, they realized that Mother was unusually fortunate.

Bessie herself had trouble performing many of the tasks she used to do. Arthritis limited her mobility, so she could no longer walk about as freely as she once did or keep up the knitting and needlepoint that she was so fond of. It proved useful to have nurses to remind her to take her medication. However, she hadn't lost her zest for life; her eyesight was strong, so she turned to books and newspapers, sometimes reading aloud to the other patients. She always felt good when she could do a little something for someone at the Home. And while she missed the independence and privacy of her own home, she enjoyed the steady companion-

ship and the freedom from worry. She was grateful for the ease her children now had, knowing that she was secure and comfortable.

One afternoon, reading quietly to herself in the lounge with several other patients, Bessie grew weak and sleepy. The words on the page blurred. She lost her grip on the book and let out a soft involuntary moan. The residents called to the nurses, alarmed when the book thumped the floor and Bessie slumped forward in the chair. When he arrived, Dr. Stead checked her vital signs, and had Bessie taken back to her room. Both pupils were dilated and the muscles of her face and extremities were paralyzed. Her pulse was weak, rapid, and its rhythm irregular. Her face was distorted by the paralysis, and her cheeks flopped passively with each breath. Her level of coma precluded the definitive neurological examination that might have precisely localized her vascular stroke, but her brainstem damage was so extensive that she would probably die quickly, unless intensive medical and nursing care kept her alive in a vegetative or, at best, severely disabled state.

"Shouldn't we give her oxygen and call 911, Doctor?" asked Janice Holder. Janice, recently hired, was unfamiliar with Dr. Stead's philosophy concerning the elderly.

"Mrs. Greene has asked that we not put her on life support of any kind," Dr. Stead replied. "If she were over there at the hospital, they would be compelled to put her in Intensive Care and keep her alive artificially. And once they started life support, they wouldn't be able to stop, even after they realized it had been a mistake. My responsibility is to Bessie, and she would not thank us for doing that."

When Elizabeth and Jim arrived by early evening, Dr. Stead explained their mother's condition. "If she survives the acute effects of the stroke, she may remain in a coma or possibly be completely paralyzed and unable to speak. The chance of recovery, even to a wheelchair existence is very slim. As it is, however, I don't expect her to regain consciousness."

Elizabeth, holding her brother's arm, cried softly on his shoulder as she watched her mother unconsciously struggle for each breath. "You might try to have a little supper and get some rest," Dr. Stead advised them. "We'll call you immediately if anything happens."

Back at their motel, Elizabeth and Jim spent a quiet evening reminiscing childhood memories. Both their parents had loved life and lived each day with vigor, so it seemed terribly hard to think of them being gone from their lives. "I suppose we really have nothing to regret," Elizabeth said, "I just hope she doesn't suffer."

Next morning they were at the Home before the sun had fully risen. Neither had slept very well but they decided they would rather be with Mother. When they entered her room, they were surprised to see how peacefully she slept. She looked different with her dentures removed and a plastic airway in her mouth to keep her tongue from blocking her throat. Elizabeth sat down beside her mother and stroked her hair; Jim stood silently over her bed watching and thinking about earlier times with her. "She's so still," Elizabeth whispered, but just as she spoke, a tremble seemed to move across her mother's body like a wave, and then a tiny gasp. "Jim," Elizabeth cried. The two crouched down beside the bed, but in a moment it was over. Jim called for a nurse and suddenly the tiny room seemed to be filled with people. Dr. Stead appeared as if from nowhere with instructions for the nurses and words of comfort for Bessie's children. Things needed to be settled, but that could be done later. Perhaps it would be best for Jim and Elizabeth to have some private moments with their Mother. Then they needed to get some air and maybe a cup of coffee.

Later, Dr. Stead led them to the door. As they reached the foyer, they were stopped by a small, grey-haired woman, bowed by the weight of years. "I'm so sorry," she said to Jim and Elizabeth. "Your mother was such a lovely person, wasn't she Dr. Stead?" He nodded in response. "She used to read to us," she continued, "and we all loved her." After pausing briefly, as though considering her next words, she added, "I hope I'm as lucky as she was when my time comes." Elizabeth was still holding her mother's wedding ring, which the nurse had given her. She began to cry.

Three days later at the weekly staff conference, Dr. Stead reviewed the events of the past week. It was his style to listen and to draw out the staff with questions before he made his own comments. Janice Holder, who had attended to Bessie during her stroke and requested that oxygen be given, listened quietly as the other staff members discussed a patient who had just been admitted to the Home:

The Case of Rupert Ferry: *Mr. Ferry, a 92 year old comatose patient, had been transferred from a small hospital the day before. He had arrived with a series of problems, including deep bedsores on his back and buttocks. Mrs. Holder was horrified to learn the extent of these infected and putrid ulcers. When the head nurse finished describing the patient's condition, Dr. Stead issued instruction to her on how to care for the patient. "I have examined the patient and agree with your findings. The family, I understand, does not want us to give him intravenous fluids, which is as it should be. We are simply to allow nature to take its course. Since Mr. Ferry is not aware of his condition, I suggest that we try to keep the smell down, but don't spend a whole lot of time on the problem."*

Mrs. Holder shifted uncomfortably in her chair, scribbling with a pen, eyes lowered to the page on the clipboard she held. She was deeply disturbed by Dr. Stead's assessment; was, in fact, having a hard time believing what she heard. The incident with Mrs. Greene had upset her. She felt that the staff had not done everything they could for the old woman. Now Mr. Ferry! She had chosen a nurs-

ing career because she wanted to save lives, not extinguish them. She had been at the Home for only a month, but Mrs. Holder now felt that she should have stayed at the Medical Center. The work schedule there had been more demanding, but the philosophy was a lot more consistent with her beliefs. Dr. Stead might have a great reputation as a doctor and educator, but she didn't think she would be able to stand another day among people who were so casual about life and death.

When the meeting broke up, Mrs. Holder requested a moment with Dr. Stead. His office was a strikingly modest room, with only enough space for a desk, a couple of chairs, and some medical books. "What a peculiar person," Mrs. Holder thought as she surveyed the small room for clues to Dr. Stead's personality but failed to find anything substantial. Most doctors had lavishly paneled offices with large desks and opulent decor. There was none of that here. She realized that this man was unlike any other she had met.

"I wondered, Dr. Stead," she began, trying to center her thoughts on her reason for being there, "if we might—that is, if the nurses might—learn cardiopulmonary resuscitation. Given the ages and diseases of many of the people here, I thought it might be useful for us to know. Also, I don't see any equipment here for resuscitation."

"Those are reasonable thoughts for a nurse coming from your background, Mrs. Holder, and I'm glad you brought them forward. I do understand why you think it would be a good idea for us to do resuscitation. But that isn't why people come here in their twilight years. My philosophy on aging and death is not quite aligned with what you might call popular thought. Of course I don't expect you to have the same belief system I have. Naturally, your experiences have been different from mine and I accept that you may not be able to appreciate my viewpoint now. But I'd like to make a suggestion, and see if perhaps you don't feel differently afterwards. Over the next six months, I would like you to observe the reactions of the other patients in the Home when residents die. Some of them will clearly be candidates for resuscitation, patients in whom the attempt would unquestionably be made in the hospital setting. After a patient dies, I would like you to find out whether their friends thought they would have wanted to die twice or three or even four times over by our resuscitating them. In my experience, nobody regrets sudden death, and I think you will come to understand that as you spend more time with these patients. Death is part of biology. It's going to happen sooner or later to all of us, and it doesn't much matter if it happens today or six weeks from now, especially in the aged and infirm. It's easier to learn that lesson as you get older. For example, I have left instructions with my own doctor that no extraordinary measures are to be used to keep me alive if my medical situation becomes irreversible. That seems only a sensible precaution to protect my own interests."

Mrs. Holder knew there was some truth in what Dr. Stead said, but it seemed so cut and dried. Did he have no compassion? she wondered. "I suppose it could be," she said, "but I hold human life sacred. It just seems wrong not to try. I've gone into this profession to help people."

"We recognize that, and that is why we hired you. There is every reason for you to continue to help your patients," Dr. Stead replied. I just don't think we're actually doing a patient any favor to retrieve them from death when they will only have to face it soon again. It's a question of degree. If people who suffer a massive stroke are resuscitated, they would only live out their remaining days as invalids with seriously limited ability to participate in the activities of life. We have several patients with terminal cancer in the Home. Some bright young doctors might put them on aggressive chemotherapy, which would cause nausea, vomiting, hair loss, and other discomfort. For what gain? These kinds of advanced cancers have never been cured, even in young people. A wise doctor knows when to stop. I try to teach that to young doctors. Aging, with its loss of independence and diminishing faculties, is difficult enough as it is. So to revive patients only to have them deteriorate beyond the point of meaningful life does not make sense to me. As I said, however, I would like you to observe for yourself."

Mrs. Holder sat quietly for a moment, not knowing what to say. On the one hand, she knew that what Dr. Stead was saying was quite true, yet she had never before met anyone who was quite so blunt about it. She thought back to the staff meeting and remembered Mr. Ferry, and that he was really the stimulus to speak to Dr. Stead in the first place. "I would like to take care of Mr. Ferry," she said.

"You can discuss your assignments with the Head Nurse," Dr. Stead said. "I certainly have no objection."

"What I mean is, I think he should be turned. I've taken care of patients suffering with severe bedsores, and had some great successes, though it does take months."

"I'm afraid it isn't going to make much difference to him whether or not he's turned. He's no longer aware of anything around him."

"But certainly we still are concerned with the dignity of the human being," Mrs. Holder said, a bit flustered now. She had tried to be accommodating but he was making it awkward.

"We are always concerned with the dignity of the human being," Dr. Stead insisted, "however, I'm afraid Mr. Ferry no longer warrants that kind of attention. He is well beyond that point. His brain is already dead and we are simply waiting for the rest of his body to catch up. It would take a skilled nurse like you almost full time to clean his sores, change the dressings, and position him. If we were to focus our attention and resources on someone who, for all intents and purposes, is already brain dead, then we would be seriously short-changing the *patients with whom we could make a difference. Our resources are limited, Mrs. Holder, as you know. We want to make a difference with the living; that's what we're here to do; we have to be intelligent in how we distribute those resources. Once the resources are spent there are no more."*

What a hard man to talk to, she thought. Whatever points she raised, he seemed to have thought about before. In spite of the anger she instinctively felt about Dr. Stead's direct and inflexible logic, Janice Holder knew she had a lot to think about. Nursing and its goals had always seemed so straightforward, now they seemed complex, even though there was nothing convoluted about Stead's opinions. Issues that had always been black and white now seemed like patches of gray. She felt challenged and, admittedly, a little threatened. It didn't seem right to leave the patient with his foul, open skin ulcers. She shuddered. Looking at Stead's office once more, she noticed what she had not seen before. In fact there was a great deal of character in the simplicity of that modest office. It was as direct and no-nonsense as the person who occupied it. If Stead was right, she would learn something new; if not, she would leave.

Shortly after Mrs. Holder left, the receptionist announced that Mrs. Weaver had arrived with her daughter and son-in-law. Mrs. Weaver was to be admitted, and Dr. Stead had arranged to interview the woman and her family prior to admission, as he did with all new incoming patients.

"Please ask Dr. Rainey join us," he instructed the receptionist.

Matthew Rainey had recently finished a Family Practice Residency. He worked at the Home part-time under Dr. Stead, and was involved in the admission evaluation of each patient. A light knock at Dr. Stead's door, and a frail, white-haired old woman appeared at the threshold, hunched so that it was difficult to make out her features. Beside her, a middle-aged man gingerly supported her elbow. Behind them was a woman of about the same age as the man. Like a back seat driver, she called out to the other two: "Don't let's just barge in there. I'm sure the doctor is a very busy man. Wait for him to invite you in so we know we're not interrupting anything." The three stopped mechanically in the doorway and the woman in back peered in over the heads of the other two.

"Come in," Dr. Stead said to the group.

As the old woman and her son-in-law shuffled into the office, the daughter called out directions to both. "Put her in the chair closest to the door. Mama, take the chair right there. Don't make her walk so far." Dr. Stead walked around from his desk to help the patient into her seat. Up close to Mrs. Weaver, he noticed a coarse tremor in her hands, but that was all he could tell about her for the time being. The woman held her head down away from all of them, fixing her gaze on the floor.

Dr. Stead introduced himself once everyone was seated. The man and woman were Charles and Catherine Porter, the responsible relatives of the patient. At that moment, Matt Rainey appeared at the door. "Have I missed much?" the young doctor said. The Porters looked up to see a red haired young man with a closely clipped beard standing in the doorway. He smiled at them as he was introduced, but when Dr. Stead introduced him to Mrs. Weaver, she responded only with a nod, keeping her eyes fixed downward. Because all of the chairs were taken, Dr. Rainey stood to the side of the crowded office. Dr. Stead sat behind his desk and asked some general questions. He systematically toyed with a pencil, moving it from point to eraser and back again.

It seemed, as the questions began, that Mrs. Porter had definite ideas about what should be discussed, addressing herself to Dr. Stead as though Mrs. Weaver were not in the room, and talking about her mother in the third person. She spoke quickly, outlining her mother's condition and her opinions on the type of care Mrs. Weaver would require. "My mother has a heart condition and is very nervous, Dr. Stead. She needs medication for these things and can't be relied on to take it on her own. She forgets doses and, since Charlie and I both work, we're not able to keep track of the medicine the way we should. We're always writing out schedules for her to follow, but she either loses them or forgets them. Her doctor explained that it's very important for her to take her pills, you know, and we thought in a place like this someone would give her medicines on a regular basis so she doesn't miss any. Charlie and I can't possibly provide her with the 24-hour care she needs. She really requires constant attention. I try to fix meals for her when I know I'll be out. I cook low-salt dishes and encourage her to drink herbal teas instead of all the caffeine in coffee. It's no good for her you know, but I get home and find the salt-shaker on the table beside her dish. I know I haven't left it out. And there are coffee grinds in the trash. She's either thrown out the tea bag or put it back in the box. Frankly, she gets resentful of me when I scold her, and I wonder why I go to the trouble to fix all those special things when she just goes and salts them anyway. In a place like this you can control that sort of thing." She stopped to take a breath before continuing, "And then there's the companionship. She needs someone with her. She gets so lonely in the house all day long by herself. Honestly, it just breaks my heart sometimes to think of her there all alone. We just can't take care of her the way she needs and so we've brought her here."

Dr. Stead listened to Mrs. Weaver's daughter, glancing over to see the patient's response to her daughter's words when she had finished. "It sounds as though you don't want to be deprived of the things you like at this point in your life, Mrs. Weaver." The old woman lifted her head for the first time, and Dr. Stead was surprised to be greeted by two clear, strikingly blue eyes and a set of aged, but noble features. However, she wore the expression of a woman whose patience had long been exhausted.

"I am an old woman. What does it matter if I sprinkle a little salt on my steak or have butter with my potatoes? They deny me everything I enjoy. I think they would prefer that I wasn't around to be such a nuisance."

"Now Mama," Mrs. Porter said, "you know that just isn't true. You know what the doctor said about the importance of your diet. I worry about you, dear."

Dr. Stead could see that the daughter's overbearing desire to 'do what was right' for mother had caused hard feelings between the two. It wasn't important who was objectively right or wrong—what mattered was the feelings involved. Perhaps the best thing for both mother and daughter would be a little distance between them. "I have to be perfectly honest with you," Dr. Stead said to the Porters, "there's no way we can police your mother's eating habits. Even if we do serve her a special salt-restricted diet, there is no way, in facilities of this type, to guarantee that she won't help herself to a serving on someone else's tray. Nor would we want to impose our will on hers—she seems to have a very sound mind. All of our patients receive basically the same meal and snack choices. We don't have the financial or personnel resources to provide otherwise. You don't have the resources either. On the other hand," Dr. Stead continued, alternating his glance among the group, "you can expect to be well cared for in a way that meets with your agreement and makes good medical sense, Mrs. Weaver. You will find good people here at the Home, both the residents and the staff. You can choose among many activities, educational opportunities and exercise programs. We will tailor these to your physical abilities and interests."

Dr. Stead recognized that Mrs. Porter genuinely wanted the best care for her mother, but she had become frustrated by her inability to reconcile what she thought her mother needed and what she could do. The inability to meet her own high demands had created stress for the entire family, particularly because there were differing opinions about what the patient really needed. Stead knew that if he didn't outline exactly what the family and patient could reasonably expect from the Home, the confusion would perpetuate the ongoing power struggles and arguments—then everyone would lose, most of all Mrs. Weaver. Dr. Stead outlined the specifics he felt the family needed to learn so that some problems would be avoided in the future.

"Exactly what medication are you on, Mrs. Weaver?" Dr. Stead asked.

"Well," the old woman began, but before she could finish, her daughter interrupted.

"She has nerve pills, sleeping pills, vitamins for strength and two different kinds of heart pills."

The old woman cast a resentful look at the younger one, but, steeling herself, continued as though the interruption had not occurred. "I have them here in my bag. They make me so sleepy during the day that I can't remember the names."

Slowly, deliberately she pulled her purse onto her lap and snapped open its clasp. Fishing inside for a moment, she extracted five bottles, one by one.

Dr. Rainey read the labels aloud, as he took one after the other from the patient's trembling hand. "Valium, 5 mg. 3 times a day; phenobarbital, 30 mg. at bed time; multi-vitamins, digoxin, 0.25 mg. daily; and quinidine 200 mg. daily. Yes, we are very familiar with such prescriptions." Of course the Porters couldn't know, as Dr. Stead did, that elderly patients often perk up considerably when tranquilizers and barbiturates are stopped, and that constant doses of digoxin and quinidine are often worthless, even dangerous. There would be time to see what Mrs. Weaver really needed.

"You'll be sure she takes those regularly, won't you?" Mrs. Porter asked. "I've tried, Lord knows, we've both tried, haven't we Charlie? But Mama just can't remember to take them." Mr. Porter nodded in response to his name, but other than that, he remained quiet. It was obvious that he would rather be elsewhere.

"I'm not sure I understand why all of these pills have been prescribed, but if she needs anything, we'll see that she gets it," Stead assured her. By observing the dynamic that had occurred in his office, Dr. Stead had learned a great deal about the patient's condition. He had a real sense of Mrs. Weaver's situation, and knew that, with the exception of her heart condition yet to be assessed, the patient would require minimal medical management. He concluded the interview by calling a nurse to show Mrs. Weaver and the Porters her new room. As the family trailed off down the hall behind the nurse, Dr. Stead motioned to Dr. Rainey to be seated.

"What is your assessment of this case, Matt?" Stead asked.

"Well, the patient seems to be quite alienated and depressed. Of course I can't fully assess her without a more complete examination, but she might benefit more from an anti-depressant than a tranquilizer. We could also check her blood digoxin level to see if the blood levels are adequate. I've been working on a schedule for the nurses to insure that patients get medications on time and in the right doses. It's a little involved, but it would eliminate missed doses. I'm sure we can handle the current irregularity of her medications. Also, she needs to have enough quiet time to deal with her level of anger about being dependent."

Dr. Stead leaned back in his chair, listening. Having worked with the elderly for some time, he knew that he was going to have to head Rainey off at the pass. He didn't want to embarrass the young man, but he knew his own years of valuable experience and practical information were not yet part of the young doctor's internal library. When Rainey had finished, Stead responded, slowly, thoughtfully. "You know, Matt," he began, "in dealing with sick old folks, you don't want to spend too much time taking their history because they get tired. And the longer you take, the more inaccurate the history is. When I first came here, the nurses took very elaborate histories, and then the doctor signed off on them. After I took *charge, I whittled it down to the few things I thought were important, most of which I could ask myself. I suggest you try that and hold all treatment until you have made a careful, independent assessment. Virtually all of our newly admitted patients are taking a long list of medicines, which their doctors have given them over the years. They keep adding prescriptions but rarely stop any. As far as I can tell, these medications either don't do anything to improve organ function, or actually cause mischief, such as paralyzing the bladder or keeping the brain from working normally, aggravating tremors, causing loss of memory or even confusion. The most obvious culprits are drugs that doctors have prescribed because the patient has been unhappy, and is being treated for some supposed psychiatric illness. My general rule is simply to stop all medications for which I cannot find a definitive and pressing reason.*

"As people age and lose agility and independence, they go to their doctor for help. However, because they don't always understand what's wrong with them, the patients may not clearly communicate the true nature of their problem. They tell the doctor they've got a headache, a backache, or that their feet are swollen, instead of the real problem, which is that they're getting old and losing control over body functions they've always taken for granted. The patient wants help, and the doctor wants to help, so he prescribes something. Many of those medications are prescribed in very small doses that really don't do any particular harm except cost money. It's easier for the doctor to add 10, 15, or 20 drugs than to get to the bottom of the patient's complaints. We often have patients admitted here who bring in a shoebox full of medicines. However, no medicine is going to give the patient what is really desired—the agility and independence of youth. The difficulty arises from patients being over-medicated or from the combination of drugs. In many instances, the patients end up feeling worse than before they went to the doctor, unless of course they forget to take their medications. If they get in a situation where they are forced to take the prescribed medications, they often become seriously over-medicated. The only thing that saved them before was that they just forgot to take it!

"Since nobody can reverse the patient's complaints, the patient often becomes paranoid. 'Someone stole my glasses or pocket book,' rather than 'I can't remember where I left it.' They need to blame somebody for what is happening to them and they usually accuse the family of things for which the family clearly is not responsible. Although that seems not to be a problem in this instance, it is evident in the way Mrs. Weaver resents her daughter. And Mrs. Porter, in spite of the fact that she's overly protective, really does want to help her mother. This is a situation in which her being here will clearly alleviate conditions at home.

"For my own learning about treating the aged, I used to sit in the lobby of the Senior Citizens High Rise Building once a week, and just make myself available

to talk to the residents. It was just very informal—and free—office hours. They could come to chat and visit or ask medical questions. They were often confused about their schedule of medications and why they were taking them, and my advice was usually to stop taking all drugs. It was remarkable how often these people would perk up, become more energetic, and sleep at night instead of napping during the day and staying awake at night. Once medications are out of the system it becomes clear which, if any, are important for their health. But taking a cardiac drug like digoxin or quinidine on a daily basis at the same dose for years, as Mrs. Weaver has done, makes absolutely no sense. That's bad medicine!

"When patients come into the Home with a suitcase full of prescriptions, I usually have one ace in the hole—I can stop the drugs. That alone usually makes a difference. But a doctor has to decide when there is an underlying problem that can be successfully treated with drugs versus a condition where a little understanding and an arm around the shoulder is needed instead. In cases of the latter, the doctor then has to accept that limitation. If the doctor cannot satisfy the demands of a patient, he cannot reject that person. The best thing is to be human with them. A doctor can't achieve any great medical triumphs with someone in that particular time of life.

"In a nursing home, psychiatrists get caught in two traps: they spend time making notes that are irrelevant to care, and they may prescribe too many drugs too quickly for an old population. In working with the elderly, one needs to appreciate that growing old and dependent are not things that make life joyful. But as far as I've been able to tell, unhappiness is totally drug resistant. Joy is a thing created within yourself, and if you can't create it within yourself, no doctor or drug can create it for you. I've always been skeptical of the ease with which psychiatrists diagnose depression in the elderly because for me it's a much more complicated situation."

The young physician listened intently. Dr. Stead finished his thoughts and sat with the fingertips of his two hands lightly pressed together and rested on an invisible point on his kneecap.

"Perhaps I need to reconsider Mrs. Weaver's treatment," Dr. Rainey said eventually.

"Perhaps," Dr. Stead replied.

One thing is for sure, Dr. Stead practiced what he preached. Some years back he was concerned about an aging relative who was seeing her world collapsing around her. He wanted her doctors not to meddle with life-support systems, if that issue ever arose, much as he had arranged for himself. He was willing to share these ideas with others, and to put them on record in print, as in the following editorial from *Medical Times*:

This is the first generation in which the majority of persons between 40 and 60 years of age are financially responsible for three generations. Each family with children has at least four grandparents and, in this day and age, at least one of the grandparents will survive and become partially or completely senile. This last week I have been shopping for a very sweet but beginning-to-be-confused grandmother. She is used to doing for herself and she does not adapt easily to having other people do for her. She tells her house-helper not to do most things, intending to do them herself. But alas, she forgets and they are never done. She likes the visiting nurse who helps her with personal cleanliness and gives her advice about cooking, eating and shopping but, again, she cannot believe that she can't go it on her own.

As I shopped in the community where she has spent her life, I found good will on all sides. The saleswoman in the department store, the assistant manager of the bank, the salesmen responsible for mattresses, pillows and linens were interested in my problem: how to keep my lady functioning and living in her community. Each of them has faced similar problems. They look on the nursing home as inevitable but each, based on his own experience, hopes that that time can be postponed. They have no good answers to old age, nor do I.

What shall we do if Grandmother slips and breaks her hip? What shall we do if she develops pneumonia? Must medical science intervene and keep her breathing but not living?

Many years ago, I wrote my own personal physician a letter to guide his hand if I became ill and my mind was not functioning normally. I quote from that letter:

"In the event of unconsciousness from an automobile accident, I do not wish to remain in a hospital for longer than two weeks without full recovery of my mental faculties. While I realize that recovery might still be possible, the risk of living without recovery is still greater. At home, I want only one practical nurse. I do not wish to be tube-fed or given intravenous fluids at home.

"In event of a cerebral accident, other than a subarachnoid hemorrhage, I want no treatment of any kind until it is clear that I will be able to think effectively. This means no stomach tube and no intravenous fluids.

"In the event of a subarachnoid hemorrhage, use your own judgment in the acute stage. If there is considerable brain damage, send me home with one practical nurse.

"If, in spite of the above care, I become mentally incapacitated and have remained in good physical condition, I do not want money spent on private care. I prefer to be institutionalized, preferably in a state hospital.

"If any other things happen, this will serve as a guide to my own thinking. Go ahead with an autopsy with as little worry to my wife as possible."

Now the time has come to write a letter to Grandmother's doctor. He is a wise man and will appreciate the support a family can give in a problem for which there is no wholly satisfactory answer. (Med Times. 1970;98:191)

Geriatric medicine is a new and rapidly growing subspecialty of medicine, reflecting the profound demographic changes characterized as the "graying of America." It also reflects the fact that the care of elderly people has many unique aspects, many special "tricks of the trade" that require specialized knowledge. No longer is it necessary for elders to be over-medicated because the doctor is unaware of how older people respond to medications, or of the non-medical things that can improve ability to function. All of that is for the good. The shortage of nursing home facilities and comprehensive health care is not good, nor is it likely to improve in the foreseeable future.

The elderly and their elected representatives are fighting hard for more and better facilities. Stead, however, held an unpopular, even a singular view among medical experts. He was convinced that the economy in this country simply cannot stand the added costs of comprehensive medical and nursing home care for everyone. Our society has not been willing to make the hard choices of whether to put more money into educating poor children or into intensive medical and nursing care of people with dementia who have no idea of who or where they are. Stead found it hard to justify the growing demand on scarce resources. His choice would clearly be to put the most money where it will do the most good. He didn't expect that people will understand the problem until it becomes much worse, far into the 21st century. Whatever else we may think, it is clear that there are no simple answers.

CHAPTER 24

STEADY THOUGHTS

The reasonable man adapts himself to the world; the unreasonable one persists in trying to adapt the world to himself. Therefore, all progress depends on the unreasonable man.

George Bernard Shaw

No simple collection of Dr. Stead's thoughts can do justice to the full array of his range and depth. He was never one to pull punches or soften the impact of his judgments. Many have (and will) disagree with his iconoclastic viewpoints. We present here some of his recorded reflections on a series of topics that seem to be universal in the medical world.

1. Health Care USA: Too Much, Too Expensive

Medicare is a striking example of a law passed without adequate information being available to the Congress or Executive branch. In the absence of a uniform federal-state system of data gathering, there was no possible way to estimate the actual impact and cost of this legislation on health care. This legislation was proposed and Congress had to pass it or not pass it. No mechanism existed to field test in advance any of the component parts.

There are already a great many laws affecting the health field, and each year there will be more. Doctors out in the field are aware of the problems created by these laws and by the operating agencies they produce. Once the laws are put into operation, they gain support at the agency level. The new agencies, and the personnel employed by them, become part of the large governmental bureaucracy. Regardless of the absurdities that develop, or the lack of progress in achieving the goals that lawmakers envisaged, the new agencies will not disappear.

E. A. Stead Jr.

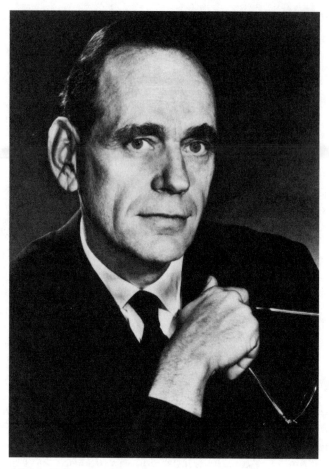

Eugene Stead in his 62nd year.

Dr. Stead:

I've never been as much of a believer in medical care as many of my colleagues are. There's no relationship between the number of doctors in a community and the quality of health in that community. Many variables determine what happens to individuals, and the doctor is only one. The difference between minimal care and the most high-priced care in the world is so small that it gets lost in the noise level. Too many important health variables (nutritional status, hygiene, motivation, education) are not controlled in the system to know what small effect the medical and nursing care has.

I've always thought that there were two kinds of medical care. One relates to treatment of short-lived phenomena that should be available to everybody. If an individual breaks his leg, I see no reason why he shouldn't have his bones put back together, or why an individual with acute pneumonia shouldn't have some antibiotics. On the other hand, we spend most of our money on treatment of disorders like severe heart or liver failure, which (regardless of their cause) are not going to go away. In those cases, it's extraordinarily easy for health care people to make prescriptions that they think will favorably affect outcomes. But the treatments they prescribe have to be carried out over many weeks, months and years. And, since that kind of compliance is extraordinarily difficult for the patient, most of the things that doctors order might as well not be done at all, because intermittent or partial compliance are usually worthless.

So, access to care for broken bones, which are simple to treat, should be universal, but I see the other kind of problems, those that require long-term treatment, as analogous to an enzyme-substrate reaction. In the absence of an enzyme, certain chemical reactions proceed so slowly that they're not even detectable; when an enzyme is mixed in, the reaction occurs quickly. Without a substrate, the enzyme is useless, and without an enzyme, the substrate is useless. The doctor can be the enzyme or catalyst, but his effectiveness depends on the substrate, which in this case is his patient.

I do think third party payments and government help are useful for short-term or emergency situations. When I was growing up, the episodes that put my family in financial straits were acute episodes. They were not the kinds of problems that required a basic change in the structure and pattern of everyday family life, but even those brief, acute episodes were difficult to afford. Most of health care money in the U.S. is spent on long-term problems, which the medical profession has relatively little chance of changing.

Decreeing that everybody with kidney failure should have government-sponsored dialysis before he dies is kind of crazy. If we shifted the economic responsibility to the family, dialysis for chronic kidney failure would largely disappear. The technology to keep people alive is entirely different from the ability to transplant kidneys, which, at times, can be quite effective. What is possible technically, and what is reasonable for society, are often at odds. For example, in a government-sponsored program like the VA, the central administration can (and has) determined that everybody with renal failure will be dialyzed. This doesn't allow the doctor to choose the course of treatment and use the available resources wisely. After all, the resources are not infinite, even if we act as though they were. The medical profession, in conjunction with the family, should determine who is dialyzed and who is not. It shouldn't be decreed by a single voice in Washington. Dialysis programs are now paid for by Social Security so that everyone is eligible to receive this costly technology.

Whenever the government sets a policy that it perceives will be good for everybody, the policy becomes ridiculous. The population is too diverse and the problems too varied to have simple legal solutions. Preferably, the family should have enough financial responsibility that no member will enter into a dialysis program if the family cannot pay for at least part of it. I have no objection to subsidizing dialysis, but to pay it entirely through tax money for everybody is a mistake. Whenever any service is available at governmental expense, whether it serves a useful purpose or not, it becomes susceptible to abuse. The patient and the patient's family have to share in the responsibility so that they cannot simply say, "I want the services because they're available and they cost me nothing."

Dean Davison had a good philosophy; he wanted decisions about payment of any welfare or social benefits to be determined by the people immediately involved with the individual receiving the payments. He said that there was no way for someone in Washington to know who was a fraud or who had the ability to take care of himself. The only people who could know these things were those in the community where the individual lived—the people who came into contact with him daily. When the money is distributed from Washington or Raleigh, it's easy to sponge off the system. The real question is what level of services should we provide, and that may be determined better by the local community than by people operating at a distance.

Aside from dialysis and services for hemophiliacs, no other type of chronic disease is yet covered through social security. Why do people with these medical problems get free assistance from the government when this is not available to people with other kinds of illnesses? That is a politically determined inequity that makes no sense. The government hasn't gone any further with public health assistance, but they haven't retracted those two programs either. Individual tragedy—and the apparent relief of that tragedy—makes such an effective television and congressional hearing appeal, and people will do for individuals in those circumstances what they will not do for anyone else. We know perfectly well that money spent in support of education of children at a very early age would be more profitable to society than the same amount of money spent to transplant an organ in a fifty-year-old. The difficulty is that if we cut off the transplant money or the dialysis money, we have no mechanism for transferring the money to the areas where it would achieve greater good for society. There is no effective opposition to bad use of national resources, because everybody knows that the money saved won't go to those children but revert back to the Treasury Department. And so, the constituency that might make meaningful choices, doesn't function. Our budgeting process doesn't permit these trade-offs to be considered in this manner, and so it seems hopeless to lobby for better utilization of limited resources.

I have run into situations of this nature, as everybody else in the health world has. I'm a Depression child and never liked to see money wasted, and so I cut down the medical expenses greatly when I operated a retirement home. I knew money was being thrown away without any benefit to the patients. I would have liked to use some of that money to brighten up the physical facilities of the institution so the people could enjoy it. There was no way, however, to transfer or redirect those funds. The people who were doing the budgeting were not connected to those doing the spending. So, the discovery of cost saving initiatives was stifled. At the retirement home I was saving the government money, and I was also saving some of the patient's money, but that didn't really help me because the Home put the saved money to other uses—they never used it for anything I wanted to use it for. Most people in my position in the Home wouldn't have saved the money, they would have said, "What the hell, why take the time and trouble to explain to this patient that he doesn't need certain things done and that we don't want to spend the money this way?" The problem is that, in the end, you can't touch the money you might save.

The cost of medical care has certainly outstripped the rate of inflation for any other part of the economic system. Health Maintenance Organizations and like mechanisms haven't affected it. In fact, one of the problems with these schemes is that, in the end, more people go to more doctors because services, once paid for, seem free. Even with a gate-keeper, a generalist who makes the decision to call in a specialist or get a second opinion, you can't indefinitely suppress the fact that many people are complainers; eventually you open the gate to unlimited access and more and more procedures are done, regardless of the outcome they achieve. For example, in the cardiovascular area, our ability to diagnose diseases far exceeds our ability to cure them, but that doesn't keep us from continually pouring money into new diagnostic tests that have a very marginal effect on outcomes.

Better diagnosis, or earlier diagnosis and detection of three-vessel coronary artery disease is not going to have much effect on dying of that heart disease. We are already good at making such diagnoses, but we still use every new diagnostic test that comes along. What's worse financially is that we usually keep using the old methods for a long time too, so essentially we double the amount of money it costs to have the studies. For example, we've made no real progress by using expensive CT scans in treating people with headaches. Very few headaches are caused by anything that the CT can identify, but nevertheless we get a lot of extremely expensive CT's for headaches. Since we're not outcome-oriented, we have a great difficulty reducing the level of expenditures for a complaining population. The more people who bring their complaints to the doctor, the more are expensive tests done. The fact that most of the population's complaints are due to the way people use or abuse their bodies, rather than to the presence of disease in the body, means that technological advances won't solve their problems or make them happy. Becoming obese from overeating or destroying the lungs or liver by smoking or drinking cause all manner of physical complaints. I find that patients usually go to see doctors because they're not happy for one reason or another—but neither technological procedures nor medications make anyone happy as far as I know! They merely cover over the symptoms for a time.

Another important determinant of the extent of health care should be the family. A doctor has a responsibility to the patient's family. I've seen many families financially destroyed because the doctor never really found out what the family wanted or whether the doctor was really going to do the patient any good. It's my contention that the doctor should at least feel out the position of the family, and not just that of the patient. Every doctor should know enough about what's going on in a family to take care of the social problems to whatever extent is needed and possible. That's part of the practice of medicine.

2. The Veteran's Administration System

Dr. Stead has worked closely with Veterans Hospitals throughout his career. After he retired as Chairman at Duke, he was awarded a VA Distinguished Professorship, an honor given to a few top clinicians in the country. In that capacity he toured the nation, speaking at many VA hospitals. Few people outside the VA system have Stead's insights into the advantages and disadvantages of this huge federal hospital system, and fewer still have spoken so candidly on the issues. As the crisis in financing health care mounts in America we should try to learn what "government medicine" can be like, though obviously the issues of health care for the nation are much larger than the scope of medicine for veterans of the armed services.

Dr. Stead:

> With some 166 hospitals, the VA system is the biggest health care system in the country. The Durham VA Hospital played an important role in the development of the Duke Medical Center, and I worked with it from the time it opened in the early 1950s. Now, having traveled extensively to other VA hospitals, I'd say the VA system served an excellent educational purpose by training doctors up to a certain level. But as the system attempts to become highly specialized and more medically sophisticated, the problem you run into is that so much of its patient population is a poor substrate for change. So we're back, in part, to the city hospital model. The other big problem with the VA is that it is required by law to determine the status of its clients who are now out of the service and not able to function in civilian society. The ex-soldier who suffers from anxiety and complains of a headache, back pain or abdominal problems is often awarded 10% disability payments for a service-related anxiety disorder. That person may spend the rest of his life trying to get the VA to award him the remaining 90%, and he does that by going back repeatedly to the VA hospital with additional complaints. Perhaps the person abuses alcohol and is hospitalized for that, then for indigestion, then for emphysema from too much smoking; each of these medical events is paid for by the taxpayer, but they also generate a request for larger and larger disability checks for life. Paying pensions at different levels is a very expensive way to go about giving services.
>
> The VA has a level of bureaucracy that is nearly unbelievable, because everybody knows that people will try to get something that is "free." So, in order to keep people from cheating the system, the VA has built a structure that requires a tremendous flow of paper records. In order to keep the system operating, they continually add more resources to the bureaucracy than to health care itself. The VA has become a system in which it's extraordinarily difficult to create move-

ment, and it's extraordinarily difficult to direct funds that will pay for actual services provided to patients by nurses and doctors rather than for administrators, monitors and lawyers.

In any program where the federal government makes money available, one has to hedge the system around with a whole series of requirements that would be ridiculous in private business. People look on government money in a somewhat different light; if they can chisel a few dollars out of the federal government or overcharge it for their services, they will. So the federal government feels that it has to build in a large number of safeguards against this kind of behavior. And the more guards they build in, the more rigid the system becomes and the harder it is to operate. There is no flexibility about what services and medications can be offered to eligible veterans, regardless of their financial status. These safeguards mean that there are more opportunities to squeeze money from the system once one learns the complexity of its operation and how to manipulate it. For this reason, people who leave the government after years in high administrative positions are in tremendous demand by private industry. They know how to work the system. It's not an easy system to make work honestly, and there's a great temptation to try to use influence. Recently, we've seen a good deal of influence peddling for profit in defense contracts, housing loans and banking, and it goes on in other area of government as well. The result is a tremendous number of regulations, which are very easy to get tangled in. Then you end up in court or before the ethics committee and whatnot. I think it's a problem that is universal to government and, to a point, the only sensible answer is to have less government. Still, it would be a very great loss to the training of doctors if there weren't any VA hospitals. Those VA Hospitals that are run by medical schools extend the teaching scope of university medical centers to all kinds of health personnel and provide faculty positions for young people starting out in academic careers.

When nearby medical schools take responsibility for managing professional appointments (that is, they name the doctors who work there), VA hospitals deliver a level of professional services far beyond what the system had before the medical schools were involved. In terms of educating doctors, and in service to its patients, the VA's record since World War II is infinitely better than it was previously, when it operated at a much lower professional level. But looking over the years I was involved in its operation, I saw the governmental bureaucracy consume more and more of the money, while less and less of the total resources went toward the goal, which is caring for sick people.

Philosophically it's a difficult question whether or not our society would be better off without VA hospitals, and I don't know the answer. I do not know what fraction of the people now going to the VA hospital are there for war- or service-connected disability. As you go through a VA hospital, you do not see a highly educated, well-off group of patients who simply don't want to pay for private health care. You really see broken-down members of society. As to the people who are there because they suffered injuries or illness directly because of their military service, I just think we have to grit our teeth and say, "We wish we were smart enough not to have wars, but we do have wars, and this is a war casualty, which we have to pay for." Undoubtedly, a considerable portion of the veteran's hospital population never would have been economically or socially useful, whether we had a war or not—they are the kind of people who would go to a city hospital if there were no VA. I'm not smart enough to know which portion of the veterans' problems society should pay for and which it shouldn't because it is the responsibility of the individual. Considering that the VA system does employ people, if you stopped all useless VA hospital activity, you would have a tremendous unemployment problem. I'm not crusading to get rid of the VA system.

I have tried to keep veterans from being involved in protracted disability quests and disputes, and to discourage their attempts to collect more than they are really due. But I don't think this problem is related just to service. It exists whenever someone is attempting to collect from other people things that are not unequivocally and clearly due them. Similarly, I've tried to prevent people from trying to collect a tremendous amount of money from automobile accidents in which the evidence is clear that they really don't deserve to collect it. In order to justify pursuing things you really don't deserve, you have to believe that all the people who don't agree with you are bad people. Not only can this result in a tremendous amount of time and effort poured into a totally unprofitable venture, but I think it leads to a kind of paranoia about everybody else. Finally, you lose sight of the truth. In the beginning you may have known that things really didn't happen as you say they did, but you expected to make a profit out of it nevertheless; in the end you may not know that anymore—you honestly believe what you hear yourself say and believe that your cause is just. All of this business of attempting to collect marginal things is very destructive, and I've always tried to keep anybody that I've had contact with, from becoming involved in that particular kind of behavior. The payoff is rarely very great, and the risk to the person's integrity and belief system is simply too high. Trying to get what doesn't belong to you is a universal temptation, and the VA stands out merely because it is a concentrated example of an opportunity ripe for the plucking.

The bureaucratic difference between VA Hospitals and Duke Hospital is that Congress has not given resources to the VA as liberally as the private sector has given to its hospitals. This allows hospitals like Duke to increase their cash flow. Private hospitals have a very large administrative structure, but they simply raise the cost of medical care to a higher level than the VA has been able to do. Given the same number of dollars, the systems might have been equally bad off. But the considerable increase in dollars to the private institutions has enabled them to keep nursing and professional services at a considerably higher level than the VA has been able to do.

3. The Education of Nurses

As long as nurses insist that nursing has a different intellectual content from medicine, the matter cannot be resolved, and nurses will become increasingly less important in the health field. The nurse is either doing menial tasks or administration or practicing medicine but by tradition cannot diagnose or treat patients.

E. A. Stead Jr.

Dr. Stead:

The Department of Medicine and all other hospital departments have had problems due to a shortage of nurses. In fact, at one point during a severe hospital nursing shortage, we actually hired nurses directly into the Department of Medicine. When World War II started there were essentially nurses and doctors—that was it for health professionals. Conventional medical practices needed an office nurse, and hospitals needed somebody to nurse on the wards. Nurses were in extremely short supply during the war because factory and other jobs gave women an opportunity for careers that were more progressive than nursing. During WWII, the medical profession grew tremendously in its technical aspects; specialization, equipment and procedures just blossomed, but the nurses were pinned down to their previous role in the system, and were extraordinarily short-handed, even for making up the beds, which they insisted on doing themselves. In that setting, when doctors came back from the war and increased the demands on the nursing service, nursing just said they couldn't meet them and wouldn't try. I was not totally unsympathetic to the predicament in which the nurses found themselves. I didn't think it was entirely of their own making, but at the same time I did not sympathize with the fact that, finding themselves in an unsatisfactory situation, they weren't very imaginative about how to get out of it. Miss [Leila] Clark, the Director of Nursing at Duke, was not a very imaginative person, and she ran a very routine service. I often asked her why nurses didn't try to make nursing at Duke more attractive, but they were absolutely inflexible. With a better record keeping system, they clearly could have arranged for nurses to work on a rotation schedule of three days one week, and five days the next week, for example. There were ways to do it, but the nurses in the main office simply weren't going to implement any "new" ideas. They blocked any movement toward change, and when we pointed out the nursing shortage, they just said it was impossible to recruit anybody. I suggested that there were devices they'd never used, but they were completely inflexible.

In the old days, nurses were really selected for their passivity, and they went through a very rigorous indoctrination in hospital nursing schools. During their training they learned that they would be penalized for making any errors. For example, a student would be thrown out of nursing school for making a medication error, whether or not the actual error was, in itself, harmful. When teachers and supervisors make the penalty for error very, very high, then immediately they destroy the intellectual growth of the student. Students become over-cautious, tentative, afraid to take initiative. They focus on the rules of their jobs instead of thinking creatively. Now, people who don't mind making errors will never be very good, but there are a great many people who really want to turn in an excellent performance. And they will succeed if, when they make an error, it is identified and they are offered a suggestion of how to avoid it the next time. When the criticism is of a positive nature and when doing something correctly elicits praise, then the person is likely to perform without error the next time. That is the way people grow.

Nursing in the old days was not attuned to the concepts of advancement and learning because, for many years, nursing was such a passive profession, and because many doctors believed that the ideal qualification in a nurse was to passively and faithfully follow orders. As nursing began to recruit a different caliber of student, conflicts between doctors and nurses became the rule, and this continues to the present time. Duke had some very bright undergraduate nurses, yet few of them found their way into the permanent work force. This is a serious nation-wide problem of course, and many factors contributed to it. One was that the students married doctors, a reasonable thing to have happen since they were thrown into such close contact during the work day. But once they married, they were no longer economically dependent upon nursing. Another factor had to do with the rigidity that was built into the system when nurses were more passive and willing to tolerate a very rigid system. The idea of sitting down with the nurses and working out a schedule that deviated from the routine that was in place in the hospital was very difficult for the older nursing administrators. They really didn't know how to plan a complex schedule; they were intolerant of change and unwilling to creatively deal with the fact that the nurses needed flexibility and opportunity if they were going to remain in the field of nursing. And since many nurses could afford not to work, we had to bear the consequences of the leaders of the nursing profession not meeting the needs of the young people working in their field. At the same time, nurses became extremely useful in a variety of non-hospital jobs, which enabled them to go to work at a fixed hour, without having weekend or night responsibilities, and have normal holidays. A great variety of interesting opportunities came with these jobs, many of which were created by new research interests and activities being conducted in medical schools or other health organizations, home care operations, or hospital bed utilization reviews; these 9:00–5:00, Monday-to-Friday jobs did not carry the rigidity of hospital schedules. They attracted nurses away from hospital nursing.

The global differences between medicine and nursing didn't really have to do with making a diagnosis or other specific skills. It really related to the fact that the doctor came in and looked wise, did certain things and then went home. By contrast, the nurse stayed on the ward taking care of the patient. The doctor collected most of the income, based on the number of patients seen, and this phenomenon interfered with the development of nursing. We've never been willing to give nurses a proportionate share of the economic rewards of taking care of patients. I don't know of a single institution that has a program designed to reward a nurse when the burden of nursing, the number of patients to be cared for, exceeds the norm. No one rewards nurses for extra effort. By contrast, doctors have always been interested in keeping the health care mills operating at full tilt, because they reap both professional satisfaction and economic rewards from it. I know of no instance in which the nursing service has not wanted to shut up the hospital or decrease the number of beds and services offered because they simply were not economically rewarded for an increase in the services they were asked to render. The old concept of the nurse as handmaiden of the doctor worked very well when they *were* handmaidens; it's turned out to be a rather considerable liability now that there are no handmaidens.

Hospital administrators never want to pay any more money than they have to, and doctors don't want to share the wealth. Yet, when I tried to create an incentive system for nurses, the nurses rejected it on the basis that any nurse who would respond to an incentive system was not really a good nurse. In spite of the fact that they could see that the profession was not going to grow, they somehow couldn't comprehend that good people can and should respond to incentive programs. So the nurses were partly responsible for the situation in which they found themselves.

In an attempt to evolve the role of nurses and change their working conditions and satisfactions we went to the nurses at Duke and offered them a variety of programs that would enable them to do things that the current nursing staff couldn't do, including the medical evaluation of patients. But they weren't interested; they said they couldn't keep their heads above water as it was, they couldn't cope. They didn't want any nurses trained to do anything that they weren't accustomed to doing, certainly not anything they perceived as doctor's work. So we have had to deal with shortages of nurses, and defects in their training programs.

The idea that nurses could learn by doing and, with enough people around, could think in addition to doing, simply didn't penetrate nursing education. At Duke, the hospital nursing service was housed in a building separated from the nursing school, and nurses' education was purely cookbook. Thelma Ingles, RN, was the first nursing instructor I met at Duke who seemed to have any sense of how people learn and how they are taught. She was in charge of teaching Medicine and Surgery to students in the School of Nursing. From time to time, I saw her on the ward with students, and I thought the

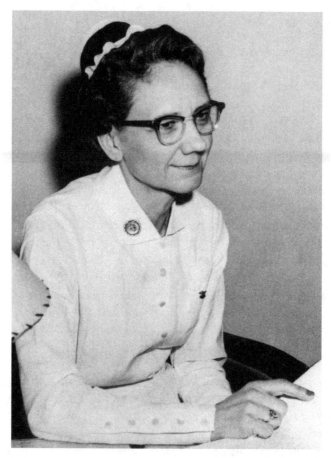

Photograph of Thelma Ingles, RN, Professor of Nursing at Duke. The original photograph is inscribed "To Gene: Who taught me that learning could be fun."

interaction she was having with her students was entirely different from what I'd seen previously in the nursing school. It caught my interest.

Thelma served on various committees with me, and one day, she told me she was going to take a sabbatical year in order to become more proficient in sociology and psychology. There was no way in which she could become more proficient in nursing, as such. I suggested instead that she break the pattern that had been established for nurses, and take a sabbatical year at the medical school. I told her we were both in the business of caring for people, both sick and well. Since there was so little communication between our two disciplines, it seemed to me that if she just came and lived in the medical school, watching the doctors at work, learning how they think and taking care of some patients with them, a whole series of vistas would open up to her that never were accessible before. So I arranged to meet with her regularly on a specified day at five o'clock, and go over all of the learning opportunities she'd had during the week. Then we'd outline how she would spend the next week and see to it that the channels of the various areas of the medical school that she really wanted opened were open to her. It would be a didactic year, but a year in which she could explore the many, many avenues of patient care that never had been open to her as a nurse. It would be like a Nursing Research Training Program. We worked together for the year, and as a result, she eventually developed a master's degree program to produce better nurses, not psychologists or sociologists. However, Thelma was ahead of her time and she couldn't get the program accredited by the National League for Nursing. They argued that she didn't have a standard because there was no precedent, that there weren't enough lectures, that the program was too patient-oriented, that there wasn't enough nursing theory. They were of the didactic school. But Thelma trained some very interesting people, such as Ruby Wilson, who later became Dean of the Nursing School at Duke, for example. Some of those nurses have done extremely well. We instituted the program because Thelma was in favor of it. The students thought it was a terrific idea, and learned a great deal from it, but I don't think Duke Hospital wanted a strong nursing service. The system died when the next year's class wasn't invited to enroll in the special program.

Nowadays, there are specialty nurses of all kinds, who act as individual units. By virtue of highly specialized training on coronary care or dialysis units or on oncology wards, they know more than their predecessors. And they aren't penalized to any greater degree than anybody else for errors. Because they're more self-confident, aggressive, and recruited on a somewhat different basis, many of those nurses are part of the care team in a way that they never were in the more general portion of the hospital. The traditional nursing role was to take vital signs, clean patients, help feed them if necessary, change dressings, administer medications, and write extensive notes in the chart (which, by the way, were rarely read). The specialty nurses of today carry out physical exams, watch cardiac monitors and provide rapid treatment for emergencies. They keep substantive records, and write to referring doctors. The last year Thelma was here, we formed an agreement with Duke Hospital, which unfortunately didn't last. We arranged to have a separate nursing service on Hanes Ward [the Hanes Ward Project], run by Ruby Wilson; we would charge different patients different amounts, depending on the amount of nursing service they received. We eliminated the use of private duty nurses who knew little about their patients, were not part of the ward team and were expensive. A patient who needed little nursing care paid much less than someone who needed full-time care. The money that was generated was intended to go back into the Nursing School, and the people who administered the money were a nurse, the superintendent of the hospital and I. However, even though we made a profit, no money ever went into the program for things like additional staff or clerical positions that the nurses determined to be necessary. The hospital kept the money. I don't know whether they needed it or they just thought that the nurses wouldn't know what to do with it.

I was convinced the Hanes program made money. It seemed to me that the one thing you couldn't buy at that time at any hospital in North Carolina was good nursing care for people with different degrees of illness, and we produced that on Hanes Ward. I didn't think there was any argument about whether we made money. Unfortunately, the hospital administration completely broke its promises, and we ran into ridiculous conflicts. For example, at Christmas time we had a number of people who needed custodial care. The families didn't want these patients at home, and doctors didn't want to go to see them at home, so they were admitted to Duke Hospital. But our nurses, who were in the master's program and had been senior students only the year before, really needed some vacation over the holidays. I knew many people in the black community in Durham needed money and were able to work as custodial care-givers, and since there was money in the budget, I decided to send the majority of our students home for three days and hire some custodial people. But we couldn't get administration to approve the temporary hiring. Then we needed an extra coffee pot, and we couldn't even get the coffee pot. There were no good reasons why we couldn't have these things. If there had not been any money, I would have understood it, but as long as we were making money from the service the nurses were rendering, I couldn't understand it.

I've always been impressed by the fact that the more patients there are in the hospital, the more disease the doctor gets to look at. This means there is the potential for more intellectual excitement and more money to be made. But none of that's ever been shared with the nurses. And as long as I was involved in administration, I tried to get the hospital administrators who make the decisions to say, "We're paying you for this amount of basic nursing, and you will receive a bonus for any nursing above that." If the hospital had more patients, the nurses should receive more money. Doctors get more money, why shouldn't the nurses? It is because the nursing profession has not been incorporated fully as a partner in the care of patients. And I think we've had troubles because they haven't been. The resistance to change in this regard has been two-fold, and interestingly enough, one of the factions opposing the change is the nurses themselves. They haven't been willing to receive bonuses. They believe there shouldn't be any relationship between money and nursing, and at the same time they complain about their low salaries. And then the hospital likes everything budgeted in advance and fixed tightly, so that at the beginning of the fiscal year, they don't have to think or use their heads; it's inertia, pure laziness

Over the years, I got grades on all the housestaff and medical students from the nurses with whom they worked, and when we were thinking about whether to keep residents and assistant residents on for the next year, the nurses were always consulted. The nurses provided me with useful information, such as whether a certain doctor was angry with them and with his patients all the time. They were one voice in the final decision of whether we should keep young doctors in the Duke system or tell them to go someplace else. If the general opinion was that a given young doctor was not really going to be very pleasant to have around next year, he usually disappeared. You've got to be worth the hassle if I'm going to keep you.

The nurses had less input into the decision about selection of Chief Residents. I never had a Chief Resident who set out to pick fights with the Head Nurses, even a guy as belligerent as Bob Whalen got along with the nurses. He knew it was in his own interest to do so. I always believed in respecting people's feelings, and I never cared whether the facts they presented to me were right or wrong. People act on their feelings and not on facts; this is important for a leader to know. Consequently, I collected a great deal of information that would give me insight into people's feeling states. For example, if someone was mad today or mad yesterday, it seemed irrelevant why they were mad or if they were right or wrong. I found that consideration of people's feelings went a long way toward helping me interact with the nurses on the general medical service.

Beginning during my early days at Duke, I ate breakfast with the nurses one morning a week and insisted that the Chief Resident and all the Ward Assistant Residents come to that breakfast. It was never my most popular meeting, but having the protagonists sit around a table helped settle a great many things. It eliminated the practice of having one person come to me and tell me one thing, and another come to me and tell me another version. I arranged these meetings with the Head Nurse as long as I was responsible for the service. Administratively, the nurses had the most contact with junior residents, and I think having a common meeting with all the key nurses, myself and all the residents, helped keep the peace between the medical housestaff and the nursing staff.

4. The Training of Medical and Paramedical Staff

Dr. Stead:

I would like to say a word about names in the health profession. They do get us in trouble. People look on MDs as a kind of a uniform product, when actually, you know, MDs are not interchangeable. They have a very wide spectrum of skills and interests, so determining the number of doctors per unit population gives you no information at all about how many people are available for any particular kind of thing that doctors do.

We are even in worse trouble in regard to nurses. You know, the word "nurse" creates a fairly uniform picture for doctors and for many consumers of health care. But, interestingly enough, these pictures are quite different from that created by the word "nurse" in a nursing educator. We would have to say, at least in our part of the world, that nursing education is a general form of education. And I would also say that we have a very attractive student body. Nurses are fun to talk to and to work with. They generally marry well and they live well. But they are not a very active force in the health field. And, because of the amount of time devoted to nursing education relative to the short half-life of active work in the field, we no longer look upon nurses as primary allies of doctors giving care. We are going to have to begin to bring into the health field people who will be more closely allied with medicine and who will, on a career basis, stay with it over a longer period of time.

As the whole world changes around us, we are tripped up just by the use of names. I think it is interesting, as a problem in communication and learning, to watch a nursing educator talk to a group of doctors and explain to them that nursing is general education and is not really closely related to activities in the hospital. Two or three weeks later, ask the group of doctors to give you the gist of what was said. They never remember the part about the hospital no longer being the central point in nurses' training.

But I think that nurses have a perfectly good point, which we had better hear. We are at the period of time when new professionals are going to have to be brought into the health field if doctors are to be able to do their jobs. I would draw a parallel again with the nursing field. Over 20 years ago, it became obvious that there were not going to be enough nurses to carry out their traditional function in the health field. The problem is highlighted by the fact that the nurse is the only person in our hospital who cannot learn. Anybody else in the hospital can be upgraded in their work by learning something new every year. But nurses are in such short supply and are so overwhelmed by their responsibilities that they frankly have no time for learning.

This same problem is beginning to confront doctors. If you watch the average doctor in practice, you discover he now has little time for learning. If we try to give medical care to the entire population, our current supply of doctors will not go around. Unless we add more workers to the health field, in 10 to 15 years doctors will find themselves in exactly the situation nurses are in. And for all I know, doctors may use the same solution—namely, to withdraw as a major factor in the health field.

There is a difference in point of view between those people who believe the past can be recreated and shored up by tinkering with the present here or there, and those who believe that a new era is beginning, an old era is ended, and that not too much time should be spent in tinkering with or shoring up what's past. It is clear that I believe one era is ended and another is started.

I would like to say just one word about the problem of putting doctors in relationship to people who haven't in the past received medical care. I was certainly a slow learner in this area. It is easy for one hand to learn something and not be able to relate it to what your other hand is doing. For years we have been concerned with what to do for people who have come from countries with a much different society and a much less developed educational system than we have. Frequently they come to this country for education. They spend four years in college, then four years in medical school. They then go through four or five years of further professional training in this country. When they return home, they find they cannot fit into the society they left; they can find no niche in which they can be useful. Having given 12 years of fairly hard work and made a large emotional commitment to one way of life, they tend to become unhappy back home or they come back here.

We now want to give modern medical care to a large section of our American citizenry who have received limited care in the past. The question is how do we get doctors to them? It is becoming obvious that those bright black students who compete well in college, who get into the Harvard Medical School, who come to Duke for four years of postgraduate training, are not any help at all with this problem. And we are dealing with exactly the same kind of situation we were dealing with when we took other people out of their culture or changed the culture for 12 years and then hoped they would go back to it.

In attempting to improve the doctor's ability to provide more service, we looked at how he should be supplied with assistants. We separated those things the doctor does that require judgment from those that require intelligence and skill but are done repetitively every day. If you break down the activities of the doctor this way, it becomes obvious that many things done by doctors can be done by non-doctors. Since specialization is now with us, it is very difficult for the hospital to produce a pool of personnel trained to fit the various needs and aspects of medical practice. It seemed to us that the physician had to define what his needs were, had to find that population which could serve those needs, and to train people to act as his helpers. We have begun to train a group of people that we call Physician Assistants, and that is exactly what they are. These are people who are recruited by doctors, trained by doctors and, in the end, paid by the doctors.

Of course, we have had the usual kind of problems expected with any new venture. We've had questions from nurses about whether we were "stealing" things that belonged to them. We've had many questions from our intern and resident staff, and our senior professional staff. Were we going to create trouble by having PAs do things traditionally done by doctors? Would PAs eventually set up as doctors? We have had trouble from the hospital administrators who want the command line to run through the nursing service up to the hospital superintendent. They wanted the duties and the financial rewards for the PAs to be determined by hospital managers rather than by doctors. We've had trouble getting support from the government, which said that you needed a college degree to work in the health field at any advanced level. Having been to college myself, I've always been skeptical about this thesis. Rather than a college education, you need dedication to the health field and a willingness to give service, some understanding of why sick people are irrational, and why they make demands that well people don't make.

Each year, the Physician Assistant learns things he didn't know the year before. This has to be a lifetime commitment. He doesn't work a few years and stop learning, but says, "This is my business," and works at it year in and year out. We have selected for training people for whom the turn of the social wheel has been such that they have gone through high school but not been in a financial position to go to college. I do not think we would gain anything by sending them for four years of college; they have already identified that they want to be in the health field and are ready to go to work.

PAs may want to become doctors. If so, they should be required to take the general education and the basic science courses required of physicians. Work as a PA could count towards the clinical training required of doctors. The amount of credit awarded for clinical experience should be determined by an appropriate examination. In practice, PAs with families and a high school education will rarely become physicians; a large number of those who are already college graduates may want to become doctors.

The point we came to quickly was that doctors had to be trained alongside PAs; otherwise, the doctors really wouldn't know how to use PAs or what to do with them. Our general plan was to give the PA student a year of didactic work, supervised by the people he was going to work with. The next year, we put the assistant into those areas of the hospital that had a high doctor-patient ratio (the Emergency Clinic, Admitting Room at the VA Hospital, Recovery Room, Respiratory Care Unit, Endocrine Clinic, Cardiac Care Unit, group and individual practices in North Carolina, state prison hospitals).

We hoped to give our PAs an open-ended certificate and, indeed, this is what we are doing at the present time. The certificate states what we have taught and what, in our opinion, the PA is able to do under the supervision of a doctor. The terms of the contract state that whenever his supervising doctor or doctors want him to do something that would be of benefit to his work, and for which he needed more training, we would train him. We then amend his certificate to say that now he is competent to do these additional procedures under the supervision of the doctor.

Most nurses work at jobs that are not heavily involved in busy hospital care. I have no objection to this, I just come back to the fact that an awful lot of the work of the health field cannot be done by this group. The reason hospital-centered nurses cannot learn is that there are not enough of them, so they cannot be released from the pressing duties of the day for new ventures. They cannot share in the continual learning process of the physician because they lack time. Time and learning are always related. If the number of interns in the hospital were to drop below a certain level, all the learning would disappear. It takes time, irrespective of the service aspect, to master new material. And nurses just simply do not have the time to put aside for learning purposes.

I think every profession can profit from what I have learned: that you cannot get too far behind in the manpower to cover the jobs you have agreed to cover without finding that you have extraordinarily little flexibility. I did not mean that an individual nurse, given time to learn, cannot learn. I meant that the system as now worked, at least in our part of the world where the numbers of nurses are sufficiently low relative to the tasks that have to be done, provides no time to learn what you might like to learn next year or the next year.

I am not advocating only one position: that the old system is ending and that we all ought to be trying new programs that we can start in our own areas. I have talked about people and now I will say a few things about machines. As you know, this is a computerized era, and the health field is developing new ways to handle data. As computerized information systems come into being, we must continually reexamine the role of the people who collect the data and put it into the computer. My guess is that a great deal of the data usually collected by doctors can be collected by non-physicians and then synthesized by the computer to the point that the computer can ask relevant questions about the patient's particular problem. And this is really the point where medical practice is the easiest to teach and the easiest to learn. So we have this problem of computer-person interface. What will the machine be like? What will the people be like? What will the practice be like? Obviously, we don't know yet.

5. Fame

Fame is a projection of time but not a biological projection. Enjoy a moment by enjoying what life has to give at that time. There are many hazards of maybe not living.

E. A. Stead Jr.

Dr. Stead:

I've always said I wouldn't walk across the street for fame, it clearly isn't worth the struggle. In the short-term view of things, I suppose what I have done is important, that my contribution will affect a few generations because my knowledge can be built on and added to. I would suspect that in a few million years, you'll have a great deal of trouble finding any traces of what we now look on as a permanent society. It's certainly true that each society has eventually built a more complex society than the one that preceded it, and that there are remnants of one society in another. My prediction is that man will disappear as man, and another life form will take our place. There are certainly many possibilities in the biological system (and it is not unthinkable that humans may develop into a form different from what we now know man to be).

I was sort of an amateur biologist before I became a doctor, and I observed that life is a system with checks and balances. In the end, nearly every species dies because it overproduces like bacteria in a test tube that can't find food, or natural disasters come along, or the species contaminates the environment with waste and can't survive. This is biology and man is essentially part of it. So I'm not as convinced that what we do on this earth in our time will have a dominant, all-pervasive effect for all time like most of my colleagues are. I don't think our present form of existence is likely to continue as most people think it will, nor do I think that's necessarily a great tragedy. The notion that we can build something which will go on forever certainly defies all past experiences.

The AIDS virus is an example of how extraordinarily potent biological forces can be and, in the face of such forces, man's power and knowledge are severely handicapped; a few more craters blown off of volcanoes will give man some notion of what physical forces can do. We know what atomic energy can do. But curiously, we haven't discussed what we're going to do with the nuclear waste from all the missiles we are getting ready to destroy. Sooner or later, we will be building waste depots that have the capacity to produce really tremendous disasters; we have already heard of several tragedies connected with radioactive waste, in fact. So while on the one hand, we think we're making progress and improving the quality and security of our lives, we're short-sighted enough as a race to miss the potentially hazardous consequences of the actions we call progress. I've no objection to living as satisfying and comfortable a life as we can, a life that is as constructive and non-destructive as possible. Supposing we do destroy most of the world with nuclear forces? In the end, I think the odds are that we will, but really what difference does it make? It's perfectly clear that when you're dead, you're dead; you don't then worry about what has happened.

I've done lots of things in my long clinical career, and there was very little that was not newly reportable, even though it wouldn't be that dramatic today. My colleagues and I spent quite a lot of time studying the various mechanisms that induce fainting; we did a lot of research on the relationship between the way you breathe and the way your brain works; and we looked at the peripheral circulation and learned a good deal about how it works in certain disease states. We played around with a very wide range of things in the total circulation, studied the flow of blood to the brain, liver and kidneys, but none of our names ever appear in modern reviews of these subjects, so we don't exist anymore in the scientific world. I looked up the work of Minot and Murphy, who won the Nobel Prize for discovering that vitamin B12 cured pernicious anemia, only to find that these great men were in the same state as Stead and Warren; they no longer appear as references in standard textbooks. There's nothing wrong with that—it's the way the world is.

Dr. Robert Whalen:

One of the problems of history is that you can read hard artifacts like papers, monuments or other evidence, but how do you divine what the human spirit has contributed to a profession or society? If you look at Stead, he's not much of a scientist. He was a great educator, but he didn't write much about education. I could pick out a few papers, which, if really read carefully, are probably seminal pieces of educational information for future readers of medicine. But there's no written record of him as an educational philosopher, so it's going to be very hard to reconstruct his role in American medicine. Obviously it has been huge because he's touched so many people in academic medicine who, in turn, have touched so many people who take care of the sick. The trickle-down effect is very large, but in another way, it's undetectable, because the source gets lost. For instance, Dr. Stead gave a talk at a party years ago. Jim Warren was expected to be there, and talk about what it's like to be a chairman of a department of medicine. Well, at the last minute Jim got sick and couldn't come, so Stead got up and spoke spontaneously about how to run a Department of Medicine. I sat there unhappy that I didn't have a tape recorder because he just ticked it off, boom, boom, boom, boom, boom. It was the best talk he gave, but it's lost on the winds now. Later I went back and told him "That's the best talk you've ever given, and why don't you write it down? It's very insightful and I think it's the sort of thing somebody would want to read." So Stead said, "I'll write it down." And I asked, "When?" and he said, "I'll think about it."

Dr. Stead:

One of the reasons that I decided early on that I was never going to do anything for fame was because it became quite obvious that fame was ephemeral, it just plainly wasn't worth messing with. So I've had total freedom from thinking that I had to be distinguished. I had fun with the work I was involved with, and I wouldn't give that up for anything. I even enjoyed going to the library to find out that something I'd just discovered in the laboratory had been discovered by 18 other people before me. We'd take the articles around the hospital, admiring ourselves and laughing at ourselves, joking about how long it took us to read the right books. We're all subject to the realities of geologic time and learning that is an important part of growing up. Once you realize it, that knowledge will cool you down.

CHAPTER 25

THE MEDICAL LEGACY OF EUGENE A. STEAD JR.

The only test of leadership is that somebody follows.
Robert K. Greenleaf

Leadership in medical sciences came late to this country. Before World War II, Europe was the place one went for the finest of medical care or for medical training. All that changed with the immigration of leading physicians and with the great leaps in focus and funding for science and technology that began during and shortly after the war. Targeted government defense initiatives like the search for a synthetic substitute for quinine as an anti-malarial for troops in the South Pacific, advances in battlefield trauma surgery, the use of blood transfusions, and the search for antibiotics became successful national priorities.

But for scientific discoveries to be medically significant, they have to be applied to sick people, and the hierarchical, Herr Professor systems of Europe did not fit the American style. New leaders were needed for the revolution in American medicine and they could be found in only a few places, predominantly along the eastern seaboard of the United States in cities like Baltimore, Philadelphia, New York and Boston.

Men like Halsted, Kelly, Osler, and Welch had started the current flowing when they formed the Johns Hopkins Hospital and medical school at the end of the 19th century. Their efforts transformed medical teaching and practice throughout the country, including at older institutions like the University of Pennsylvania, Columbia and Harvard. Just as the 20th century was reaching its mid-point, one extraordinary man emerged, almost out of nowhere, out of the woefully backward South of the time: that man was Eugene A. Stead Jr. He assumed the chair in Medicine at Duke University in 1947, and before he gave up the reins twenty years later, he had forged of one of the most successful departments of medicine in this country, had created an entirely new kind of medical practitioner (the Physician Assistant), had begun the computer-based collection of clinical information, and had served as mentor guide

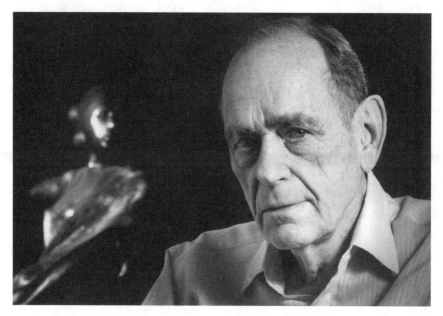

Eugene Stead at his Kerr Lake house, 1995. Isadora Duncan (sculpture) in background.

to more future Chairmen of Medicine than any contemporary. It is unlikely that his record will be equaled again.

German medicine, which had reached its zenith at the end of the 19th century, emphasized teaching through lectures, textbook assignments, and laboratory exercises; Stead, on the other hand, caught the spirit that Osler had introduced at Hopkins: he insisted that medical teaching take place at the bedside of the patient. He imbued students with the recognition that each patient is one-of-a-kind, therefore treatments need to be individualized. Textbooks describe only the similarities in a thousand patients diagnosed with the same "disease"; Stead emphasized to his students the uniqueness of each patient, and did this in front of the patient himself. He demonstrated to young doctors the value of taking a careful medical history, one that included past occupational exposure and the observations of other doctors, as well as the environment to which the patient would return after the hospitalization ended. He continually emphasized two points at the bedside: how do we know what we think we know, and how can the doctor help this patient in trouble. He insisted that his protégés be able to define and defend the words they used to describe those under their care. Many are the house officers who have begun a case presentation by saying something like "This is a 40 year-old man from Stumpy Point..." only to be interrupted, "Where is Stumpy Point?" and then realize that they have been using words whose definitions they did not know. None of those at the bedside (probably even including Stead) would have called this the asking of fundamental epistemological questions, but all participants came away the wiser for being subjected to Stead's burning queries. We always think we know so much more than we do about the many different disorders covered under terms like "heart attack" or "stroke," or that we are not doing a disservice to patients *and* ourselves to think of symptoms as "psychosomatic" rather than the result of different brains responding in different ways to different inputs. Stead probed all these issues, over and over, to students, residents, faculty and visiting professors.

Stead knew that *every* patient deserved the doctor's respect and careful attention, regardless of social or economic standing. Those who worked to achieve this goal, he called "doctor" as in his most famous aphorism, "What this patient needs is a doctor!" There were lots of MDs, Stead said, but only a few were doctors. These were hard lessons for a tired young resident faced with a middle-of-the-night emergency admission of someone who had already been hospitalized more than twenty times for alcoholic liver disease. To Stead each patient was a fresh opportunity—a chance to go to the library to learn what was new, what could explain an unusual finding, what would be a reasonable plan for *this* patient, now. Not the least was the opportunity to discover something, something that could not be explained by citation of the literature, a chance to find a new solution by calling in a specialist or by taking the problem to an experimental laboratory. In other words, as Osler emphasized, the medical "text" was the patient, and answers to the questions posed by the patient should be sought from all possible sources.

A critical Stead lesson was that so-called "functional disorders," such as unexplained but seemingly incapacitating headaches, fixation on bowel function, or recurrent or mysterious abdominal complaints that did not fit known diseases, were signs of brain dysfunction that called for a new kind of understanding and treatment. Often such patients were passed off unkindly as "crocks" by weary house officers, but Stead insisted that by trying to understand their own feelings, residents could begin to understand and treat even the most demanding patients, and with better outcomes than treating delightful persons with terminal illnesses. This all became apparent in bedside teaching and in careful follow-up of each patient. The lessons were so self-evident that they seldom needed repeating.

Another crucial lesson to be mastered under Stead was that devoting the time to hear and comprehend the patient's story, to carefully examine the patient, to personally review all laboratory and x-ray data (including those from past admissions) led to more rapid and accurate and less expensive diagnoses than new panels of laboratory tests and the advice of a bevy of consultants. Developing self-reliance and the confidence and perseverance to do whatever was needed for the care of the patient is what colleagues and pupils learned from Dr. Stead. In turn, when these doctors left their training to practice or to teach, the reputations of Duke and Stead grew to legendary proportions.

Stead made singular contributions to our understanding of what happens to the circulation when the heart begins to fail, and to many other perplexing scientific questions in medicine. But his even greater impact on research was to stimulate original work by his staff. He did this by giving them enough time to really work in the laboratory, away from routine patient care and teaching duties, and by starting them up with research funds until they could compete for grants on their own. Scientific research contributions, presented at national and international meetings, built the reputation of Duke. And when the best and brightest of his young staff got job offers elsewhere, Stead encouraged them to go and build their programs. His was a training ground, and he knew that the success of his alumni would recruit great new students and faculty to Duke.

When colleagues, no matter how senior, were stumped by clinical or personal problems, they went to Gene Stead for help. They knew they would get from him a fresh approach, one that cut straight to the heart of the problem and led to original solutions. It is only fitting for friends and associates to refer to him as the doctors' Doctor, whose "doctoring" stretched far beyond the mere treatment of disease.

Stead's ideas and standards, his reflections about patient care and how to achieve academic success, reach far beyond medicine; they are applicable to those who seek excellence in any field of endeavor. Deep commitment and a single-minded dedication are traits commonly found in hard-driving executives, politicians, coaches, parents, teachers, scientists and artists. To be a positive influence on the development of young people and to show pride in their success are attributes that all educators must have if they are to succeed in their profession. The ability to empathize with students, patients, colleagues, with the aged or the disadvantaged as well as the bright and the gifted, was used by Stead as an important ingredient for building successful and trusting relationships.

Opinions honestly stated regardless of consequences can be universally respected, if not always appreciated. This is especially so when the message is not always delivered with tact. For example, Dr. Stead at age 96 preached that medical schools had become "evil" institutions because they were far too expensive, did not take advantage of modern ways to store and retrieve information, and had a monopoly on the production of doctors. The substance of his message may have merit but it was painful to the ears of medical school deans and administrators. Stead's technique was, as always, to articulate the problem, in this case, the high cost of medical education, and propose original solutions that would involve major shifts in thinking about—and by—medical schools. Having spent much time constructing such analyses, he impatiently assumed that others should rally to his unorthodox approach, something that rarely happens in any walk of life. Institutions adopt "paradigm shifts" in their operation only after long, hard fights to maintain the status quo before recognizing that change is the key to survival. Those who begin the change often do not themselves survive the process. But Stead never worried about fame or self-aggrandizement; none of these is of consequence in the context of glacial time.

Eugene Stead was not the first American physician to teach about how to properly care for patients. Francis Weld Peabody's *The Care of the Patient* summarizes his idea that "the secret of the care of the patient is in caring for the patient." And William Osler, perhaps the most famous English-speaking doctor of all time, wrote that in "the natural method of teaching the student begins with the patient, continues with the patient, and ends his studies with the patient, using books and lectures as tools, as means to an end." He said, further, that "to study the phenomena of disease without books is to sail an uncharted sea, while to study books without patients is not to go to sea at all." This emphasis on the centrality of the patient in the education of doctors was an integral part, if not the fundamental cause, of the rise of American medicine in the 20th century.

One can construct a list of outstanding educators, *the* "Professors of Medicine" at school after school; an American list would include Osler, Loeb, Bean, Dock, Weiss, and many others, finally to Stead. There the line ends. Over the last third of the 20th century, the notion of a *Professor*, an identifiable comprehensive figure, whose shadow would fall across an entire department, who was abreast of and guiding what his faculty did, who touched the lives of student after student throughout the school, has faded from view and from memory. Now those christened with the title of "professor" or "department head" have nominal control of vastly larger faculties and budgets than Stead had, but they have no time for any real teaching presence on the wards, know only a small fraction of the students and trainees that come through their departments, survive only briefly as chair, and have almost no public persona outside the narrow confines of their own school and department. Today, no one knows the name of any professor outside his or her own department, no house officers come, as they did to Stead, to work under that specific professor, at great sacrifice of time and money, because of the publicly acknowledged value of sitting at the foot of the master.

Why is it unlikely that we will ever again see such medical leader? Why do we say that Stead is the last American doctor to carry the mantle of Osler and

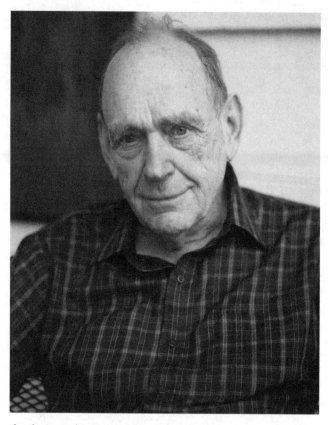

Eugene Stead, relaxing at his Kerr Lake house, circa 2000.

Peabody? One factor is the continuing fragmentation of medicine into smaller and smaller sub-specialties, where greater reverence is given to those with deep comprehension of narrower and narrower disciplines rather than to those with breadth of vision and an abiding interest in how medical information can help us understand and care for the sick. Chairs of departments are now usually chosen from the ranks of candidates with highly impressive scientific credentials. These individuals are often much more at ease with test tubes than with bronchial tubes, and tend to avoid the bedside where a lack of certainty can wound the pride of those who have made a reputation by knowing things. A second reason is that medical trainees are no longer permitted by law to be in the hospital for long hours, no matter their interest or devotion. And, very sadly, the day-to-day focus of most hospital and medical school leaders is now on the financial bottom line rather than on excellence in medical care and training. With all of these constraints, it seems unlikely that a socially unpolished genius like Eugene Stead could ever gain sufficient foothold within a medical school to have a dramatic impact on teaching medicine as it should be taught.

A final question for the reader: would you want to give up so much family life and other activities to rise to the top of your profession? That is a question that each of us must answer for ourselves, one that cannot be answered by anyone else.

INDEX

Finn, Davis, 102
Fisher, Morris, 5
Five out of seven Nights, 105, 195,
  197–199, 211
Flexibility, 103, 165, 272, 312, 316,
  326
Forbus, Wiley, 110
Free Money, 103–104, 159,
  164–165, 182–183, 187, 189,
  236, 252, 280
Fulton, Marshall, 58

G
Galveston (University of Texas
  Medical Branch at), 139, 265
Georgia Pharmacy Association, 6
Gibson, Jack, 53
Glaser, Robert (Bob), 57
Gleason, Bill, 161
Grand Rounds, 56–57, 60, 80–81,
  167, 261, 269
Grant, Robert, 225–227
Graves, Robert, 131
Greenfield, Joseph C. (Joe), 154, 279
Gunnells, J. Caulie, 285

H
Hamburger, Morton, 41
Hammond, William E. (Ed), 281,
  287
Handler, Philip, 165, 169–170, 207
Hanes Ward Project, 320
Hanes, Elizabeth Peck, 101, 184
Hanes, Frederic M., 101, 102, 104,
  108, 110, 184
Harlan, Bill, 205
Harrison, Hartwell, 32, 35
Harrison, Tinsley, 236–237
Hart, Deryl, 123, 164

Harvard Medical School, 26–28,
  35–36, 52, 57–58, 67–69,
  73–74, 79, 96, 117, 119, 140,
  170, 238, 257–258, 260,
  268–269, 331, 324
Harvard University, 57, 139, 180,
Hawkins, Ralph, 281
Heart Failure, 53, 86–90, 93,
  184–185, 258–259, 262, 270
Heyman, Albert, 78–83, 91–93,
  131–132
Heyman, Dorothy, 91
Hickam, John, 46, 56, 62, 69–70,
  73, 75, 81, 92, 96, 102, 104, 106,
  119–121, 147, 180, 193–194,
  207, 257, 260–262, 265–269,
  281, 285–286
History Meeting, 197–198, 211
History, Patient, 24, 76, 91,
  133–134, 136, 141–142, 167,
  173, 211, 227, 283, 299, 332
Hodgson, Patricia K. (Penny), 220,
  222
Hohman, Leslie, 261
Holland, Bernard C., 262
Hospitals
  Boston City, 41, 47–49, 56,
    58–59, 117, 155, 258
  Cincinnati General, 35–42, 46,
    71, 153, 268
  Emory, 22, 68, 72–73, 79, 81,
    99, 103, 262
  Grady, 22–26, 28, 36–37, 46,
    70–73, 75, 77–82, 84–86, 89,
    91–99, 103, 139, 225–226,
    261–262, 265, 269–270,
    275–276
    Black, 23, 71–72, 261–262
    White, 23, 71–72, 261–262

Master's Degree Program (nursing), 319
Mau, James C. (Jim), 281
McCord, Dr., 24
McDermott, Walsh, 74–75
McGeachy, English, 21, 23, 27
McIntosh, Henry, 113–114, 149, 160–163, 174–175, 182, 213, 236–237
McKee, Patrick A., 220
Medical, Outpatient Clinic 150, 157–158, 262
Medicare, 233, 284, 305
Merrill, Arthur, 26, 30, 67, 69, 270
Methemoglobinemia, 96
Methodist Church, 107–108
Methodist Retirement Home, 281, 289–303
Mickeljohn, Mike, 65
Miller, Eddie, 69, 75, 79, 93
Minot, George, 47, 328
Mitchell, Margaret, 61
Moonlighting, 148, 174, 197
Morning Report, 79–80, 137, 259, 263
Murphy, William, 58, 328
Myers, Jack, 46, 54, 56–58, 69, 95–96, 102, 104, 106, 117, 119–121, 146, 180–181, 229, 237–238, 259
Myocardial Infarction Research Unit (MIRU), 227–228
Myocardial infarction, 26, 77, 219, 226–227, 230–232

N

National Institutes of Health (NIH), 118, 148, 159, 166–167, 170–172, 187–188, 227–228

Neural Network, 76
Nicholson, William (Bill), 106, 130, 185
Nickel Bet, 142–144
Noon Conference, 195
Nursing Homes, 284, 289–303
Nursing, 39–40, 138, 174–175, 306, 314–324
Nursing, School of, 315, 317, 319–320

O

O'Hare, James P., 58
Ohio State University (College of Medicine), 139, 180, 194, 265
Orgain, Edward, 185
Osler Ward, 133, 136, 138, 142, 152, 202–204
Osler, William, 193, 273, 331–333, 335

P

Paddock, Franklin, 57
Parran, Thomas, 188
Patient care, 25, 37–38, 40, 53, 58, 72, 76, 79, 84, 91, 94, 97–98, 104, 132, 141–142, 144–146, 153–158, 175–177, 184, 186, 195, 197, 199–203, 206, 209, 215, 217–219, 222, 226, 230, 233, 247, 251, 253, 267, 269, 271, 283–285, 290–293, 295, 297–298, 301–303, 305–310, 313–314, 316–317, 319–324, 326, 329, 331–332, 334–336
Paullin, James, 13–14, 22–24, 67, 70–71
Peete, Billy, 247